Genetics of Endocrine Disorders

Editor

CONSTANTINE A. STRATAKIS

ENDOCRINOLOGY AND METABOLISM CLINICS OF NORTH AMERICA

www.endo.theclinics.com

Consulting Editors
ANAT BEN-SHLOMO
MARIA FLESERIU

June 2017 • Volume 46 • Number 2

ELSEVIER

1600 John F. Kennedy Boulevard • Suite 1800 • Philadelphia, Pennsylvania, 19103-2899

http://www.theclinics.com

ENDOCRINOLOGY AND METABOLISM CLINICS OF NORTH AMERICA Volume 46, Number 2
June 2017 ISSN 0889-8529, ISBN 13: 978-0-323-53005-7

Editor: Stacy Eastman
Developmental Editor: Meredith Madeira

Endocrinology and Metabolism Clinics of North America (ISSN 0889-8529) is published quarterly by Elsevier Inc., 360 Park Avenue South, New York, NY 10010-1710. Months of issue are March, June, September, and December. Periodicals postage paid at New York, NY and additional mailing offices. Subscription prices are USD 337.00 per year for US individuals, USD 674.00 per year for US institutions, USD 100.00 per year for US students and residents, USD 423.00 per year for Canadian individuals, USD 834.00 per year for Canadian institutions, USD 490.00 per year for international individuals, USD 834.00 per year for international institutions, and USD 245.00 per year for international and Canadian and foreign students/residents. To receive student/resident rate, orders must be accompanied by name of affiliated institution, date of term, and the signature of program/ residency coordinator on institution letterhead. Orders will be billed at individual rate until proof of status is received. Foreign air speed delivery is included in all *Clinics* subscription prices. All prices are subject to change without notice. **POSTMASTER:** Send address changes to *Endocrinology and Metabolism Clinics of North America*, Elsevier Health Sciences Division, Subscription Customer Service, 3251 Riverport Lane, Maryland Heights, MO 63043. **Customer Service: Telephone: 1-800-654-2452** (U.S. and Canada); **1-314-447-8871** (outside U.S. and Canada). **Fax: 1-314-447-8029. E-mail: journalscustomerservice-usa@elsevier.com (for print support); journalsonlinesupport-usa@elsevier.com (for online support).**

Reprints. For copies of 100 or more, of articles in this publication, please contact the Commercial Rights Department, Elsevier Inc., 360 Park Avenue South, New York, NY 10010-1710; phone: +1-212-633-3874; fax: +1-212-633-3820; E-mail: reprints@elsevier.com.

Endocrinology and Metabolism Clinics of North America is covered in *MEDLINE/PubMed (Index Medicus)*, *EMBASE/Excerpta Medica, Current Contents/Clinical Medicine, Current Contents/Life Sciences, Science Citation Index, ISI/BIOMED, BIOSIS,* and *Chemical Abstracts.*

Contributors

CONSULTING EDITORS

ANAT BEN-SHLOMO, MD
Pituitary Center, Division of Endocrinology, Diabetes, and Metabolism, Cedars Sinai Medical Center, Los Angeles, California

MARIA FLESERIU, MD, FACE
Northwest Pituitary Center, Departments of Medicine (Endocrinology) and Neurological Surgery, Oregon Health and Science University, Portland, Oregon

EDITOR

CONSTANTINE A. STRATAKIS, MD, D(med)Sci
Senior Investigator and Head, Section on Endocrinology and Genetics, Scientific Director, Eunice Kennedy Shriver National Institute of Child Health and Human Development, National Institutes of Health, Bethesda, Maryland

AUTHORS

ANENISIA C. ANDRADE, MD, PhD
Division of Pediatric Endocrinology, Department of Women's and Children's Health, Karolinska Institutet, Karolinska University Hospital, Solna, Sweden

JEFFREY BARON, MD
Program in Developmental Endocrinology and Genetics, Eunice Kennedy Shriver National Institute of Child Health and Human Development, National Institutes of Health, Bethesda, Maryland

ANDREW J. BAUER, MD
Director, Division of Endocrinology and Diabetes, The Thyroid Center, The Children's Hospital of Philadelphia, Associate Professor of Pediatrics, The Perelman School of Medicine, The University of Pennsylvania, Philadelphia, Pennsylvania

REBECCA J. BROWN, MD, MHSc
National Institute of Diabetes and Digestive and Kidney Diseases, National Institutes of Health, Bethesda, Maryland

WUYAN CHEN, PhD
Human Molecular Geneticist, Clinical DNA Testing and DNA Banking, PreventionGenetics, Marshfield, Wisconsin

GILBERT J. COTE, PhD
Professor, Department of Endocrine Neoplasia and Hormonal Disorders, University of Texas MD Anderson Cancer Center, Houston, Texas

EMMANUÈLE C. DÉLOT, PhD
Associate Adjunct Professor, Departments of Human Genetics and Pediatrics, David Geffen School of Medicine, University of California, Los Angeles, Los Angeles, California

CHARIS ENG, MD, PhD, FACP
Genomic Medicine Institute, Cleveland Clinic; Lerner Research Institute, Cleveland Clinic; Taussig Cancer Institute, Cleveland Clinic; Department of Genetics and Genome Sciences, Case Western Reserve University School of Medicine; Germline High Risk Focus Group, CASE Comprehensive Cancer Center, Case Western Reserve University, Cleveland, Ohio

MARIAM GANGAT, MD
Assistant Professor, Department of Pediatrics, Child Health Institute of New Jersey, Rutgers-Robert Wood Johnson Medical School, Rutgers, The State University of New Jersey, New Brunswick, New Jersey

LETICIA FERREIRA GONTIJO SILVEIRA, MD, PhD
Unidade de Endocrinologia do Desenvolvimento, Laboratório de Hormônios e Genética Molecular/LIM42, Hospital das Clínicas, Disciplina de Endocrinologia, Faculdade de Medicina da Universidade de São Paulo, São Paulo, Brasil

ELIZABETH G. GRUBBS, MD, MS
Associate Professor, Department of Surgical Oncology, University of Texas MD Anderson Cancer Center, Houston, Texas

FADY HANNAH-SHMOUNI, MD
Associate Investigator, Section on Endocrinology and Genetics, Eunice Kennedy Shriver National Institute of Child Health and Human Development, National Institutes of Health, Bethesda, Maryland

ZEINA C. HANNOUSH, MD
Department of Medicine, University of Miami Miller School of Medicine, Miami, Florida

SAMUEL M. HYDE, MS, CGC
Departments of Surgical Oncology and Clinical Cancer Genetics, University of Texas MD Anderson Cancer Center, Houston, Texas

YOUN HEE JEE, MD
Program in Developmental Endocrinology and Genetics, Eunice Kennedy Shriver National Institute of Child Health and Human Development, National Institutes of Health, Bethesda, Maryland

MÁRTA KORBONITS, MD, PhD
Professor of Endocrinology, Centre for Endocrinology, William Harvey Research Institute, Barts and the London School of Medicine and Dentistry, Queen Mary University of London, London, United Kingdom

ANA CLAUDIA LATRONICO, MD, PhD
Unidade de Endocrinologia do Desenvolvimento, Laboratório de Hormônios e Genética Molecular/LIM42, Hospital das Clínicas, Disciplina de Endocrinologia, Faculdade de Medicina da Universidade de São Paulo, São Paulo, Brasil

MARISSA LIGHTBOURNE, MD, MPH
Eunice Kennedy Shriver National Institute of Child Health and Human Development, National Institutes of Health, Bethesda, Maryland

LORENA GUIMARAES LIMA AMATO, MD
Unidade de Endocrinologia do Desenvolvimento, Laboratório de Hormônios e Genética Molecular/LIM42, Hospital das Clínicas, Disciplina de Endocrinologia, Faculdade de Medicina da Universidade de São Paulo, São Paulo, Brasil

MAYA LODISH, MD, MHSc
Director, Pediatric Endocrinology Fellowship, Staff Clinician, Eunice Kennedy Shriver National Institute of Child Health and Human Development, National Institutes of Health, Bethesda, Maryland

ANTON LUGER, MD
Clinical Division of Endocrinology and Metabolism, Department of Internal Medicine III, Medical University of Vienna, Vienna, Austria

PEDRO MARQUES, MD
Clinical Fellow, Centre for Endocrinology, William Harvey Research Institute, Barts and the London School of Medicine and Dentistry, Queen Mary University of London, London, United Kingdom

DEBORAH P. MERKE, MD, MS
Senior Investigator, Section on Endocrinology and Genetics, Eunice Kennedy Shriver National Institute of Child Health and Human Development, National Institutes of Health; Department of Pediatrics, National Institutes of Health Clinical Center, Bethesda, Maryland

JOANNE NGEOW, MBBS, MRCP, MPH
Cancer Genetics Service, Division of Medical Oncology, National Cancer Centre, Singapore, Singapore; Genomic Medicine Institute, Cleveland Clinic, Cleveland, Ohio

OLA NILSSON, MD, PhD
Division of Pediatric Endocrinology, Department of Women's and Children's Health, Karolinska Institutet, Karolinska University Hospital, Solna, Sweden; University Hospital, Örebro University, Örebro, Sweden

JEANETTE C. PAPP, PhD
Adjunct Professor, Department of Human Genetics, David Geffen School of Medicine, University of California, Los Angeles, Los Angeles, California

SALLY RADOVICK, MD
Senior Associate Dean for Clinical and Translational Research; Professor, Department of Pediatrics, Child Health Institute of New Jersey, Rutgers-Robert Wood Johnson Medical School, Rutgers, The State University of New Jersey, New Brunswick, New Jersey

MARIE HELENE SCHERNTHANER-REITER, MD, PhD, MSci
Clinical Division of Endocrinology and Metabolism, Department of Internal Medicine III, Medical University of Vienna, Vienna, Austria; Section on Endocrinology and Genetics, Eunice Kennedy Shriver National Institute of Child Health and Human Development, National Institutes of Health, Bethesda, Maryland

DAVID E. SANDBERG, PhD
Professor, Division of Pediatric Psychology, Department of Pediatrics & Communicable Diseases, Child Health Evaluation and Research Center, University of Michigan Medical School, Ann Arbor, Michigan

KAITLIN SESOCK, MSc
Genomic Medicine Institute, Cleveland Clinic; Lerner Research Institute, Cleveland Clinic; Taussig Cancer Institute, Cleveland Clinic, Cleveland, Ohio

WILLIAM F. SIMONDS, MD
Metabolic Diseases Branch, National Institute of Diabetes and Digestive and Kidney Diseases, National Institutes of Health, Bethesda, Maryland

CONSTANTINE A. STRATAKIS, MD, D(med)Sci
Senior Investigator and Head, Section on Endocrinology and Genetics, Scientific Director, Eunice Kennedy Shriver National Institute of Child Health and Human Development, National Institutes of Health, Bethesda, Maryland

RODRIGO ALMEIDA TOLEDO, PhD
Division of Hematology and Medical Oncology, Department of Medicine, Cancer Therapy and Research Center, University of Texas Health Science Center at San Antonio (UTHSCSA), San Antonio, Texas; Clinical Research Program, Spanish National Cancer Research Centre, CNIO, Madrid, Spain

ERIC VILAIN, MD, PhD
Professor, Departments of Human Genetics, Urology, and Pediatrics, David Geffen School of Medicine, University of California, Los Angeles, Los Angeles, California

ROY E. WEISS, MD, PhD
Kathleen and Stanley Glaser Distinguished Chair, Professor and Chairman, Department of Medicine, University of Miami Miller School of Medicine, Miami, Florida

Contents

the great advances of molecular genetics of IHH and pointed up the heterogeneity and complexity of the genetic basis of this condition.

Diabetes insipidus is a disease characterized by polyuria and polydipsia due to inadequate release of arginine vasopressin from the posterior pituitary gland (neurohypophyseal diabetes insipidus) or due to arginine vasopressin insensitivity by the renal distal tubule, leading to a deficiency in tubular water reabsorption (nephrogenic diabetes insipidus). This article reviews the genetics of diabetes insipidus in the context of its diagnosis, clinical presentation, and therapy.

Although most of pituitary adenomas are benign, they may cause significant burden to patients. Sporadic adenomas represent the vast majority of the cases, where recognized somatic mutations (eg, *GNAS* or *USP8*), as well as altered gene-expression profile often affecting cell cycle proteins have been identified. More rarely, germline mutations predisposing to pituitary adenomas -as part of a syndrome (eg, MEN1 or Carney complex), or isolated to the pituitary (*AIP* or *GPR101*) can be identified. These alterations influence the biological behavior, clinical presentations and therapeutic responses, and their full understanding helps to provide appropriate care for these patients.

Congenital hypothyroidism (CH) is the most common inborn endocrine disorder and causes significant morbidity. To date, we are only aware of the molecular basis responsible for the defects in a small portion of patients with CH. A better understanding of the pathophysiology of these cases at the genetic and molecular basis provides useful information for proper counseling to patients and their families a well as for the development of better targeted therapies. This article provides a succinct outline of the pathophysiology and genetics of the known causes of thyroid dysgenesis, dyshormonogenesis, and syndrome of impaired sensitivity to thyroid hormone.

There has been a steady incorporation of powerful new molecular tools into the evaluation and management of thyroid nodules and thyroid cancer. With an increasing incidence of nodules and differentiated thyroid cancer (DTC) being diagnosed in children and adolescents, oncogene data are providing insight into the clinical differences between pediatric and adult patients with histologically similar DTC. However, additional investment and efforts are needed to define the genomic landscape for pediatric DTC with the goal of improving preoperative diagnostic accuracy as well as stratifying treatment in an effort to reduce complications of therapy.

Primary hyperparathyroidism (HPT) is a metabolic disease caused by the excessive secretion of parathyroid hormone from 1 or more neoplastic parathyroid glands. HPT is largely sporadic, but it can be associated with a familial syndrome. The study of such families led to the discovery of tumor suppressor genes whose loss of function is now recognized to underlie the development of many sporadic parathyroid tumors. Heritable and acquired oncogenes causing parathyroid neoplasia are also known. Studies of somatic changes in parathyroid tumor DNA and investigation of kindreds with unexplained familial HPT promise to unmask more genes relevant to parathyroid neoplasia.

This article links the understanding of developmental physiology of the adrenal cortex to adrenocortical tumor formation. Many molecular mechanisms that lead to formation of adrenocortical tumors have been discovered via next-generation sequencing approaches. The most frequently mutated genes in adrenocortical tumors are also factors in normal adrenal development and homeostasis, including those that alter the p53 and Wnt/β-catenin pathways. In addition, dysregulated protein kinase A signaling and ARMC5 mutations have been identified as key mediators of adrenocortical tumorigenesis. The growing understanding of genetic changes that orchestrate adrenocortical development and disease pave the way for potential targeted treatment strategies.

Congenital adrenal hyperplasia (CAH) refers to a group of autosomal recessive disorders due to single-gene defects in the various enzymes required for cortisol biosynthesis. CAH represents a continuous phenotypic spectrum with more than 95% of all cases caused by 21-hydroxylase deficiency. Genotyping is an important tool in confirming the diagnosis or carrier state, provides prognostic information on disease severity, and is essential for genetic counseling. In this article, the authors provide an in-depth discussion on the genetics of CAH, including genetic diagnosis, molecular analysis, genotype-phenotype relationships, and counseling of patients and their families.

Genomic studies conducted by different centers have uncovered various new genes mutated in pheochromocytomas and paragangliomas (PPGLs) at germline, mosaic, and/or somatic levels, greatly expanding our knowl-edge of the genetic events occurring in these tumors. The current review focuses on very new findings and discusses the previously not recognized role of *MERTK*, *MET*, *fibroblast growth factor receptor 1*, and *H3F3A* genes in syndromic and nonsyndromic PPGLs. These 4 new genes were selected because although their association with PPGLs is very recent, mounting evidence was generated that rapidly consolidated the prominence of these genes in the molecular pathogenesis of PPGLs.

Multiple endocrine neoplasia syndromes types 1 and 2 represent well-characterized yet clinically heterogeneous hereditary conditions for which diagnostic and management recommendations exist; genetic testing for these inherited endocrinopathies is included in these guidelines and is an important part of identifying affected patients and their family members. Understanding of these mature syndromes is challenged as more individ-uals undergo genetic testing and genetic data are amassed, with the po-tential to create clinical conundrums that may have an impact on individualized approaches to management and counseling. Clinicians who diagnose and treat patients with MEN syndromes should be aware of these possibilities.

Patients with *PTEN* hamartoma tumor syndrome (PHTS) may present to a variety of different subspecialties with benign and malignant clinical fea-tures. They have increased lifetime risks of breast, endometrial, thyroid, renal, and colon cancers, as well as neurodevelopmental disorders such as autism spectrum disorder. Patients and affected family members can be offered gene-directed surveillance and management. Patients who are unaffected can be spared unnecessary investigations. With longitudi-nal follow-up, we are likely to identify other non-cancer manifestations associated with PHTS such as metabolic, immunologic, and neurologic features.

Although many next-generation sequencing platforms are being created around the world, implementation is facing multiple hurdles. A strong hur-dle to the full adherence of clinical teams to the Disorders of Sex Develop-ment Translational Research Network (DSD-TRN) guidelines for standardization of reporting and practice is the current lack of integration of the standardized clinical forms into the various electronic medical re-cords at different sites. Time allocated to research is also limited. In spite of these hurdles, genetic information for half the enrolled patients is already available in the DSD-TRN registry, and early results demonstrate the value of such an infrastructure.

Marissa Lightbourne and Rebecca J. Brown

Lipodystrophy disorders are characterized by selective loss of fat tissue with metabolic complications including insulin resistance, hypertriglyceridemia, and nonalcoholic liver disease. These complications can be life-threatening, affect quality of life, and result in increased health care costs. Genetic discoveries have been particularly helpful in understanding the pathophysiology of these diseases, and have shown that mutations affect pathways involved in adipocyte differentiation and survival, lipid droplet formation, and lipid synthesis. In addition, genetic testing can identify patients whose phenotypes are not clearly apparent, but who may still be affected by severe metabolic complications.

ENDOCRINOLOGY AND METABOLISM CLINICS OF NORTH AMERICA

VISIT THE CLINICS ONLINE!
Access your subscription at:
www.theclinics.com

Foreword

Updates in the Genetics of Endocrine Disorders

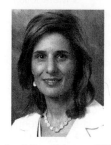 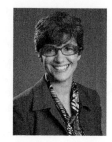

Anat Ben-Shlomo, MD   Maria Fleseriu, MD, FACE
Consulting Editors

This issue of *Endocrinology and Metabolism Clinics of North America* presents to our readers an overview on Genetics in Endocrine Disorders. This exciting issue was edited by Dr Constantine A. Stratakis, an internationally renowned investigator in the field of Genetics in Endocrine Disorders at the National Institute of Child Health and Human Development. Dr Stratakis assembled a group of excellent physician-scientists from around the world to review current knowledge in the genetics of endocrine disease and its relevant application to our medical diagnostic and treatment approach.

Endocrine genetics evolved from a single disease—single mutation discovery to an accumulation of big data from next-generation sequencing technologies, enabling us to accelerate identification of new genes involved in endocrine diseases and to shed light on their underlying molecular mechanisms.

The authors discuss mutations causing a variety of endocrine diseases, including short stature, diabetes insipidus, congenital hypothyroidism, pituitary hypoplasia, congenital hypogonadotropic hypogonadism, disorders of sex development, congenital adrenal hyperplasia, and lipodystrophy. Genetic syndromes involving multiple organs, including MEN1 and MEN2 syndromes and PTEN-spectrum disorders, are reviewed, as are mutations causing endocrine cancers in the pituitary, thyroid, parathyroid, and adrenal cortex and neuroendocrine tumors such as pheochromocytoma and paraganglioma.

We hope you will find this issue on Genetics in Endocrine Disorders of the *Endocrinology and Metabolism Clinics of North America* useful in your practice. We thank

Endocrinol Metab Clin N Am 46 (2017) xiii–xiv
http://dx.doi.org/10.1016/j.ecl.2017.03.002
0889-8529/17/© 2017 Published by Elsevier Inc.

endo.theclinics.com

Dr Constantine A. Stratakis for guest-editing this exciting and highly relevant issue, and the Elsevier editorial staff for their valuable assistance.

Anat Ben-Shlomo, MD
Pituitary Center
Division of Endocrinology Diabetes
& Metabolism
Cedars Sinai Medical Center
8700 Beverly Boulevard
Los Angeles, CA 90048, USA

Maria Fleseriu, MD, FACE
Northwest Pituitary Center
Departments of Medicine (Endocrinology) and Neurological Surgery
Oregon Health & Science University
3303 Southwest Bond Avenue
Portland, OR 97239, USA

E-mail addresses:
benshlomoa@cshs.org (A. Ben-Shlomo)
fleseriu@ohsu.edu (M. Fleseriu)

Preface

Genetics and the New (Precision) Medicine and Endocrinology: In Medias Res or Ab Initio?

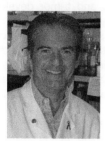

Constantine A. Stratakis, MD, D(med)Sci
Editor

As medicine is poised to be transformed by incorporating personalized and genetic data in its daily practice, it is essential that clinicians familiarize themselves with the information that is now available from more than 50 years of genetic discoveries that continue unabated and increase by the day. Endocrinology always stood at the forefront of what is called today "precision medicine": genetic disorders of the pituitary and the adrenal were among the first to be molecularly elucidated in the 1980s. Among the first oncogenes whose discovery contributed greatly in the understanding of cancer and its progression were two "endocrine" genes: *GNAS* and *RET*, that were both identified in the late 1980s. The use of *RET* mutation testing for the prevention or treatment of medullary thyroid cancer was among the first and, to date, most successful applications of genetics in informing clinical decisions in an individualized manner, preventing cancer or guiding the choice of tyrosine kinase inhibitors in cancer treatment.

Today, there is tremendous volume of new information emerging every day in the genetics or system biology of endocrine disorders. In this issue, we attempted to capture what we think is a useful compendium of the new developments in the genetics of the pituitary (hypoplasia, hypogonadotropic hypogonadism, diabetes insipidus, and pituitary adenomas), thyroid (thyroid hormone synthesis and action, thyroid cancer), parathyroid (genetics of hyperparathyroidism and cancer), and adrenal glands (adrenocortical hyperplasia and tumors, steroidogenic defects affecting adrenal function and pheochromocytomas and related lesions). We also included the highly relevant but nonspecific gland-based genetic updates on the investigation of short stature, multiple endocrine neoplasias and related disorders (PTEN-spectrum), sex development, and lipodystrophy. We selected the latter as areas of Endocrine genetics that have been transformed by new and exciting developments in the last decade or so.

Endocrinol Metab Clin N Am 46 (2017) xv–xvi
http://dx.doi.org/10.1016/j.ecl.2017.03.001
0889-8529/17/© 2017 Published by Elsevier Inc.

endo.theclinics.com

It is a reflection of the nature of the field and the rapid pace of discoveries that a number of these articles will not include the latest genetic updates in their respective areas by the time they are published. However, each article included in this issue is written in such a way that I hope will make it useful for years to come. Each review provides the framework of developmental and system biology of the endocrine gland (pituitary, thyroid, parathyroid, adrenal) or disease (short stature, multiple endocrine neoplasias, sex development, lipodystrophy) that is covered. Unlike in the first years of genetic medicine, we now understand a lot about what signaling pathways guide development of a gland, its hypoplasia or hyperplasia, and tumor development. And, thus, most of the time, a new gene fits into this framework nicely.

Furthermore, these articles are written by clinicians (all senior authors are clinically active, while simultaneously being leading researchers in their respective field) for clinicians: thus, beyond attempting to cover all that is new in their areas, these articles provide information that can be used by the clinician in daily practice. This issue aspires to be of help in practicing state-of-the-art medicine, as a lot of genetics finds its way in our clinics by the day.

Many would say that in media res (in the middle of the story) genetics is hard to incorporate in our practice; genetics is by definition ab initio (at the start of it all). This issue argues that a new Endocrinology is also being set up now, ab initio, like in many other medical disciplines. In this era of precision medicine, clinicians need to be familiar with the main molecular pathways governing glandular development, growth, function, and tumor formation, such as what is presented in this issue.

This work is supported by the intramural program of the *Eunice Kennedy Shriver* National Institute of Child Health and Human Development, National Institutes of Health.

Constantine A. Stratakis, MD, D(med)Sci
Section on Endocrinology & Genetics
Eunice Kennedy Shriver National Institute of Child Health
and Human Development
National Institutes of Health
31 Center Drive, Room 2A46
Bethesda, MD 20892, USA

E-mail address:
stratakc@mail.nih.gov

Pituitary Hypoplasia

Mariam Gangat, MD[a],*, Sally Radovick, MD[b]

KEYWORDS

- Pituitary development • Transcription factor
- Combined pituitary hormone deficiency • Hypopituitarism

KEY POINTS

- Coordinated temporal and spatial expression of several transcription factors is essential for normal pituitary gland development and function.
- The pituitary gland is responsible for the production of hormones that play a crucial role in growth, metabolism, puberty and reproduction, lactation, and stress response.
- Several mutations in patients with hypopituitarism have been identified; however, the vast majority of patients remain labeled idiopathic.
- Next-generation sequencing technology is expanding our understanding of the underlying genetic mechanisms of hypopituitarism, and has the potential of revolutionizing clinical care.

INTRODUCTION AND CLINICAL PRESENTATION OF HORMONE DEFICIENCIES

The pituitary gland lies in the hypophyseal fossa, the deepest part of the sella turcica, located in the sphenoid bone of the neurocranium. It is composed of 2 distinct structures, the adenohypophysis (anterior and intermediate lobes) and neurohypophysis (posterior lobe), which differ in embryologic origin. The anterior originates from the Rathke pouch, an invagination of the oral ectoderm, and the posterior lobe arises from the neuroectoderm. Multiple transcription factors act in a coordinated temporal and spatial sequence during pituitary development, and ultimately result in the differentiation of specific pituitary cell lineages (**Table 1**). The anterior lobe has 5 distinct cell types that produce 6 hormones: somatroph (growth hormone [GH]), thyrotroph (thyrotropin [TSH]), gonadotroph (luteinizing hormone [LH] and follicle-stimulating hormone [FSH]), lactotroph (prolactin), and corticotroph (adrenocorticotropin [ACTH]). These

The authors have nothing to disclose.
[a] Department of Pediatrics, Child Health Institute of New Jersey, Rutgers-Robert Wood Johnson Medical School, Rutgers, The State University of New Jersey, 89 French Street, Room 1360, New Brunswick, NJ 08901, USA; [b] Department of Pediatrics, Child Health Institute of New Jersey, Rutgers-Robert Wood Johnson Medical School, Rutgers, The State University of New Jersey, 89 French Street, Room 4212, New Brunswick, NJ 08901, USA
* Corresponding author.
E-mail address: gangatma@rwjms.rutgers.edu

Table 1
Mutations causing abnormal pituitary development and function

Gene	Chromosome	Pituitary Deficiencies	Associated Syndromes/ Malformations	Inheritance
HESX1	3p21	IGHD, CPHD (GH, TSH, LH, FSH, Prolactin, ACTH)	SOD	AR, AD
LHX3	9q34	CPHD (GH, TSH, LH, FSH, Prolactin)	Rigid cervical spine, limited neck rotation, sensorineural hearing loss	AR
LHX4	1q25	CPHD (GH, TSH, ACTH)	Cerebellar defects	AD
PROP1	5q35	CPHD (GH, TSH, LH, FSH, Prolactin, ACTH)		AR
POU1F1	3p11	CPHD (GH, TSH, Prolactin)		AR, AD
OTX2	14q22	CPHD (GH, TSH, LH, FSH, Prolactin, ACTH)	Microphthalmia, retinal dystrophy	AD

Abbreviations: ACTH, adrenocorticotropin; AD, autosomal dominant; AR, autosomal recessive; CPHD, combined pituitary hormone deficiency; FSH, follicle-stimulating hormone; GH, growth hormone; LH, luteinizing hormone; SOD, septo-optic dysplasia; TSH, thyrotropin.

hormones play a crucial role in growth, metabolism, puberty and reproduction, lactation, and stress response.

Combined pituitary hormone deficiency (CPHD), involvement of more than 1 anterior pituitary hormone, is associated with severe morbidity and can be life-threatening. The clinical presentation varies depending on age as well as the number and severity of hormone deficiencies. Many findings are nonspecific, especially in the newborn period, mandating a high index of suspicion, particularly in patients with midline defects.

Newborns with growth hormone deficiency (GHD) may not show overt growth failure; however, may present with hypoglycemia and prolonged jaundice. When combined with gonadotropin deficiency, genitourinary abnormalities such as microphallus and cryptorchidism are seen. Children present with growth failure evidenced by poor growth velocity, short stature, and increased weight-to-height ratio. Pulsatile secretion of GH limits the use of random serum GH levels. However, insulin-like growth factor 1 (IGF-1), the primary mediator of the actions of GH, and its most abundant carrier protein IGF-BP3, are stable throughout the day and therefore are useful screening laboratory tests. Growth hormone stimulation testing, although flawed,[1] can be performed using several protocols,[2] and can aid in establishing the diagnosis of GHD. Recombinant GH is the treatment of choice, and commonly administered once daily via subcutaneous injections.

Although congenital hypothyroidism (CH) due to TSH deficiency is rare, early diagnosis and treatment are critical to prevent adverse neurologic outcomes.[3] Infants can present with myxedema, hypotonia, hoarse cry, poor feeding, macroglossia, umbilical hernia, large fontanels, hypothermia, and prolonged jaundice. Some symptoms overlap with those seen in childhood, such as lethargy, constipation, and dry skin. Additional features seen in children include poor linear growth, cold intolerance, brittle hair, and a decline in academic performance. Newborn screening protocols for CH vary by state, and central hypothyroidism can be missed with primary TSH with backup thyroxine (T4) measurements.[3] If suspected, free or total T4 should be assessed; TSH is not useful, as it can be inappropriately normal. Levothyroxine (synthetic form of T4) is the treatment of choice.

Hypogonadotropic hypogonadism resulting from deficient section of LH and FSH can lead to genitourinary abnormalities as discussed previously in boys; however, newborn girls have normal-appearing genitalia. Failure to undergo pubertal development and associated growth spurt is seen later in childhood and adolescence. Prepubertal serum concentrations of sex-steroid hormones (testosterone in male individuals and estradiol in female individuals), along with low or "normal" serum LH and FSH concentrations are seen. Sex-steroid treatment goals include attainment of secondary sex characteristics, normal growth spurt, and fertility preservation.

The main physiologic role of prolactin is for lactation. Isolated prolactin deficiency is rare, and therefore patients often have manifestations of other pituitary hormone deficiencies.[4]

ACTH deficiency (secondary adrenal insufficiency) results in cortisol deficiency, the primary glucocorticoid secreted by the adrenal cortex. Cortisol is essential for stress response, has significant effects on carbohydrate, protein, and fat metabolism, as well as anti-inflammatory effects. Generally, the presentation of anterior pituitary hormone deficiencies is similar to primary deficiencies of the target organs they control; however, there are 2 distinct differences between primary and secondary adrenal insufficiency. ACTH deficiency does not lead to mineralocorticoid deficiency, as this pathway is primarily regulated by the renin-angiotensin-aldosterone system, and therefore does not result in salt wasting, hyperkalemia, and volume contraction. However, hyponatremia can be seen in secondary adrenal insufficiency due to inappropriate secretion of vasopressin.[5] Second, ACTH deficiency is not associated with hyperpigmentation, which results from high circulating ACTH and other melanocyte-stimulating hormone levels. Initial laboratory studies should include cortisol (measured at approximately 8 AM once diurnal patterns are established) and ACTH levels. Low-dose (1 μg) Cortrosyn (synthetic ACTH) stimulation testing can aid in confirming the diagnosis. In an adrenal crisis, emergency treatment is crucial, starting with fluid resuscitation, intravenous glucose, and parenteral hydrocortisone. Chronic treatment requires maintenance oral hydrocortisone, with additional doses at times of increased physiologic stress.

HOMEOBOX EXPRESSED IN ES CELLS 1

Homeobox expressed in ES cells 1 (HESX1), a member of the class of homeobox genes, is one of the earliest markers of pituitary development. HESX1 has been mapped to 3p21.1 to 21.2 and contains a highly conserved 185-amino acid open reading frame with 4 coding exons.[6] HESX1 transcripts are initially expressed in the anterior midline visceral endoderm and neural ectoderm; however, are ultimately restricted to the Rathke pouch, the primordium of the anterior pituitary.[7] In addition to pituitary development, HESX1 plays a broad role in the development of other placodally derived anterior structures, including the eye, olfactory epithelium, and forebrain.[6]

HESX1 functions as a promoter-specific transcriptional repressor with a minimal 36-amino acid repression domain that can suppress the activity of homeodomain-containing activator proteins.[8] The attenuation of HESX1 expression coincides with the rise of PROP1, one its downstream targets.[9] The sequential repressive actions of HESX1 followed by the activating effects of PROP1 are critical steps in pituitary organogenesis.[10] Involvement of other factors, including TLE1 and TLE3, Groucho-related corepressors, shown to enhance HESX1 regression of PROP1 activity,[11] have expanded our knowledge of the complex interactions involved in pituitary development.

The functional effects of mutations in HESX1 vary depending on the gene defect studied. Decreased DNA binding of the mutant HESX1 protein has been described.[6,12] Absent DNA binding due to the introduction of a premature stop codon, resulting in the generation of a protein lacking the carboxyl-terminal homeobox domain,[13] as well as increased DNA binding resulting in enhancement of PROP1 regression[14] also have been reported. Interestingly, in a patient with CPHD, a homozygous missense mutation (I26T) did not affect the DNA-binding ability of HESX1, but rather led to an impaired ability to recruit Groucho-related corepressors (TLE1), thereby leading to partial loss of repression.[9]

A broad range of phenotypes ranging from isolated GHD,[12] CPHD,[12] to septo-optic dysplasia (SOD),[6] along with variable neuro-radiologic findings, have been described in patients with HESX1 mutations. The reported incidence of SOD is 1 in 10,000 live births, and the diagnosis of this rare disorder is made when at least 2 features of the classic triad, optic nerve hypoplasia, pituitary hormone abnormalities, and midline brain defects including agenesis of the septum pellucidum and/or corpus callosum, are present.[15] Generally, heterozygous mutations are associated with milder phenotypes.[12] A recent study highlighted the phenotypic variability and lack of genotype-phenotype correlation, suggesting the influence of modifier genes or environmental factors. A homozygous pR160C mutation initially described almost 20 years ago in a patient with CPHD, SOD, and ectopic posterior pituitary (EPP) was recently identified in 2 patients with only CPHD without SOD, and a normally positioned posterior pituitary.[16] Further, HESX1 mutation carriers can be clinically unaffected, a recently described novel heterozygous mutation (pArg109Gln) was found in a young girl with CPHD, whereas her father carrying the same mutation was clinically normal including normal height.[17]

LHX3/LHX4

LHX3 is a member of the LIM family of homeodomain genes, which are characterized by 2 tandemly repeated unique cysteine/histidine LIM motifs located between the N-terminus and the homeodomain.[18] LHX3 maps to the subtelomeric region of chromosome 9 at band 9q34.3, and contains 7 coding exons. It encodes a transcription factor important for motor neuron specification and pituitary development.[19]

Earlier studies of LHX3 mutations have shown associations with hypopituitarism with or without cervical abnormalities. A young boy with CPHD, hypointense pituitary lesion, and rigid cervical spine limiting head rotation was found to be homozygous for a single base pair (bp) deletion in exon 2.[20] In a study of 366 patients with pituitary insufficiency, 7 patients from 4 families were found to have 4 novel recessive mutations: a deletion of the entire gene, 2 causing truncated proteins (E173ter, W224ter), and a mutation causing a substitution in the homeodomain (A210V). The investigators concluded that LHX3 mutations are a rare cause of CPHD and limited neck rotation is not a universal feature.[21] More recent studies have expanded the phenotypic spectrum. In a consanguineous family, 3 patients with hypopituitarism, anterior pituitary hypoplasia, skeletal abnormalities, and sensorineural hearing loss were found to have a homozygous 3088-bp deletion in the LHX3 gene resulting in complete loss of exons 2 to 5.[22] Further, the investigators showed that SOX2 is capable of binding and activating transcription of the LHX3 proximal promoter, suggesting an interaction between SOX2 and LHX3 may play a role in pituitary embryonic development. Sensorineural hearing loss also was identified as a key feature in a study of 6 patients with CPHD, restricted neck rotation, and scoliosis found to have a recessive, splice-acceptor site mutation in intron 3.[23]

The LHX4 gene, another member of the LIM family of homeodomain genes, is located at chromosomal location 1q25 and contains 6 exons encoding 390 amino acids.[24,25] The LHX4 protein is highly homologous to the LHX3 protein, except in the N-terminal region.[25] Studies of LHX3 and LHX4 mutations have shown that both genes direct formation of the pituitary gland. Although LHX4 is required for the proliferation of lineage precursors, LHX3 is necessary to establish the fate of pituitary precursor cells.[26]

In an early study of a consanguineous family with short stature and pituitary and cerebellar defects, as well as abnormalities of the sella turcica and central skull base, an LHX4 germline splice-site mutation was found. The investigators highlighted the pleiotropic role of LHX4 in brain development and skull shaping during head morphogenesis.[24] In a study of a young girl with severe CPHD, pituitary hypoplasia, EPP, poorly developed sella turcica, and Chiari malformation (structural defects in the cerebellum), a heterozygous missense mutation (P366T) in exon 6 was present. Further studies have expanded the range of phenotypes associated with LHX4 mutations. In a study of 253 patients with CPHD, 3 heterozygous missense mutations in LHX4 were identified in 5 patients. In 1 family with 2 affected female siblings and father, a mutation in the homeodomain (A210P) was found. One sibling was deficient in GH, TSH, ACTH, and gonadotropins; however, her sibling only had partial GH and TSH deficiencies. Further, the father only had GHD and normal MRI imaging. Another homeodomain mutation (L190R) was found in a patient with CPHD involving the GH, TSH, and ACTH axes. The final patient who had GH, TSH, and gonadotropin deficiencies was found to have a substitution between the LIM domains (R84C). Despite previous associations with LHX4 mutations and cerebellar abnormalities, MRI revealed only aberrant pituitary imaging, including small anterior pituitary, EPP, and pituitary cyst; none of the patients were found to have abnormalities in other regions of the brain.[27] Another large study, involving 136 patients with congenital hypopituitarism associated with brain malformations revealed 3 allelic variants of LHX4; however, based on functional studies, 2 were deemed polymorphisms. A C insertion into the third exon of LHX4, resulting in an early stop codon (pThr99fs) was responsible for the following phenotypes in 1 family: 2 brothers with CPHD with pituitary hypoplasia, and poorly developed sella turcica (the younger brother also had corpus callosum hypoplasia and EPP), and the father with only GHD and pituitary hyperplasia. Functional studies of the mutant LHX4 demonstrated a complete loss of transcriptional activity on the POU1F1 promoter and a lack of DNA binding.[28] A recent study identified a novel homozygous missense variant (pT126M), located within the LIM2 domain, absent in more than 65,000 controls, in 2 deceased male patients with severe panhypopituitarism associated with anterior pituitary aplasia and posterior pituitary ectopia.[29]

PROPHET OF PIT1

The human Prophet of Pit1 (PROP1) gene, located at chromosomal position 5q35, has at least 3 exons encoding 226 amino acid proteins, and contains both a paired-like DNA-binding protein and a C-terminal transactivation domain.[30] PROP1 precedes and plays a critical role in the expression of PIT1 and the development of PIT1-dependent cell lineages (somatotroph, lactotroph, and thyrotroph) in early pituitary organogenesis.[31] Further, PROP1 involvement in gonadotropin and ACTH deficiencies has been explored; however, the mechanisms remain unclear.[32]

Mutations in the PROP1 gene are the most frequent genetic defects in patients with CPHD,[33] with a 2-bp deletion (301delAG) in exon 2 reported as the most common, based on an analysis of 10 unrelated CPHD kindreds.[33] The identification of a tightly linked polymorphic marker, D5S408, led the investigators to conclude that these deletions may be independent recurring mutations rather than being inherited from a common founder mutation.[33] Mutations typically involve the DNA-binding homeodomain; however, a mutation affecting the transactivating domain resulting in a truncated protein with only 34% activity of that of the wild-type PROP1 has been reported, suggesting a critical functional role of the C-terminal end of the transcription factor in protein-DNA interaction.[34]

Abnormalities in PROP1 typically result in GH, PRL, TSH, and LH/FSH deficiencies[35]; however, a retrospective analysis of 9 patients with CPHD with known PROP1 mutations found that all patients developed adrenal insufficiency requiring hydrocortisone treatment.[36] Phenotypic variability, even among patients with the same mutation, has been described. A study of 5 patients with CPHD, homozygous for the R120C mutation, showed that each patient followed a different pattern and time scale in the development of pituitary hormone deficiencies; the age at diagnosis was dependent on the severity of symptoms. Although all 5 patients eventually presented with gonadotropin deficiency, they all entered pubertal development, and 2 female patients experienced menarche.[37] The most consistent feature is short stature; however, normal growth and attainment of normal adult height has been reported.[34,38] One such patient was a female individual with expected hypogonadotropic hypogonadism, who continued to grow until age 20 years at which time she reached a normal adult height. The lack of circulating estrogen delaying epiphyseal fusion and resulting in a prolonged period of growth was noted among the contributing factors.[38] On MRI, most patients exhibit some degree of anterior pituitary hypoplasia with a normal-appearing stalk and posterior pituitary; however, normal, and even enlarged, pituitary gland imaging has been reported.[39,40]

POU1F1 (PIT1)

POU1F1 (also known as PIT1) is a founding member of the POU family of transcription factors, characterized by 2 protein domains, POU-homeodomain and POU-specific, both necessary for high-affinity DNA binding.[41] The human POU1F1 gene, located on chromosome 3p11, containing 6 exons,[42] is essential for the development of somatotroph, lactotroph, and thyrotroph cell lineages.[41]

The first mutation within POU1F1 was described in a child with "cretinism" born to consanguineous unaffected parents. She was found to have TSH, GH, and prolactin deficiency, secondary to a homozygous nonsense mutation resulting in a truncated peptide lacking the POU-homeodomain region.[43] This triad of hormone deficiencies has been well described in association with POU1F1 gene mutations, with variable phenotypic presentations and inheritance patterns.[44] Most patients present with growth failure, whereas fewer than half present with hypothyroidism as the first clinical manifestation.[45] Occasional preservation of TSH secretion has been described.[46] Most patients are homozygous for a recessive mutation or have a dominant negative mutation in codon 271, a well-recognized hotspot[46]; however, compound heterozygosity also has been described.[44,45] MRI demonstrates a small or normal anterior pituitary, with a normal posterior pituitary.[44]

Mutations result in altered DNA binding and/or transactivation of target genes. In a previously described patient with severe mental retardation and short stature found to have a dominant negative point mutation in codon 271,[47] a recent study showed that this mutation results in loss of POU1F1 association with beta-catenin and SATB1. This association is required for binding of POU1F1-occupied enhancers to a nuclear matrin-3-rich network/architecture, which is a key event in effective activation of gene transcription.[48]

ORTHODENTICLE HOMEOBOX 2

Orthodenticle homeobox 2 (OTX2), mapped to 14q22.3,[49] is organized into 5 exons, 3 of which are translated, and contains an N-terminal paired type homeodomain, SIW-SPA conserved motif, and 2 tandem tail motifs within a C-terminal transactivation domain.[50] OTX2 has a well-established role in ocular development[51]; however, recent studies have demonstrated a role in pituitary development. One study reported abnormal pituitary structure/function in 30% of patients with mutations in OTX2.[52]

In 2 unrelated children with CPHD (GH, TSH, LH, FSH, and ACTH), anterior pituitary hypoplasia, and EPP, without any midline or optic nerve abnormalities, a heterozygous missense mutation (N233S) was identified. Despite preserved binding to target genes, the mutant was shown to act as a dominant negative inhibitor of HESX1 gene expression, suggesting that hypopituitarism may be due to diminished expression of HESX1.[53] In a recent study of 94 patients with varied ocular or pituitary abnormalities, 3 heterozygous truncation mutations in 4 patients and a microdeletion in 1 patient were identified. One patient had CPHD, 2 patients had isolated GH deficiency, and 2 patients had normal pituitary function. Abnormal pituitary imaging (pituitary hypoplasia and/or EPP) was seen in all 3 affected patients. All 5 patients had ocular anomalies. The wild-type OTX2 protein transactivated GNRH1, HESX1, POU1F1, and IRBP (interstitial retinoid-binding protein) promoters, whereas the mutated proteins had reduced or loss of transactivation for the 4 promoters. The investigators highlighted the variable pituitary phenotype, and lack of genotype-phenotype correlations in OTX2 mutations.[50]

FUTURE CONSIDERATIONS/SUMMARY

Pituitary gland development is a complex orchestrated process that results in essential hormone production. Advances in molecular genetics have identified mutations within genes encoding pituitary transcription factors in patients with isolated or syndromic hypopituitarism, expanding our understanding of the underlying molecular basis. However, the vast majority of affected patients remain labeled idiopathic, presumably due to mutations yet to be identified, as well as modifier genes and environmental factors. Next-generation sequencing, including whole-genome sequencing (WGS) and whole-exome sequencing (WES), are now being used in clinical care.[54] The less expensive of the two, WES, provides coverage of more than 95% of the exons, which contains 85% of disease-causing mutations in Mendelian disorders.[55] High costs, ethical concerns including the assessment of significance and the need for user-friendly software in the analysis of the raw sequence, are limiting factors.[55] Nonetheless, WES, and eventually WGS, hold the potential of exponentially increasing our knowledge of the genetic basis of hypopituitarism and personalizing preventive, diagnostic, and therapeutic patient care.

REFERENCES

1. Rosenfeld RG, Albertsson-Wikland K, Cassorla F, et al. Diagnostic controversy: the diagnosis of childhood growth hormone deficiency revisited. J Clin Endocrinol Metab 1995;80(5):1532–40.

2. Biller BM, Samuels MH, Zagar A, et al. Sensitivity and specificity of six tests for the diagnosis of adult GH deficiency. J Clin Endocrinol Metab 2002;87(5): 2067–79.

3. American Academy of Pediatrics, Rose SR, Section on Endocrinology and Committee on Genetics, American Thyroid Association, et al. Update of newborn screening and therapy for congenital hypothyroidism. Pediatrics 2006;117(6): 2290–303.

4. Mukherjee A, Murray RD, Columb B, et al. Acquired prolactin deficiency indicates severe hypopituitarism in patients with disease of the hypothalamic-pituitary axis. Clin Endocrinol 2003;59(6):743–8.

5. Oelkers W. Hyponatremia and inappropriate secretion of vasopressin (antidiuretic hormone) in patients with hypopituitarism. N Engl J Med 1989;321(8):492–6.

6. Dattani MT, Martinez-Barbera JP, Thomas PQ, et al. Mutations in the homeobox gene HESX1/Hesx1 associated with septo-optic dysplasia in human and mouse. Nat Genet 1998;19(2):125–33.

7. Hermesz E, Mackem S, Mahon KA. Rpx: a novel anterior-restricted homeobox gene progressively activated in the prechordal plate, anterior neural plate and Rathke's pouch of the mouse embryo. Development 1996;122(1):41–52.

8. Brickman JM, Clements M, Tyrell R, et al. Molecular effects of novel mutations in Hesx1/HESX1 associated with human pituitary disorders. Development 2001; 128(24):5189–99.

9. Carvalho LR, Woods KS, Mendonca BB, et al. A homozygous mutation in HESX1 is associated with evolving hypopituitarism due to impaired repressor-corepressor interaction. J Clin Invest 2003;112(8):1192–201.

10. Dasen JS, Martinez Barbera JP, Herman TS, et al. Temporal regulation of a paired-like homeodomain repressor/TLE corepressor complex and a related activator is required for pituitary organogenesis. Genes Dev 2001;15(23):3193–207.

11. Carvalho LR, Brinkmeier ML, Castinetti F, et al. Corepressors TLE1 and TLE3 interact with HESX1 and PROP1. Mol Endocrinol 2010;24(4):754–65.

12. Thomas PQ, Dattani MT, Brickman JM, et al. Heterozygous HESX1 mutations associated with isolated congenital pituitary hypoplasia and septo-optic dysplasia. Hum Mol Genet 2001;10(1):39–45.

13. Tajima T, Hattorri T, Nakajima T, et al. Sporadic heterozygous frameshift mutation of HESX1 causing pituitary and optic nerve hypoplasia and combined pituitary hormone deficiency in a Japanese patient. J Clin Endocrinol Metab 2003;88(1): 45–50.

14. Cohen RN, Cohen LE, Botero D, et al. Enhanced repression by HESX1 as a cause of hypopituitarism and septooptic dysplasia. J Clin Endocrinol Metab 2003; 88(10):4832–9.

15. Webb EA, Dattani MT. Septo-optic dysplasia. Eur J Hum Genet 2010;18(4):393–7.

16. Fang Q, Benedetti AF, Ma Q, et al. HESX1 mutations in patients with congenital hypopituitarism: variable phenotypes with the same genotype. Clin Endocrinol 2016;85(3):408–14.

17. Takagi M, Takahashi M, Ohtsu Y, et al. A novel mutation in HESX1 causes combined pituitary hormone deficiency without septo optic dysplasia phenotypes. Endocr J 2016;63(4):405–10.

18. Zhadanov AB, Bertuzzi S, Taira M, et al. Expression pattern of the murine LIM class homeobox gene Lhx3 in subsets of neural and neuroendocrine tissues. Dev Dyn 1995;202(4):354–64.

19. Sloop KW, Showalter AD, Von Kap-Herr C, et al. Analysis of the human LHX3 neuroendocrine transcription factor gene and mapping to the subtelomeric region of chromosome 9. Gene 2000;245(2):237–43.
20. Bhangoo AP, Hunter CS, Savage JJ, et al. Clinical case seminar: a novel LHX3 mutation presenting as combined pituitary hormonal deficiency. J Clin Endocrinol Metab 2006;91(3):747–53.
21. Pfaeffle RW, Savage JJ, Hunter CS, et al. Four novel mutations of the LHX3 gene cause combined pituitary hormone deficiencies with or without limited neck rotation. J Clin Endocrinol Metab 2007;92(5):1909–19.
22. Rajab A, Kelberman D, de Castro SC, et al. Novel mutations in LHX3 are associated with hypopituitarism and sensorineural hearing loss. Hum Mol Genet 2008; 17(14):2150–9.
23. Kristrom B, Zdunek AM, Rydh A, et al. A novel mutation in the LIM homeobox 3 gene is responsible for combined pituitary hormone deficiency, hearing impairment, and vertebral malformations. J Clin Endocrinol Metab 2009;94(4):1154–61.
24. Machinis K, Pantel J, Netchine I, et al. Syndromic short stature in patients with a germline mutation in the LIM homeobox LHX4. Am J Hum Genet 2001;69(5): 961–8.
25. Kawamata N, Sakajiri S, Sugimoto KJ, et al. A novel chromosomal translocation t(1;14)(q25;q32) in pre-B acute lymphoblastic leukemia involves the LIM homeodomain protein gene, Lhx4. Oncogene 2002;21(32):4983–91.
26. Sheng HZ, Moriyama K, Yamashita T, et al. Multistep control of pituitary organogenesis. Science 1997;278(5344):1809–12.
27. Pfaeffle RW, Hunter CS, Savage JJ, et al. Three novel missense mutations within the LHX4 gene are associated with variable pituitary hormone deficiencies. J Clin Endocrinol Metab 2008;93(3):1062–71.
28. Castinetti F, Saveanu A, Reynaud R, et al. A novel dysfunctional LHX4 mutation with high phenotypical variability in patients with hypopituitarism. J Clin Endocrinol Metab 2008;93(7):2790–9.
29. Gregory LC, Humayun KN, Turton JP, et al. Novel lethal form of congenital hypopituitarism associated with the first recessive LHX4 mutation. J Clin Endocrinol Metab 2015;100(6):2158–64.
30. Duquesnoy P, Roy A, Dastot F, et al. Human Prop-1: cloning, mapping, genomic structure. Mutations in familial combined pituitary hormone deficiency. FEBS Lett 1998;437(3):216–20.
31. Sornson MW, Wu W, Dasen JS, et al. Pituitary lineage determination by the Prophet of Pit-1 homeodomain factor defective in Ames dwarfism. Nature 1996; 384(6607):327–33.
32. Nakamura Y, Usui T, Mizuta H, et al. Characterization of Prophet of Pit-1 gene expression in normal pituitary and pituitary adenomas in humans. J Clin Endocrinol Metab 1999;84(4):1414–9.
33. Cogan JD, Wu W, Phillips JA 3rd, et al. The PROP1 2-base pair deletion is a common cause of combined pituitary hormone deficiency. J Clin Endocrinol Metab 1998;83(9):3346–9.
34. Reynaud R, Barlier A, Vallette-Kasic S, et al. An uncommon phenotype with familial central hypogonadism caused by a novel PROP1 gene mutant truncated in the transactivation domain. J Clin Endocrinol Metab 2005;90(8):4880–7.
35. Rosenbloom AL, Almonte AS, Brown MR, et al. Clinical and biochemical phenotype of familial anterior hypopituitarism from mutation of the PROP1 gene. J Clin Endocrinol Metab 1999;84(1):50–7.

36. Bottner A, Keller E, Kratzsch J, et al. PROP1 mutations cause progressive deterioration of anterior pituitary function including adrenal insufficiency: a longitudinal analysis. J Clin Endocrinol Metab 2004;89(10):5256–65.

37. Fluck C, Deladoey J, Rutishauser K, et al. Phenotypic variability in familial combined pituitary hormone deficiency caused by a PROP1 gene mutation resulting in the substitution of Arg–>Cys at codon 120 (R120C). J Clin Endocrinol Metab 1998;83(10):3727–34.

38. Arroyo A, Pernasetti F, Vasilyev VV, et al. A unique case of combined pituitary hormone deficiency caused by a PROP1 gene mutation (R120C) associated with normal height and absent puberty. Clin Endocrinol 2002;57(2):283–91.

39. Fofanova O, Takamura N, Kinoshita E, et al. MR imaging of the pituitary gland in children and young adults with congenital combined pituitary hormone deficiency associated with PROP1 mutations. AJR Am J Roentgenol 2000;174(2):555–9.

40. Mendonca BB, Osorio MG, Latronico AC, et al. Longitudinal hormonal and pituitary imaging changes in two females with combined pituitary hormone deficiency due to deletion of A301,G302 in the PROP1 gene. J Clin Endocrinol Metab 1999; 84(3):942–5.

41. Andersen B, Rosenfeld MG. POU domain factors in the neuroendocrine system: lessons from developmental biology provide insights into human disease. Endocr Rev 2001;22(1):2–35.

42. Ohta K, Nobukuni Y, Mitsubuchi H, et al. Characterization of the gene encoding human pituitary-specific transcription factor, Pit-1. Gene 1992;122(2):387–8.

43. Tatsumi K, Miyai K, Notomi T, et al. Cretinism with combined hormone deficiency caused by a mutation in the PIT1 gene. Nat Genet 1992;1(1):56–8.

44. Radovick S, Cohen LE, Wondisford FE. The molecular basis of hypopituitarism. Horm Res 1998;49(Suppl 1):30–6.

45. Hendriks-Stegeman BI, Augustijn KD, Bakker B, et al. Combined pituitary hormone deficiency caused by compound heterozygosity for two novel mutations in the POU domain of the Pit1/POU1F1 gene. J Clin Endocrinol Metab 2001; 86(4):1545–50.

46. Turton JP, Reynaud R, Mehta A, et al. Novel mutations within the POU1F1 gene associated with variable combined pituitary hormone deficiency. J Clin Endocrinol Metab 2005;90(8):4762–70.

47. Radovick S, Nations M, Du Y, et al. A mutation in the POU-homeodomain of Pit-1 responsible for combined pituitary hormone deficiency. Science 1992;257(5073): 1115–8.

48. Skowronska-Krawczyk D, Ma Q, Schwartz M, et al. Required enhancer-matrin-3 network interactions for a homeodomain transcription program. Nature 2014; 514(7521):257–61.

49. Wyatt A, Bakrania P, Bunyan DJ, et al. Novel heterozygous OTX2 mutations and whole gene deletions in anophthalmia, microphthalmia and coloboma. Hum Mutat 2008;29(11):E278–83.

50. Dateki S, Kosaka K, Hasegawa K, et al. Heterozygous orthodenticle homeobox 2 mutations are associated with variable pituitary phenotype. J Clin Endocrinol Metab 2010;95(2):756–64.

51. Hever AM, Williamson KA, van Heyningen V. Developmental malformations of the eye: the role of PAX6, SOX2 and OTX2. Clin Genet 2006;69(6):459–70.

52. Schilter KF, Schneider A, Bardakjian T, et al. OTX2 microphthalmia syndrome: four novel mutations and delineation of a phenotype. Clin Genet 2011;79(2): 158–68.

53. Diaczok D, Romero C, Zunich J, et al. A novel dominant negative mutation of OTX2 associated with combined pituitary hormone deficiency. J Clin Endocrinol Metab 2008;93(11):4351–9.
54. Bick D, Dimmock D. Whole exome and whole genome sequencing. Curr Opin Pediatr 2011;23(6):594–600.
55. Rabbani B, Tekin M, Mahdieh N. The promise of whole-exome sequencing in medical genetics. J Hum Genet 2014;59(1):5–15.

Genetics of Short Stature

Youn Hee Jee, MD[a,*], Anenisia C. Andrade, MD, PhD[b],
Jeffrey Baron, MD[a], Ola Nilsson, MD, PhD[b,c]

KEYWORDS

- Short stature • Genetic causes • Growth plate • Genome-wide association study
- Exome sequencing

KEY POINTS

- Over the past decades, advances in clinical genetics, including exome sequencing, have accelerated the identification of new genetic growth disorders and thereby greatly contributed to the understanding of the underlying molecular mechanisms of longitudinal bone growth and growth failure.
- This new knowledge will help the individual patient seeking medical attention due to severe short stature, as it will improve the chances of an exact mechanistic diagnosis, which in turn enables individualized diagnosis/management, prognostic accuracy, and better genetic counseling and may also help avoid unnecessary testing for endocrine and other disorders.
- As more genetic causes become identified, better classifications of growth disorders will become possible.

INTRODUCTION

Short stature is a common medical concern that pediatricians and pediatric endocrinologists often evaluate in their daily practice because poor growth may be a symptom of an underlying, treatable medical condition.[1] Linear growth is the result of

Disclosure: This work was supported by the Intramural Research Program of the *Eunice Kennedy Shriver* National Institute of Child Health and Human Development (ZIA HD000640), NIH (ZIA HD000640). Dr O. Nilsson was supported by grants from the Swedish Research Council (Grant no. 521-2014-3063 and 2015-02227), the Swedish Governmental Agency for Innovation Systems (Vinnova) (2014-01438), Marianne and Marcus Wallenberg Foundation (2014.0096), the Stockholm County Council (2015-0442), Byggmästare Olle Engkvist's Foundation (2015/27), Stiftelsen Frimurare Barnhuset i Stockholm, and Karolinska Institutet. Dr A.C. Andrade was supported by grants from Sällskapet Barnavård.
 a Program in Developmental Endocrinology and Genetics, *Eunice Kennedy Shriver* National Institute of Child Health and Human Development, National Institutes of Health, CRC, Room 1-3330, 10 Center Drive MSC 1103, Bethesda, MD 20892-1103, USA; b Division of Pediatric Endocrinology, Department of Women's and Children's Health, Karolinska Institutet, Karolinska University Hospital, Solnavägen 1, Solna 171 77, Sweden; c University Hospital, Örebro University, Södra Grev Rosengatan, Örebro 701 85, Sweden
* Corresponding author. National Institutes of Health, CRC, Room 1-3330, 10 Center Drive MSC 1103, Bethesda, MD 20892-1103.
E-mail address: jeeyh@mail.nih.gov

Endocrinol Metab Clin N Am 46 (2017) 259–281
http://dx.doi.org/10.1016/j.ecl.2017.01.001
0889-8529/17/Published by Elsevier Inc.

endo.theclinics.com

chondrogenesis at the growth plate and all forms of short stature are therefore due to decreased chondrogenesis at the growth plates.[2] Growth plate chondrogenesis and therefore linear growth are regulated by multiple systemic factors, including nutritional intake, hormones, and inflammatory cytokines.[3] Consequently, systemic diseases, such as hypothyroidism, celiac disease, and other chronic disorders impair childhood growth. In addition, growth plate chondrogenesis is regulated by multiple local factors, including intracellular regulatory mechanisms in the growth plate chondrocytes, cartilage extracellular matrix components, and paracrine factors in the growth plate. As a result, genetic defects in these local growth plate systems can also result in short stature (**Fig. 1**).

Height variation within the normal range involves similar mechanisms. In 2010, a genome-wide association (GWA) study revealed 180 loci that explain approximately 10% of height variation[4] and a more recent GWA study identified approximately 400 loci that are associated with adult height in the general population.[5] It is likely that many children have mild short stature because they have inherited multiple polymorphisms, each of which tends to slightly inhibit growth plate chondrogenesis and in fact, the loci implicated by GWA studies are shown enriched in genes that are expressed and important for growth plate function.[4–6] Taken together, these findings suggest that normal growth is modulated by several hundred or maybe even thousands of genes that affect growth plate function. Therefore, polymorphism and mild mutations in these identified genes may modulate height within the normal range and perhaps cause mild polygenic short stature, whereas mutations with a stronger effect on protein function and/or biallelic mutations may cause significant monogenic short stature or skeletal dysplasias.

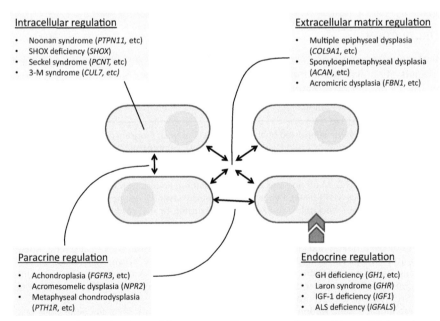

Fig. 1. Molecular mechanisms of short stature. Short stature is caused by multiple molecular defects, including intracellular signaling, extracellular matrix, and paracrine and endocrine regulation. Ovoid shapes represent growth plate chondrocytes. Arrows indicate mechanisms regulating chondrocytes. Examples of clinical syndrome and the genetic cause under different molecular mechanisms are shown in each box.

The high-throughput sequencing and bioinformatics approaches have enabled identification of genetic causes for many human disorders.[7,8] In particular, exome sequencing has been successfully applied to reveal genetic variants responsible for unknown causes of rare diseases.[7,8] Consequently, exome sequencing has become a powerful research tool to identify the etiology of disorders with a monogenic pattern of inheritance. Using this approach, an increasing number of monogenic causes of growth disorders are being identified, thereby gradually diminishing the number of children who receive the unhelpful diagnosis of "idiopathic" short stature. The GWA studies on height variation as well as the expanding genetic diagnoses of growth disorders indicate that childhood growth disorders are highly genetically heterogeneous[1,2] and that a large fraction of the genes important for growth are involved in cellular processes previously not implicated in regulation of growth. These findings will likely affect the way we diagnose childhood growth disorders. Previously, the approach to short stature was primarily focused on clinical manifestations; for example, primordial dwarfism, syndromic short stature, or skeletal dysplasia to categorize them by similar clinical features. Currently, the combination of the clinical approach and improved genetic diagnosis is advancing our understanding of genetic growth disorders and has helped to further widen the understanding of the clinical variability and genetic heterogeneity of short stature syndromes.

Identifying and understanding the genetic basis of short stature will have significant impact on the care of children seeking medical attention for severe short stature. An accurate genetic diagnosis will guide management and help limit unnecessary testing, recognize associated health risks, enable proper genetic counseling, and improve basic understanding of skeletal development and growth and may eventually lead to the development of new treatment approaches.[1,2] Therefore, we here review genetic causes of growth disorders by the molecular mechanisms (see **Fig. 1**; **Table 1**), emphasizing recently discovered causes of childhood growth disorders.

GENETICS OF SHORT STATURE
Defects in Intracellular Pathways

Mutations causing loss-of-function or gain-of-function of proteins important for fundamental cellular processes often result in severe short stature with or without an obvious skeletal dysplasia. The mutations also may be associated with microcephaly, intellectual disability, distinctive facial features, or other clinical abnormalities (see **Table 1**).

Intracellular signaling pathways

Depending on the pathway affected, defects in intracellular signaling cause a wide spectrum in the degree of growth failure, as well as in the conditions associated with each defect. The intracellular defects are highly heterogeneous, such as the RAS (rat sarcoma)-MAPK (mitogen-activated protein kinase) pathway,[9–20] guanine nucleotide exchange factor,[21–23] cyclic AMP (cAMP)-dependent regulatory subunit of protein kinase A,[24] and other signaling proteins.[25–32] Especially, altered RAS-MAPK signaling has been identified as a key pathway in regulation of growth plate chondrogenesis and is affected in several disorders, referred to as RASopathies.[33] These conditions include Coffin-Lowry syndrome,[9,10] Costello (faciocutaneoskeletal syndrome),[11] multiple lentigines syndrome (LEOPARD syndrome),[12–16] neurofibromatosis type 1,[17,18] and Noonan syndrome or Noonan-like syndrome.[11,19,20] Patients with these disorders have overlapping phenotypes of short stature, skin manifestation, cardiovascular abnormalities, and variable degree of learning disability/cognitive dysfunction and/or predisposition to cancers. RAS cycles between a guanosine

Table 1
Genetics of short stature

Genes	Function	Disorder	Key Clinical Features	[a]GWA List
1. Defects in intracellular pathways				
Intracellular signaling pathways				
FGD1	Guanine nucleotide exchange factor	Aarskog-Scott (faciogenital dysplasia)	IUGR, hyperteloʻism, ptosis, everted lower lip vermilion, joint hyperextension, finger abnormalities, shawl scrotum[21–23]	No
PRKAR1A	cAMP-dependent regulatory subunit of protein kinase A	Acrodysostosis, type 1	IUGR, skeletal dysplasia, severe brachydactyly, facial dysostosis, nasal hypoplasia, advanced bone age, obesity, hormone resistance[24]	No
PDE4D	cAMP-specific 3′, 5′-cyclic phospho-diesterase 4D	Acrodysostosis, type 2	IUGR (variable), skeletal dysplasia, accelerated bone age progression, variable hormone resistance[25]	No
GNAS	G protein alpha subunit	Albright hereditary osteodystrophy	IUGR, obesity, round-shaped face, subcutaneous ossifications and brachymetacarpal bone (4th and 5th)[26–28]	Yes
RPS6KA3	Serine/threonine kinase in RAS-MAPK pathway	Coffin-Lowry syndrome	No IUGR, microcephaly, facial dysmorphism, skeletal abnormalities intellectual disability, hypotonia, X-linked disorder[9,10]	No
HRAS	Signal transduction with GTPase activity in RAS-MAPK pathway	Costello (faciocutaneoskeletal syndrome)	No IUGR, delayed development, intellectual disability, distinctive facial features, loose folds of extra skin (especially, hands and feet), flexible joints[11]	No
PTPN11, RAF1, BRAF	Protein-tyrosine phosphatase/RAS-MAPK regulation	Multiple lentigines syndrome (LEOPARD syndrome)	No IUGR, lentig nes, hypertrophic myopathy, electro-cardiographic conduction abnormalities, ocular hypertelorism, pulmonic stenosis, abnormalities of genitalia, sensorineural deafness[12–16]	Yes (*RAF1*)

Gene(s)	Function	Syndrome	Clinical features	
NF1	RAS signal transduction	Neurofibromatosis type 1	No IUGR, cafe-au-lait spot, malignancy (pheochromocytoma and gastrointestinal stromal tumor), Lisch nodules, osteoporosis[17,18]	No
PTPN11, BRAF, SOS1, KRAS, RAF1, NRAS, RASA2, SHOC2, CBL, RIT1 (activating)	Protein-tyrosine phosphatase/RAS-MAPK regulation	Noonan syndrome or Noonan-like syndrome	No IUGR, distinctive facial appearance, a broad or webbed neck, congenital heart defects, coagulopathy, skeletal malformations, developmental delay[11,19,20]	Yes (RAF1)
ROR2, WNT5A, DVL1	Cell surface receptor, secreted signaling protein	Robinow syndrome (acral dysostosis with facial and genital abnormalities)	IUGR (variable), short-limb dwarfism, costovertebral segmentation defects, abnormalities of head, face and external genitalia, chest deformities, rib fusions, scoliosis, brachydactyly, aplasia/hypoplasia of the phalanges and metacarpal/metatarsal bones[29-32]	Yes (WNT5A)
Transcriptional regulation				
LARP7	Transcriptional regulator of polymerase II genes	Alazami syndrome	IUGR (variable), facial dysmorphism (triangular face), intellectual disability, tendon or skeletal abnormalities[48,49]	No
SOX9	Chondrocyte differentiation factor	Campomelic dysplasia	IUGR, born with bowing of the long bones, short legs, dislocated hips, ambiguous genitalia, distinctive facial features[39-41]	Yes
BRF1	RNA polymerase III transcription initiation factor	Cerebello-facio-dental syndrome	IUGR, facial dysmorphism, hypoplastic cerebellum, markedly delayed bone age[50,150]	No
SOX11	Transcriptional regulation of GDF5	Coffin-Siris syndrome	IUGR (variable), mental retardation, facial dysmorphism, hearing or vision impairment, severe scoliosis[51]	No

(continued on next page)

Table 1
(continued)

Genes	Function	Disorder	Key Clinical Features	[a]GWA List
MLL2 (KMT2D), KDM6A	Histone methyltransferase/ Histone demethylase	Kabuki syndrome	IUGR (variable), facial features that resemble the make-up worn by actors of Kabuki (long eye openings slanting upwards, arched eyebrows, prominent ears, and corners of the mouth turning downward), mild to moderate intellectual disability, problems involving heart, skeleton, teeth, and immune system[45–47]	No
ANKRD11	Transcription regulator	KBG syndrome	IUGR (variable), facial dysmorphism, hearing loss, congenital heart defect, skeletal anomalies, global developmental delay, seizures, intellectual disability[52,53]	No
SHOX	Transcription factor	Leri-Weill dyschondrosteosis, mesomelic dysplasia (Langer type)	No IUGR, skeletal dysplasia, Madelung deformity[42–44]	No
CREBBP, EP300	Transcriptional coactivator	Rubinstein-Taybi syndrome	IUGR (variable), facial dysmorphism, moderate to severe intellectual disability, broad thumbs and first toes[54,55]	Yes (CREBBP)
DNA repair				
BLM	DNA repair enzyme	Bloom syndrome	IUGR (as case report), increased risk of cancer, sun-sensitive skin changes on face, hands and/or arms, a high-pitched voice, distinctive facial features, including a long, narrow face, small lower jaw, large nose, and prominent ears[72,73]	No
ERCC6, ERCC8	DNA repair	Cockayne syndrome	IUGR (variable), microcephaly, photosensitivity progeroid appearance, progressive pigmentary retinopathy, sensorineural deafness[74,75]	No
FANCA, FANCC, FANCG	DNA repair	Fanconi anemia	IUGR, absence of thumb, hyperpigmentation, early-onset bone marrow failure, predisposition to cancers[56]	Yes (FANCA)
LIG4	DNA repair	LIG 4 syndrome	No IUGR, distinctive facial features, microcephaly, pancytopenia, various skin abnormalities, immune deficiency[69]	No

Genetics of Short Stature 265

Gene(s)	Biological process	Syndrome	Clinical features	Mouse model
NSMCE2	DNA repair	Microcephalic primordial dwarfism–insulin resistance syndrome	No IUGR reported, microcephaly, insulin resistance[76]	No
NBN (NBS1)	DNA repair	Nijmegen breakage syndrome	No IUGR, microcephaly, distinctive facial features, immunodeficiency, and cancer predisposition[70,71]	No
SMARCAL1	DNA repair	Schimke immunoosseous dysplasia	IUGR, kidney disease, immune deficiency, stroke, bone marrow failure, kidney failure[77]	No
ATR, ATRIP, CENPJ, CEP152, CEP63, DNA2, PCNT, PLK4, RBBP8, XRCC4	DNA repair, centrosome maintenance, DNA stability	Seckel syndrome	IUGR, microcephaly, beaklike protrusion of nose, facial dysmorphism[56-66]	Yes (DNA2)
Other fundamental cellular processes				
CUL7, OBSL1, CCDC8	Microtubule stabilization and genome stability	3-M syndrome	IUGR, facial dysmorphism (triangular face), relatively large head circumference, prominent fleshy heels[78-80]	No
ALMS1	Microtubule organization	Alström syndrome	No IUGR, vision and hearing abnormalities, childhood obesity, diabetes mellitus, heart disease, and slowly progressive kidney dysfunction[96]	No
SMARCB1, SMARCE1, SMARCA4, ARID1A, ARID1B	Chromatin remodeling	Coffin-Siris syndrome	IUGR (variable), mental retardation, facial dysmorphism, hearing or vision impairment, severe scoliosis[89]	Yes (ARD1B)
NIPBL (50%), SMC1A, HDAC8, RAD21, SMC3	Cohesin pathway (sister chromatid cohesion)	Cornelia de Lange syndrome	IUGR, dysmorphic facial features (facial hirsutism), microcephaly, limb reduction defects, cardiac defect, and intellectual disability[81]	Yes (NIPBL)

(continued on next page)

Table 1
(continued)

Genes	Function	Disorder	Key Clinical Features	[a]GWA List
SRCAP	Chromatin remodeling	Floating-Harbor syndrome	IUGR (variable), facial dysmorphism, abnormal thumb, delayed bone age, early puberty, delay in expressive language[86–88]	No
LMNA	Nuclear stability	Hutchinson-Gilford Progeria	No IUGR, failure to thrive, distinctive facial features (aged-looking skin), alopecia, loss of subcutaneous fat, joint abnormalities[32,83]	No
RNU4ATAC	Minor intron splicing	MOPD I	IUGR, microcephaly, dysmorphic face, skin and skeletal abnormalities developmental delay[90,91]	No
PCNT	Mitotic spindle/ chromosome segregation	MOPD II	IUGR, facial dysmorphism, microcephaly, near normal intelligence, cancer susceptibility[67,68]	No
TRIM37	Persoxisomal protein, possibly ubiquitin-dependent degradation	Mulibrey nanism	IUGR, dysmorphic craniofacial features, heart disease (constrictive pericardium), hepatomegaly, Wilms tumor[92–94]	No
CRIPT	Interaction with cytoskeleton	Primordial dwarfism	IUGR (not established), facial dysmorphism, microcephaly, ophthalmologic abnormalities, intellectual disabilities, skeletal abnormalities, pigmentation abnormalities[95]	No
POC1A	Centriole assembly/ ciliogenesis	SOFT syndrome	IUGR, disproportionate short stature, onychodysplasia, facial dysmorphism, and hypotrichosis[84,85]	No
DHCR7	Steroid biosynthesis	Smith-Lemli-Opitz syndrome	IUGR, distinctive facial features, microcephaly, intellectual disability or learning problems, behavioral problems, and malformations of heart, lungs, kidneys, gastrointestinal tract, and genitalia[97]	No

2. Defects in cartilage extracellular matrix

Gene	Protein/matrix	Disorder	Phenotype	Heterozygous
COL2A1	Extracellular matrix, collagen	Achondrogenesis (Type II), hypochondrogenesis, Kniest dysplasia, Spondylo-epiphyseal dysplasia congenita, Stickler syndrome type 1	IUGR, skeletal abnormalities and problems with vision and hearing[101,102]	No
FBN1	Extracellular matrix, fibrillin 1	Acromicric dysplasia, Geleophysic dysplasia 2	No IUGR, short hands and feet, thickened skin and joint contractures, limited range of motion in fingers, toes, wrists, and elbows, cardiac issue[109]	Yes
COL11A1	Extracellular matrix, collagen 11	Fibrochondrogenesis	IUGR (variable), skeletal dysplasia, broad long bone metaphyses, pear-shaped vertebral bodies, flat midface with a small nose and anteverted nares, significant shortening of all limb segments[103]	Yes
COL10A1	Extracellular matrix, collagen 10	Metaphyseal dysplasia, Schmid type	No IUGR, coxa vara, relatively short limbs, bow legs, waddling gait[104]	No
MATN3, COL9A1, COL9A2, COL9A3	Extracellular matrix, cartilage oligomeric matrix protein, collagen, matrillin-3	Multiple epiphyseal dysplasia	No IUGR, skeletal dysplasia, joint pain, joint deformity, waddling gait[105–108,112]	Yes (COL9A2)
COMP	Extracellular matrix, cartilage oligomeric matrix protein	Multiple epiphyseal dysplasia, pseudoachondroplasia	No IUGR, short arms and legs, a waddling walk, early-onset joint pain (osteoarthritis), limited range of motion at elbows and hips[110,111]	No
HSPG2	Extracellular matrix, perlecan	Schwartz-Jampel syndrome	IUGR (not established), permanent myotonia (prolonged failure of muscle relaxation), skeletal dysplasia, kyphoscoliosis, bowing of diaphyses and irregular epiphyses[115]	No

(continued on next page)

Table 1
(continued)

Genes	Function	Disorder	Key Clinical Features	[a]GWA List
ACAN	Extracellular matrix, aggrecan	Spondyloepimetaphyseal dysplasia, aggrecan/ Kimberly type	IUGR, macrocephaly, severe midface hypoplasia, short neck, barrel chest, brachydactyly, advanced bone age[113,114]	Yes
3. Defects in paracrine signaling				
FGFR3 (activating)	Fibroblast growth factor receptor	Achondroplasia, hypochondroplasia	IUGR, short upper arms and thighs, limited range of motion at elbows, relative macrocephaly with a prominent forehead, trident hand[119–121]	No
IHH	Secreted signaling molecule, Indian hedgehog	Acrocapitofemoral dysplasia, brachydactyly, type A1	No IUGR, brachydactyly[129]	No
NPR2 (inactivating)	CNP receptor	Acromesomelic dysplasia, Maroteaux type	IUGR (variable), short limbs and hand/foot malformations[126]	Yes
BMPR1B, GDF5	BMP receptor/ interacting protein (ligand)	Brachydactyly, type A1 and A2	No IUGR, brachydactyly[135,136]	Yes (GDF5)
PTHLH	Secreted signaling molecules (PTH-related protein)	Brachydactyly, type E2	No IUGR, shortening of fingers mainly in metacarpals and metatarsals[130,131]	No
IGF2	Secreted signaling molecule (insulinlike growth factor-II)	IGF2 deficiency	IUGR, Silver-Russel like facies[137]	No

Gene	Protein/pathway	Condition	Phenotype	Yes/No
PTH1R	PTH and PTHrP receptor	Metaphyseal chondrodysplasia (Jansen type), Eikan dysplasia, chondrodysplasia (Blomstrand type)	No IUGR, skeletal dysplasia, micrognathia, failure of tooth eruption, low-set/posteriorly rotated ears, proptosis[132,133]	No
4. Defects in endocrine ligands, receptors, and signaling pathways				
IGFALS	Acid labile subunit	ALS deficiency	IUGR (variable), low IGF-1 and IGF-BP3[148,149]	No
GH1, GHRHR, SOX3, BTK	GH production	GH deficiency	No IUGR, GH deficiency[138]	No
IGF1	IGF-1	IGF-1 deficiency	IUGR, microcephaly, mental retardation, low IGF-1 level[143,144]	No
IGF1R	Insulin-like growth factor receptor	IGF-1 insensitivity	IUGR, normal to high IGF-1 level[145-147]	Yes
STAT5B	Growth hormone signaling	Immune deficiency and GH resistance	No IUGR, elevated random GH but low IGF-1 or IGFBP-3, immunodeficiency[142]	No
GHR	Growth hormone receptor	Laron syndrome	IUGR, elevated GH and low IGF-1[139-141]	No

Abbreviations: ALS, acid labile subunit; BMP, bone morphogenetic protein; cAMP, cyclic AMP; CNP, C-type natriuretic peptide; GH, growth hormone; GTP, guanosine triphosphate; GWA, genome-wide association; IGF-1, insulin-like growth factor 1; IUGR, intrauterine growth restriction; MAPK, mitogen-activated protein kinase; MOPD, microcephalic osteodysplastic primordial dwarfism; PTH, parathyroid hormone; PTHrP, PTH-related protein; RAF, rapidly accelerated fibrosarcoma; RAS, rat sarcoma.

[a] 670 height–associated single-nucleotide polymorphisms according to GWA study by Wood et al.[5]

diphosphate-bound form (inactive) and GTP-bound form (active),[34] and RAS-GTP activates a large number of effector pathways facilitating downstream signaling taking an important role in cell proliferation and differentiation.[35,36] Moreover, RAS-MAPK is downstream of fibroblast growth factor (FGF) signaling, which is another major pathway involved in skeletal disease.[37] Some of the conditions caused by defects in the RAS-MAPK pathway carry higher risks of malignancies, including mutations in neurofibromin (NF1), RAS, or RAFs.[38] Mutations in FGD1, which encodes a protein similar to small GTP-binding proteins, cause Aarskog-Scott syndrome presenting with disproportionate short stature, skeletal and urogenital anomalies.[21–23]

Interestingly, impairment of signaling through the cAMP-protein kinase A also causes skeletal dysplasias with growth failure associated with accelerated bone age progression and/or poor pubertal growth spurts that include Acrodysostosis, type 1 (caused by mutations in PRKAR1A that encodes cAMP-dependent protein kinase type I-alpha regulatory subunit[24]), Acrodysostosis, type 2 (caused by mutations in PDE4D that encodes cAMP-specific 3', 5'-cyclic phosphodiesterase 4D[25]), and Albright hereditary osteodystrophy (caused by mutations in GNAS that encodes guanine nucleotide-binding protein stimulatory G subunit alpha protein[26–28]). Mutations in these genes may not only result in skeletal dysplasias but also variable hormone resistance, thus demonstrating the important role of this pathway both in the regulation of growth plate chondrogenesis and in signaling of the G-protein–coupled hormone receptors.[25] In addition, defects in the WNT5A/JNK signaling pathway, including mutations in ROR2, DVL1, as well as Wnt5a, the ligand of ROR2, cause skeletal dysplasia and Robinow syndrome, characterized by dysmorphic facial features, frontal bossing, hypertelorism, broad nose, short-limbed dwarfism, vertebral segmentation, and genital hypoplasia.[29–32]

Transcriptional regulation

Mutations in transcriptional factors or genes that are involved in transcription repression can cause short stature. Mutations in SOX9, an important transcription factor for sex development and chondrocyte differentiation, cause Campomelic dysplasia, which can cause sex reversal, ambiguous genitalia, chondrodysplasia, and bent bones.[39–41] SHOX is another transcription factor that is important in growth plate chondrocytes.[42] Homozygous mutations cause severe short stature in Langer mesomelic dysplasia, whereas heterozygous mutations can present either as a milder skeletal dysplasia, Leri-Weill dyschondrosteosis, or as isolated short stature.[43,44] Mutations in MLL2 (KMT2D) and KDM6A cause abnormal histone methylation and demethylation, respectively, resulting in short stature and unique facial features of Kabuki syndrome.[45–47] Mutations in transcriptional regulator of polymerase II genes (LARP7) cause Alazami syndrome,[48,49] whereas mutations in the transcription initiator factor for RNA polymerase III (BRF1) cause the newly identified cerebello-facio-dental syndrome.[50,150] Mutations in SOX11 can cause an autosomal dominant mental retardation 27, a form of Coffin-Siris syndrome presenting with relatively mild mental retardation, microcephaly, short stature, and hypoplastic fifth toenails.[51] Similarly, the ankyrin repeat domain-containing protein 11 (ANKRD11) interacts with nuclear receptor complexes to modify transcriptional activation, and mutations in this gene cause short stature, developmental delay, and seizures, as well as other features of the KBG syndrome, including macrodontia of the upper central incisors, and skeletal anomalies.[52,53] In addition, heterozygous mutations in transcription coactivators (CREBBP and EP300) cause Rubinstein-Taybi syndrome, characterized by severe short stature, intellectual disability, microcephaly, hearing loss, broad thumbs/halluces, and distinct facial features.[54,55]

DNA repair

Impairment of DNA repair can result in severe short stature (often primordial dwarfism), microcephaly, photosensitivity, and/or predisposition to leukemia/other cancers. Skeletal abnormalities may not be prominent (see **Table 1**). Especially, Seckel syndrome has many subtypes that are caused by mutations in several genes but mostly involved in DNA repair processes.[56–66] Pericentrin (PCNT) encodes a centrosomal protein in the microtubule network and the mutations cause microcephalic osteodysplastic primordial dwarfism type 2 (MOPD II), but also Seckel syndrome.[66] Moreover, clinical overlaps may occur among Seckel syndrome,[56,66] MOPD II,[56,66–68] Fanconi anemia (FANC),[56] LIG4 syndrome (LIG4),[56,69] and Nijimegen breakage syndrome (NBS1).[56,70,71] Mutations in BLM cause Bloom syndrome, which manifests as sun-sensitive skin and increased risk of malignancies, including leukemia, lymphoma, adenocarcinoma, and squamous cell carcinoma.[72,73] Due to the increased risk of malignancy, growth hormone treatment in children with Bloom syndrome is not recommended.[73] Impaired DNA repair mechanisms may also cause short stature and microcephaly without an increased risk of malignancies. For example, no cancer predisposition has been demonstrated for Cockayne syndrome.[74,75] In addition, recent reports show that heterozygous mutation in NSMCE2 causes microcephalic primordial dwarfism with severe insulin resistance[76] and homozygous mutation in SMARCAL1 causes Schimke immuno-osseous dysplasia, characterized by severe growth restriction, immune deficiency, and renal and bone marrow failure,[77] but no known increased risk of malignancies.

Other fundamental cellular processes

This group of syndromes can be caused by mutations in genes important for genome or nuclear stability (3M syndrome,[78–80] Cornelia de Lange syndrome,[81] Hutchinson-Gilford Progeria,[82,83] MOPD II,[67,68] SOFT syndrome[84,85]), chromatin remodeling (Floating-Harbor syndrome,[86–88] Coffin-Siris syndrome[89]), RNA processing (microcephalic osteodysplastic primordial dwarfism type 1, MOPD I[90,91]), ubiquitination (Mulibrey nanism[92–94]), cytoskeletal interaction (primordial dwarfism due to CRIPT mutation[95]), microtubule organization (Alström syndrome[96]), or cholesterol biosynthesis (Smith-Lemli-Opitz syndrome[97]) (see **Table 1**). The patients are often born small for gestational age indicating that growth is affected during intrauterine life. Interestingly, although the molecular mechanisms are different, the clinical phenotype may have significant overlap. For example, Cornelia de Lange syndrome caused by mutation in the NIPBL has similar features with Rubinstein-Taybi syndrome caused by EP300,[98] although their molecular mechanisms are different.

Defects in Cartilage Extracellular Matrix Defect

Growth plate chondrocytes also secrete a characteristic extracellular matrix rich in collagens and proteoglycans that are critical to maintain structure and function of the growth plate.[99] The extracellular matrix does not only provide support, but also interacts with paracrine signaling molecules regulating chondrocyte proliferation and differentiation.[99,100] Therefore, mutations in genes that encode matrix collagens, proteoglycans, noncollagenous proteins, and their processing enzymes affect growth plate chondrogenesis by several mechanisms and cause growth failure with a wide phenotypic spectrum (see **Table 1**). For example, mutations in collagens,[101–108] fibrillin 1,[109] cartilage oligomeric matrix protein,[110,111] matrillin-3,[112] aggrecan,[113,114] and perlecan[115] have been reported to cause short stature of variable severity. Mutations in genes encoding extracellular matrix proteins also may affect connective tissue beyond the growth plate, causing various degrees of skeletal and joint problems, as well as some conditions with low bone mineral density (see **Table 1**).

Abnormal Paracrine Signaling

In the growth plate, paracrine factors coordinate sequential changes in chondrocyte morphology, proliferation, differentiation, and matrix assembly.[116] The understanding of the paracrine mechanisms acting in the growth plate has advanced substantially during the past decade. Some of the identified factors include FGFs, C-type natriuretic peptide (CNP), Indian hedgehog (IHH), parathyroid hormone–related protein (PTHrP) encoded by *PTHLH*, and bone morphogenetic factors (BMPs). FGF receptor-3 (*FGFR3*) signals through several pathways, including the MAPK and JAK/STAT pathways, and acts as a negative regulator of growth plate chondrogenesis.[117,118] Consequently, activating mutations in *FGFR3* result in inhibition of growth,[119] which can result in skeletal dysplasias ranging from moderate disproportionate short stature (hypochondroplasia) to severe short stature and bone malformation (achondroplasia), and to the most severe form (thanatophoric dysplasia), a perinatal lethal skeletal dysplasia with very short limbs and underdeveloped ribs.[120] In addition, several families with autosomal dominant proportionate short stature were recently reported to have mild activating mutations of *FGFR3*, further expanding the phenotype.[121] Interestingly, both heterozygous and homozygous inactivating mutations in *FGFR3* have been reported in patients with a tall stature syndrome, including scoliosis, camptodactyly, and hearing loss.[122,123]

Despite its name, CNP acts as an important paracrine factor in the growth plate. Homozygous knockout of CNP causes dwarfism in mice.[124] In humans, overexpression of CNP results in overgrowth,[125] whereas homozygous inactivating mutations of its receptor, *NPR2,* cause a skeletal dysplasia with short stature and heterozygous inactivating mutations present as isolated short stature.[126] Conversely, activating mutation in *NPR2* can cause tall stature.[127] CNP inhibits MAPK signaling and thus antagonizes *FGFR3* signaling, and has therefore been proposed as a potential treatment for achondroplasia.[128]

PTHrP and IHH form a negative feedback loop critical to the spatial coordination of proliferation and differentiation of growth plate chondrocytes.[116] Consequently, mutations in the genes for IHH,[129] PTHrP,[130,131] and PTH1R (the receptor for both PTH and PTHrP),[132,133] as well as mutations in their signaling pathway cause specific skeletal dysplasias. Disorders of linear growth also can result from genetic defects in other paracrine signaling systems. For example, BMP signaling is important for endochondral ossification and growth plate regulation,[134] and defects in BMP family members or the receptors cause skeletal dysplasia,[135,136] characterized by brachydactyly. Mutation in *IGF2*, which encodes insulinlike growth factor-II, a paracrine factor that is important for intrauterine growth, was recently reported to cause prenatal and postnatal growth failure.[137]

Abnormal Hormone, Receptor, or Signaling Pathway

Growth hormone (GH) plays a major role in childhood growth and has, especially since the development of recombinant GH, been the main therapeutic approach available to treat patients with short stature. It is therefore common that children presenting with suboptimal growth are subjected to clinical testing for GH deficiency or resistance even though true GH deficiency or resistance is a rare cause of short stature.[2] Patients with mutations in *GH1, GHRHR, SOX3*, and *BTK* present with isolated GH deficiency.[138] On the other hand, mutations in *GHR*[139–141] and *STAT5B*[142] cause GH resistance. GHR encodes the growth hormone receptor. Because an extracellular cleavage fragment of the GH receptor circulates as a growth hormone binding protein (GHBP), mutations in the extracellular domain of *GHR* tend to cause low GHBP, whereas mutations in intracellular (signaling) domain cause normal or high GHBP.[139-141] STAT5 proteins contribute to the common pathway of GH and interleukin-2 cytokine family signaling; therefore, mutations in *STAT5B* cause growth failure and immune deficiency.[142] Mutations in *IGF1* or *IGF1R* cause intrauterine growth restriction (because IGF-1 signaling is important for intrauterine growth, whereas GH is not required), postnatal growth failure, microcephaly, and other various anomalies, including developmental delay.[143-147] Mutations in a gene that stabilizes IGF-1, *IGFALS*, forming an IGF-1-IGFBP3-ALS complex, cause growth deficiency, insulin resistance, and osteoporosis.[148,149]

MUTATIONS IN THE SAME GENE MAY CAUSE A WIDE PHENOTYPIC SPECTRUM

For many genes that support growth plate chondrogenesis, homozygous and/or severe mutations cause bones to be markedly short and malformed, presenting clinically as a chondrodysplasia, whereas heterozygous and/or milder mutations may cause "isolated" short stature, with no or only subtle signs of a skeletal dysplasia. For example, *SHOX*,[43] *NPR2*,[125] *ACAN*,[114] *IGF1*,[143] *IGF1R*,[146] or *FGFR3*[120] have been associated with "isolated" short stature without other prominent phenotypic features. There are likely numerous genetic causes still remaining to be discovered to fully explain the molecular mechanism of "isolated" growth disorders. It is likely that there soon will be a large number of genetically characterized monogenic short stature syndromes with no or only minor associated abnormalities. A suitable term for this group of patients would be "isolated" short stature.

SUMMARY AND FUTURE CONSIDERATIONS

Over the past decades, advances in clinical genetics, including exome sequencing, have accelerated the identification of new genetic growth disorders and thereby greatly contributed to the understanding of the underlying molecular mechanisms of longitudinal bone growth and growth failure. This new knowledge will help the individual patient seeking medical attention due to severe short stature, as it will improve the chances of an exact mechanistic diagnosis, which in turn enables individualized management, improved prognosis, and better genetic counseling, and may also help avoid unnecessary testing for endocrine and other disorders. As more genetic causes become identified, better classifications of growth disorders become possible. Fewer children will receive the unhelpful diagnosis of "idiopathic" short stature, and instead will be categorized clinically as having a skeletal dysplasia, syndromic short stature, or isolated short stature, will be categorized genetically as having polygenic or monogenic short stature, and will be categorized mechanistically depending on how their specific genetic defects diminish growth plate chondrogenesis and therefore linear growth.

REFERENCES

1. Jee YH, Baron J. The biology of stature. J Pediatr 2016;173:32–8.
2. Baron J, Sävendahl L, De Luca F, et al. Short and tall stature: a new paradigm emerges. Nat Rev Endocrinol 2015;11(12):735–46.
3. Nilsson O, Marino R, De Luca F, et al. Endocrine regulation of the growth plate. Horm Res 2005;64(4):157–65.
4. Lango Allen H, Estrada K, Lettre G, et al. Hundreds of variants clustered in genomic loci and biological pathways affect human height. Nature 2010; 467(7317):832–8.
5. Wood AR, Esko T, Yang J, et al. Defining the role of common variation in the genomic and biological architecture of adult human height. Nat Genet 2014; 46(11):1173–86.

6. Lui JC, Nilsson O, Chan Y, et al. Synthesizing genome-wide association studies and expression microarray reveals novel genes that act in the human growth plate to modulate height. Hum Mol Genet 2012;21(23):5193–201.

7. Gahl WA, Markello TC, Toro C, et al. The National Institutes of Health Undiagnosed Diseases Program: insights into rare diseases. Genet Med 2012;14(1): 51–9.

8. Gahl WA, Adams DR, Markello TC, et al. Genetic approaches to rare and undiagnosed diseases. Chapter 83. In: Kliegman R, Stanton, St. Gene, et al, editors. Nelson's textbook of pediatrics. 20th edition. Philadelphia: Elsevier; 2015. p. 629–33.

9. Delaunoy J, Abidi F, Zeniou M, et al. Mutations in the X-linked RSK2 gene (RPS6KA3) in patients with Coffin-Lowry syndrome. Hum Mutat 2001;17(2): 103–16.

10. Rogers RC, Abidi FE. Coffin-Lowry syndrome. Seattle (WA): University of Washington, Seattle; 2002.

11. Noonan JA. Noonan syndrome and related disorders: alterations in growth and puberty. Rev Endocr Metab Disord 2006;7(4):251–5.

12. Kalev I, Muru K, Teek R, et al. LEOPARD syndrome with recurrent PTPN11 mutation Y279C and different cutaneous manifestations: two case reports and a review of the literature. Eur J Pediatr 2010;169(4):469–73.

13. Sarkozy A, Digilio MC, Dallapiccola B. Leopard syndrome. Orphanet J Rare Dis 2008;3:13.

14. Martínez-Quintana E, Rodríguez-González F. LEOPARD syndrome: clinical features and gene mutations. Mol Syndromol 2012;3(4):145–57.

15. Pandit B, Sarkozy A, Pennacchio LA, et al. Gain-of-function RAF1 mutations cause Noonan and LEOPARD syndromes with hypertrophic cardiomyopathy. Nat Genet 2007;39(8):1007–12.

16. Sarkozy A, Carta C, Moretti S, et al. Germline BRAF mutations in Noonan, LEOPARD, and cardiofaciocutaneous syndromes: molecular diversity and associated phenotypic spectrum. Hum Mutat 2009;30(4):695–702.

17. Dunning-Davies BM, Parker AP. Annual review of children with neurofibromatosis type 1. Arch Dis Child Educ Pract Ed 2016;101(2):102–11.

18. Bizzarri C, Bottaro G. Endocrine implications of neurofibromatosis 1 in childhood. Horm Res Paediatr 2015;83(4):232–41.

19. Roberts AE, Allanson JE, Tartaglia M, et al. Noonan syndrome. Lancet 2013; 381(9863):333–42.

20. Aoki Y, Niihori T, Banjo T, et al. Gain-of-function mutations in RIT1 cause Noonan syndrome, a RAS/MAPK pathway syndrome. Am J Hum Genet 2013;93(1): 173–80.

21. Pasteris NG, Cadle A, Logie LJ, et al. Isolation and characterization of the faciogenital dysplasia (Aarskog-Scott syndrome) gene: a putative Rho/Rac guanine nucleotide exchange factor. Cell. 1994;79(4):669–78.

22. Shalev SA, Chervinski E, Weiner E, et al. Clinical variation of Aarskog syndrome in a large family with 2189delA in the FGD1 gene. Am J Med Genet A 2006; 140(2):162–5.

23. Orrico A, Galli L, Cavaliere ML, et al. Phenotypic and molecular characterisation of the Aarskog-Scott syndrome: a survey of the clinical variability in light of FGD1 mutation analysis in 46 patients. Eur J Hum Genet 2004;12(1):16–23.

24. Linglart A, Menguy C, Couvineau A, et al. Recurrent PRKAR1A mutation in acrodysostosis with hormone resistance. N Engl J Med 2011;364(23):2218–26.

25. Lindstrand A, Grigelioniene G, Nilsson D, et al. Different mutations in PDE4D associated with developmental disorders with mirror phenotypes. J Med Genet 2014;51(1):45–54.
26. Ahrens W, Hiort O, Staedt P, et al. Analysis of the GNAS1 gene in Albright's hereditary osteodystrophy. J Clin Endocrinol Metab 2001;86(10):4630–4.
27. Lemos MC, Thakker RV. GNAS mutations in pseudohypoparathyroidism type 1a and related disorders. Hum Mutat 2015;36(1):11–9.
28. Mantovani G, Ferrante E, Giavoli C, et al. Recombinant human GH replacement therapy in children with pseudohypoparathyroidism type Ia: first study on the effect on growth. J Clin Endocrinol Metab 2010;95(11):5011–7.
29. Afzal AR, Rajab A, Fenske CD, et al. Recessive Robinow syndrome, allelic to dominant brachydactyly type B, is caused by mutation of ROR2. Nat Genet 2000;25(4):419–22.
30. Person AD, Beiraghi S, Sieben CM, et al. WNT5A mutations in patients with autosomal dominant Robinow syndrome. Dev Dyn 2010;239(1):327–37.
31. Roifman M, Marcelis CL, Paton T, et al, FORGE Canada Consortium. De novo WNT5A-associated autosomal dominant Robinow syndrome suggests specificity of genotype and phenotype. Clin Genet 2015;87(1):34–41.
32. Bunn KJ, Daniel P, Rösken HS, et al. Mutations in DVL1 cause an osteosclerotic form of Robinow syndrome. Am J Hum Genet 2015;96(4):623–30.
33. Aoki Y, Niihori T, Inoue S, et al. Recent advances in RASopathies. J Hum Genet 2016;61(1):33–9.
34. Takai Y, Sasaki T, Matozaki T. Small GTP-binding proteins. Physiol Rev 2001; 81(1):153–208.
35. Giehl K. Oncogenic Ras in tumour progression and metastasis. Biol Chem 2005; 386(3):193–205.
36. Santarpia L, Lippman SM, El-Naggar AK. Targeting the MAPK-RAS-RAF signaling pathway in cancer therapy. Expert Opin Ther Targets 2012;16(1): 103–19.
37. Teven CM, Farina EM, Rivas J, et al. Fibroblast growth factor (FGF) signaling in development and skeletal diseases. Genes Dis 2014;1(2):199–213.
38. Cizmarova M, Kostalova L, Pribilincova Z, et al. Rasopathies—dysmorphic syndromes with short stature and risk of malignancy. Endocr Regul 2013;47(4): 217–22.
39. Foster JW, Dominguez-Steglich MA, Guioli S, et al. Campomelic dysplasia and autosomal sex reversal caused by mutations in an SRY-related gene. Nature 1994;372(6506):525–30.
40. Meyer J, Südbeck P, Held M, et al. Mutational analysis of the SOX9 gene in campomelic dysplasia and autosomal sex reversal: lack of genotype/phenotype correlations. Hum Mol Genet 1997;6(1):91–8.
41. Gimovsky M, Rosa E, Tolbert T, et al. Campomelic dysplasia: case report and review. J Perinatol 2008;28(1):71–3.
42. Beiser KU, Glaser A, Kleinschmidt K, et al. Identification of novel SHOX target genes in the developing limb using a transgenic mouse model. PLoS One 2014;9(6):e98543.
43. Binder G. Short stature due to SHOX deficiency: genotype, phenotype, and therapy. Horm Res Paediatr 2011;75(2):81–9.
44. Ambrosetti F, Palicelli A, Bulfamante G, et al. Langer mesomelic dysplasia in early fetuses: two cases and a literature review. Fetal Pediatr Pathol 2014; 33(2):71–83.

45. Ng SB, Bigham AW, Buckingham KJ, et al. Exome sequencing identifies MLL2 mutations as a cause of Kabuki syndrome. Nat Genet 2010;42(9):790–3.

46. Dentici ML, Di Pede A, Lepri FR, et al. Kabuki syndrome: clinical and molecular diagnosis in the first year of life. Arch Dis Child 2015;100(2):158–64.

47. Lederer D, Grisart B, Digilio MC, et al. Deletion of KDM6A, a histone demethylase interacting with MLL2, in three patients with Kabuki syndrome. Am J Hum Genet 2012;90(1):119–24.

48. Alazami AM, Al-Owain M, Alzahrani F, et al. Loss of function mutation in LARP7, chaperone of 7SK ncRNA, causes a syndrome of facial dysmorphism, intellectual disability, and primordial dwarfism. Hum Mutat 2012;33(10):1429–34.

49. Hollink IH, Alfadhel M, Al-Wakeel AS, et al. Broadening the phenotypic spectrum of pathogenic LARP7 variants: two cases with intellectual disability, variable growth retardation and distinct facial features. J Hum Genet 2016;61(3):229–33.

50. Borck G, Hög F, Dentici ML, et al. BRF1 mutations alter RNA polymerase III-dependent transcription and cause neurodevelopmental anomalies. Genome Res 2015;25(2):155–66.

51. Tsurusaki Y, Koshimizu E, Ohashi H, et al. De novo SOX11 mutations cause Coffin-Siris syndrome. Nat Commun 2014;5:4011.

52. Sirmaci A, Spiliopoulos M, Brancati F, et al. Mutations in ANKRD11 cause KBG syndrome, characterized by intellectual disability, skeletal malformations, and macrodontia. Am J Hum Genet 2011;89(2):289–94.

53. Ockeloen CW, Willemsen MH, de Munnik S, et al. Further delineation of the KBG syndrome phenotype caused by ANKRD11 aberrations. Eur J Hum Genet 2015; 23(9):1176–85.

54. Menke LA, van Belzen MJ, Alders M, et al, DDD Study. CREBBP mutations in individuals without Rubinstein-Taybi syndrome phenotype. Am J Med Genet A 2016;170(10):2681–93.

55. Negri G, Magini P, Milani D, et al. From whole gene deletion to point mutations of EP300-positive Rubinstein-Taybi patients: new insights into the mutational spectrum and peculiar clinical hallmarks. Hum Mutat 2016;37(2):175–83.

56. Khetarpal P, Das S, Panigrahi I, et al. Primordial dwarfism: overview of clinical and genetic aspects. Mol Genet Genomics 2016;291(1):1–15.

57. O'Driscoll M, Ruiz-Perez VL, Woods CG, et al. A splicing mutation affecting expression of ataxia-telangiectasia and Rad3-related protein (ATR) results in Seckel syndrome. Nat Genet 2003;33(4):497–501.

58. Ogi T, Walker S, Stiff T, et al. Identification of the first ATRIP-deficient patient and novel mutations in ATR define a clinical spectrum for ATR-ATRIP Seckel syndrome. PLoS Genet 2012;8(11):e1002945.

59. Al-Dosari MS, Shaheen R, Colak D, et al. Novel CENPJ mutation causes Seckel syndrome. J Med Genet 2010;47(6):411–4.

60. Kalay E, Yigit G, Aslan Y, et al. CEP152 is a genome maintenance protein disrupted in Seckel syndrome. Nat Genet 2011;43(1):23–6.

61. Marjanović M, Sánchez-Huertas C, Terré B, et al. CEP63 deficiency promotes p53-dependent microcephaly and reveals a role for the centrosome in meiotic recombination. Nat Commun 2015;6:7676.

62. Shaheen R, Faqeih E, Ansari S, et al. Genomic analysis of primordial dwarfism reveals novel disease genes. Genome Res 2014;24(2):291–9.

63. Griffith E, Walker S, Martin CA, et al. Mutations in pericentrin cause Seckel syndrome with defective ATR-dependent DNA damage signaling. Nat Genet 2008; 40(2):232–6.

64. Martin CA, Ahmad I, Klingseisen A, et al. Mutations in PLK4, encoding a master regulator of centriole biogenesis, cause microcephaly, growth failure and retinopathy. Nat Genet 2014;46(12):1283–92.
65. Qvist P, Huertas P, Jimeno S, et al. CtIP mutations cause Seckel and Jawad syndromes. PLoS Genet 2011;7(10):e1002310.
66. Willems M, Geneviève D, Borck G, et al. Molecular analysis of pericentrin gene (PCNT) in a series of 24 Seckel/microcephalic osteodysplastic primordial dwarfism type II (MOPD II) families. J Med Genet 2010;47(12):797–802.
67. Rauch A, Thiel CT, Schindler D, et al. Mutations in the pericentrin (PCNT) gene cause primordial dwarfism. Science 2008;319(5864):816–9.
68. Bober MB, Niiler T, Duker AL, et al. Growth in individuals with Majewski osteodysplastic primordial dwarfism type II caused by pericentrin mutations. Am J Med Genet A 2012;158A(11):2719–25.
69. Chistiakov DA, Voronova NV, Chistiakov AP. Ligase IV syndrome. Eur J Med Genet 2009;52(6):373–8.
70. Pastorczak A, Szczepanski T, Mlynarski W. International Berlin-Frankfurt-Munster (I-BFM) ALL host genetic variation working group. Clinical course and therapeutic implications for lymphoid malignancies in Nijmegen breakage syndrome. Eur J Med Genet 2016;59(3):126–32.
71. Berardinelli F, di Masi A, Antoccia A. NBN gene polymorphisms and cancer susceptibility: a systemic review. Curr Genomics 2013;14(7):425–40.
72. Ellis NA, Lennon DJ, Proytcheva M, et al. Somatic intragenic recombination within the mutated locus BLM can correct the high sister-chromatid exchange phenotype of Bloom syndrome cells. Am J Hum Genet 1995;57(5):1019–27.
73. Renes JS, Willemsen RH, Wagner A, et al. Bloom syndrome in short children born small for gestational age: a challenging diagnosis. J Clin Endocrinol Metab 2013;98(10):3932–8.
74. Troelstra C, van Gool A, de Wit J, et al. ERCC6, a member of a subfamily of putative helicases, is involved in Cockayne's syndrome and preferential repair of active genes. Cell. 1992;71(6):939–53.
75. Bregman DB, Halaban R, van Gool AJ, et al. UV-induced ubiquitination of RNA polymerase II: a novel modification deficient in Cockayne syndrome cells. Proc Natl Acad Sci U S A 1996;93(21):11586–90.
76. Payne F, Colnaghi R, Rocha N, et al. Hypomorphism in human NSMCE2 linked to primordial dwarfism and insulin resistance. J Clin Invest 2014;124(9):4028–38.
77. Boerkoel CF, Takashima H, John J, et al. Mutant chromatin remodeling protein SMARCAL1 causes Schimke immuno-osseous dysplasia. Nat Genet 2002;30(2):215–20.
78. Huber C, Dias-Santagata D, Glaser A, et al. Identification of mutations in CUL7 in 3-M syndrome. Nat Genet 2005;37(10):1119–24.
79. Hanson D, Murray PG, Sud A, et al. The primordial growth disorder 3-M syndrome connects ubiquitination to the cytoskeletal adaptor OBSL1. Am J Hum Genet 2009;84(6):801–6.
80. Hanson D, Murray PG, O'Sullivan J, et al. Exome sequencing identifies CCDC8 mutations in 3-M syndrome, suggesting that CCDC8 contributes in a pathway with CUL7 and OBSL1 to control human growth. Am J Hum Genet 2011;89(1):148–53.
81. Boyle MI, Jespersgaard C, Brøndum-Nielsen K, et al. Cornelia de Lange syndrome. Clin Genet 2015;88(1):1–12.
82. Eriksson M, Brown WT, Gordon LB, et al. Recurrent de novo point mutations in lamin A cause Hutchinson-Gilford Progeria syndrome. Nature 2003;423(6937):293–8.

83. Gonzalo S, Kreienkamp R, Askjaer P. Hutchinson-Gilford Progeria syndrome: a premature aging disease caused by LMNA gene mutations. Ageing Res Rev 2017;33:18–29.

84. Sarig O, Nahum S, Rapaport D, et al. Short stature, onychodysplasia, facial dysmorphism, and hypotrichosis syndrome is caused by a POC1A mutation. Am J Hum Genet 2012;91(2):337–42.

85. Shaheen R, Faqeih E, Shamseldin HE, et al. POC1A truncation mutation causes a ciliopathy in humans characterized by primordial dwarfism. Am J Hum Genet 2012;91(2):330–6.

86. Hood RL, Lines MA, Nikkel SM, et al, FORGE Canada Consortium. Mutations in SRCAP, encoding SNF2-related CREBBP activator protein, cause floating-Harbor syndrome. Am J Hum Genet 2012;90(2):308–13.

87. Nikkel SM, Dauber A, de Munnik S, et al, FORGE Canada Consortium. The phenotype of Floating-Harbor syndrome: clinical characterization of 52 individuals with mutations in exon 34 of SRCAP. Orphanet J Rare Dis 2013;8:63.

88. Messina G, Atterrato MT, Dimitri P. When chromatin organisation floats astray: the Srcap gene and Floating-Harbor syndrome. J Med Genet 2016;53(12): 793–7.

89. Kosho T, Okamoto N, Coffin-Siris Syndrome International Collaborators. Genotype-phenotype correlation of Coffin-Siris syndrome caused by mutations in SMARCB1, SMARCA4, SMARCE1, and ARID1A. Am J Med Genet C Semin Med Genet 2014;166C(3):262–75.

90. He H, Liyanarachchi S, Akagi K, et al. Mutations in U4atac snRNA, a component of the minor spliceosome, in the developmental disorder MOPD I. Science 2011; 332(6026):238–40.

91. Nagy R, Wang H, Albrecht B, et al. Microcephalic osteodysplastic primordial dwarfism type I with biallelic mutations in the RNU4ATAC gene. Clin Genet 2012;82(2):140–6.

92. Hämäläinen RH, Avela K, Lambert JA, et al. Novel mutations in the TRIM37 gene in Mulibrey Nanism. Hum Mutat 2004;23(5):522.

93. K1 Avela, Lipsanen-Nyman M, Idänheimo N, et al. Gene encoding a new RING-B-box-Coiled-coil protein is mutated in Mulibrey Nanism. Nat Genet 2000;25(3): 298–301.

94. Kallijärvi J, Lahtinen U, Hämäläinen R, et al. TRIM37 defective in Mulibrey Nanism is a novel RING finger ubiquitin E3 ligase. Exp Cell Res 2005;308(1):146–55.

95. Leduc MS, Niu Z, Bi W, et al. CRIPT exonic deletion and a novel missense mutation in a female with short stature, dysmorphic features, microcephaly, and pigmentary abnormalities. Am J Med Genet A 2016;170(8):2206–11.

96. Collin GB, Marshall JD, Ikeda A, et al. Mutations in ALMS1 cause obesity, type 2 diabetes and neurosensory degeneration in Alström syndrome. Nat Genet 2002; 31(1):74–8.

97. Nowaczyk MJ, Irons MB. Smith-Lemli-Opitz syndrome: phenotype, natural history, and epidemiology. Am J Med Genet C Semin Med Genet 2012;160C(4): 250–62.

98. Woods SA, Robinson HB, Kohler LJ, et al. Exome sequencing identifies a novel EP300 frame shift mutation in a patient with features that overlap Cornelia de Lange syndrome. Am J Med Genet A 2014;164A(1):251–8.

99. Dierker T, Bachvarova V, Krause Y, et al. Altered heparan sulfate structure in Glce(−/−) mice leads to increased Hedgehog signaling in endochondral bones. Matrix Biol 2016;49:82–92.

100. Melrose J, Shu C, Whitelock JM, et al. The cartilage extracellular matrix as a transient developmental scaffold for growth plate maturation. Matrix Biol 2016; 52-54:363–83.
101. Terhal PA, Nievelstein RJ, Verver EJ, et al. A study of the clinical and radiological features in a cohort of 93 patients with a COL2A1 mutation causing spondyloe-piphyseal dysplasia congenita or a related phenotype. Am J Med Genet A 2015; 167A(3):461–75.
102. Terhal PA, van Dommelen P, Le Merrer M, et al. Mutation-based growth charts for SEDC and other COL2A1 related dysplasias. Am J Med Genet C Semin Med Genet 2012;160C(3):205–16.
103. Tompson SW, Bacino CA, Safina NP, et al. Fibrochondrogenesis results from mutations in the COL11A1 type XI collagen gene. Am J Hum Genet 2010;87(5): 708–12.
104. Bonaventure J, Chaminade F, Maroteaux P. Mutations in three subdomains of the carboxy-terminal region of collagen type X account for most of the Schmid metaphyseal dysplasias. Hum Genet 1995;96(1):58–64.
105. Czarny-Ratajczak M, Lohiniva J, Rogala P, et al. A mutation in COL9A1 causes multiple epiphyseal dysplasia: further evidence for locus heterogeneity. Hum Genet 2001;69(5):969–80.
106. Spayde EC, Joshi AP, Wilcox WR, et al. Exon skipping mutation in the COL9A2 gene in a family with multiple epiphyseal dysplasia. Matrix Biol 2000;19(2): 121–8.
107. Paassilta P, Lohiniva J, Annunen S, et al. COL9A3: A third locus for multiple epiphyseal dysplasia. Am J Hum Genet 1999;64(4):1036–44.
108. Jackson GC, Mittaz-Crettol L, Taylor JA, et al. Pseudoachondroplasia and multiple epiphyseal dysplasia: a 7-year comprehensive analysis of the known disease genes identify novel and recurrent mutations and provides an accurate assessment of their relative contribution. Hum Mutat 2012;33(1):144–57.
109. Le Goff C, Mahaut C, Wang LW, et al. Mutations in the TGFβ binding-protein-like domain 5 of FBN1 are responsible for acromicric and geleophysic dysplasias. Am J Hum Genet 2011;89(1):7–14.
110. Briggs MD, Hoffman SM, King LM, et al. Pseudoachondroplasia and multiple epiphyseal dysplasia due to mutations in the cartilage oligomeric matrix protein gene. Nat Genet 1995;10(3):330–6.
111. Hecht JT, Nelson LD, Crowder E, et al. Mutations in exon 17B of cartilage oligomeric matrix protein (COMP) cause pseudoachondroplasia. Nat Genet 1995; 10(3):325–9.
112. Chapman KL, Mortier GR, Chapman K, et al. Mutations in the region encoding the von Willebrand factor A domain of matrilin-3 are associated with multiple epiphyseal dysplasia. Nat Genet 2001;28(4):393–6.
113. Gleghorn L, Ramesar R, Beighton P, et al. A mutation in the variable repeat region of the aggrecan gene (AGC1) causes a form of spondyloepiphyseal dysplasia associated with severe, premature osteoarthritis. Am J Hum Genet 2005;77(3):484–90.
114. Nilsson O, Guo MH, Dunbar N, et al. Short stature, accelerated bone maturation, and early growth cessation due to heterozygous aggrecan mutations. J Clin Endocrinol Metab 2014;99(8):E1510–8.
115. Nicole S, Davoine CS, Topaloglu H, et al. Perlecan, the major proteoglycan of basement membranes, is altered in patients with Schwartz-Jampel syndrome (chondrodystrophic myotonia). Nat Genet 2000;26(4):480–3.

116. Kronenberg HM. Developmental regulation of the growth plate. Nature 2003; 423(6937):332–6.
117. Matsushita T, Wilcox WR, Chan YY, et al. FGFR3 promotes synchondrosis closure and fusion of ossification centers through the MAPK pathway. Hum Mol Genet 2009;18(2):227–40.
118. Li M, Seki Y, Freitas PH, et al. FGFR3 down-regulates PTH/PTHrP receptor gene expression by mediating JAK/STAT signaling in chondrocytic cell line. J Electron Microsc (Tokyo) 2010;59(3):227–36.
119. Webster MK, Donoghue DJ. Constitutive activation of fibroblast growth factor receptor 3 by the transmembrane domain point mutation found in achondroplasia. EMBO J 1996;15(3):520–7.
120. Foldynova-Trantirkova S, Wilcox WR, Krejci P. Sixteen years and counting: the current understanding of fibroblast growth factor receptor 3 (FGFR3) signaling in skeletal dysplasias. Hum Mutat 2012;33(1):29–41.
121. Kant SG, Cervenkova I, Balek L, et al. A novel variant of FGFR3 causes proportionate short stature. Eur J Endocrinol 2015;172(6):763–70.
122. Toydemir RM, Brassington AE, Bayrak-Toydemir P, et al. A novel mutation in FGFR3 causes camptodactyly, tall stature, and hearing loss (CATSHL) syndrome. Am J Hum Genet 2006;79(5):935–41.
123. Makrythanasis P, Temtamy S, Aglan MS, et al. A novel homozygous mutation in FGFR3 causes tall stature, severe lateral tibial deviation, scoliosis, hearing impairment, camptodactyly, and arachnodactyly. Hum Mutat 2014;35(8): 959–63.
124. Chusho H, Tamura N, Ogawa Y, et al. Dwarfism and early death in mice lacking C-type natriuretic peptide. Proc Natl Acad Sci U S A 2001;98(7):4016–21.
125. Moncla A, Missirian C, Cacciagli P, et al. A cluster of translocation breakpoints in 2q37 is associated with overexpression of NPPC in patients with a similar overgrowth phenotype. Hum Mutat 2007;28(12):1183–8.
126. Olney RC, Bükülmez H, Bartels CF, et al. Heterozygous mutations in natriuretic peptide receptor-B (NPR2) are associated with short stature. J Clin Endocrinol Metab 2006;91(4):1229–32.
127. Miura K, Namba N, Fujiwara M, et al. An overgrowth disorder associated with excessive production of cGMP due to a gain-of-function mutation of the natriuretic peptide receptor 2 gene. PLoS One 2012;7(8):e42180.
128. Lorget F, Kaci N, Peng J, et al. Evaluation of the therapeutic potential of a CNP analog in a Fgfr3 mouse model recapitulating achondroplasia. Am J Hum Genet 2012;91(6):1108–14.
129. Hellemans J, Coucke PJ, Giedion A, et al. Homozygous mutations in IHH cause acrocapitofemoral dysplasia, an autosomal recessive disorder with cone-shaped epiphyses in hands and hips. Am J Hum Genet 2003;72(4):1040–6.
130. Klopocki E, Hennig BP, Dathe K, et al. Deletion and point mutations of PTHLH cause brachydactyly type E. Am J Hum Genet 2010;86(3):434–9.
131. Pereda A, Garin I, Garcia-Barcina M, et al. Brachydactyly E: isolated or as a feature of a syndrome. Orphanet J Rare Dis 2013;8:141.
132. Savoldi G, Izzi C, Signorelli M, et al. Prenatal presentation and postnatal evolution of a patient with Jansen metaphyseal dysplasia with a novel missense mutation in PTH1R. Am J Med Genet A 2013;161A(10):2614–9.
133. Jobert AS, Zhang P, Couvineau A, et al. Absence of functional receptors for parathyroid hormone and parathyroid hormone-related peptide in Blomstrand chondrodysplasia. J Clin Invest 1998;102(1):34–40.

134. Nilsson O, Parker EA, Hegde A, et al. Gradients in bone morphogenetic protein-related gene expression across the growth plate. J Endocrinol 2007;193(1): 75–84.
135. Lehmann K, Seemann P, Stricker S, et al. Mutations in bone morphogenetic protein receptor 1B cause brachydactyly type A2. Proc Natl Acad Sci U S A 2003; 100(21):12277–82.
136. Seemann P, Schwappacher R, Kjaer KW, et al. Activating and deactivating mutations in the receptor interaction site of GDF5 cause symphalangism or brachydactyly type A2. J Clin Invest 2005;115(9):2373–81.
137. Begemann M, Zirn B, Santen G, et al. Paternally inherited IGF2 mutation and growth restriction. N Engl J Med 2015;373(4):349–56.
138. Alatzoglou KS, Webb EA, Le Tissier P, et al. Isolated growth hormone deficiency (GHD) in childhood and adolescence: recent advances. Endocr Rev 2014; 35(3):376–432.
139. Laron Z. Lessons from 50 years of study of Laron syndrome. Endocr Pract 2015; 21(12):1395–402.
140. Ross RJ. The GH receptor and GH insensitivity. Growth Horm IGF Res 1999; 9(Suppl B):42–5.
141. Iida K, Takahashi Y, Kaji H, et al. Growth hormone (GH) insensitivity syndrome with high serum GH-binding protein levels caused by a heterozygous splice site mutation of the GH receptor gene producing a lack of intracellular domain. J Clin Endocrinol Metab 1998;83(2):531–7.
142. Bernasconi A, Marino R, Ribas A, et al. Characterization of immunodeficiency in a patient with growth hormone insensitivity secondary to a novel STAT5b gene mutation. Pediatrics 2006;118(5):e1584–92.
143. Fuqua JS, Derr M, Rosenfeld RG, et al. Identification of a novel heterozygous IGF1 splicing mutation in a large kindred with familial short stature. Horm Res Paediatr 2012;78(1):59–66.
144. van Duyvenvoorde HA, van Setten PA, Walenkamp MJ, et al. Short stature associated with a novel heterozygous mutation in the insulin-like growth factor 1 gene. J Clin Endocrinol Metab 2010;95(11):E363–7.
145. Gannagé-Yared MH, Klammt J, Chouery E, et al. Homozygous mutation of the IGF1 receptor gene in a patient with severe pre- and postnatal growth failure and congenital malformations. Eur J Endocrinol 2012;168(1):K1–7.
146. Kansra AR, Dolan LM, Martin LJ, et al. IGF receptor gene variants in normal adolescents: effect on stature. Eur J Endocrinol 2012;167(6):777–81.
147. Juanes M, Guercio G, Marino R, et al. Three novel IGF1R mutations in microcephalic patients with prenatal and postnatal growth impairment. Clin Endocrinol (Oxf) 2015;82(5):704–11.
148. Domené HM, Scaglia PA, Martínez AS, et al. Heterozygous IGFALS gene variants in idiopathic short stature and normal children: impact on height and the IGF system. Horm Res Paediatr 2013;80(6):413–23.
149. Högler W, Martin DD, Crabtree N, et al. IGFALS gene dosage effects on serum IGF-I and glucose metabolism, body composition, bone growth in length and width, and the pharmacokinetics of recombinant human IGF-I administration. J Clin Endocrinol Metab 2014;99(4):E703–12.
150. Jee YH, Sowada N, Markello TC, et al. BRF1 mutations in a family with growth failure, markedly delayed bone age, and central nervous system anomalies. Clin Genet, in press.

Molecular and Genetic Aspects of Congenital Isolated Hypogonadotropic Hypogonadism

Lorena Guimaraes Lima Amato, MD,
Ana Claudia Latronico, MD, PhD*,
Leticia Ferreira Gontijo Silveira, MD, PhD*

KEYWORDS

- Hypogonadotropic hypogonadism • Kallmann syndrome • GnRH
- Neuronal migration • Sense of smell and genes

KEY POINTS

- Congenital isolated hypogonadotropic hypogonadism (IHH) is a rare reproductive disorder caused by the deficient production, secretion or action of gonadotropin-releasing hormone (GnRH).
- Kallmann syndrome, a disorder that combines congenital IHH and anosmia or hyposmia, is caused by abnormal embryonic migration of GnRH and olfactory neurons.
- Congenital IHH is clinically and genetically heterogeneous with different modes of inheritance and several causative genes.
- Spontaneous recovery of reproductive function can occur in 10% of patients with IHH, independent of the genetic defects.

INTRODUCTION

Congenital isolated hypogonadotropic hypogonadism (IHH) is a clinical syndrome characterized by failure of gonadal function secondary to defects on the synthesis, secretion or action of the gonadotropin-releasing hormone (GnRH), an essential neuropeptide for

The authors have nothing to disclose.
This work was supported by grants from Conselho Nacional de Desenvolvimento Científico e Tecnológico (CNPq # 302849/2015-7); Fundação de Amparo à Pesquisa do Estado de São Paulo (FAPESP # 2013/03236-5) to A.C. Latronico.
Division of Endocrinology, Development Endocrinology Unit, Laboratory of Hormones and Molecular Genetics/LIM42, Clinical Hospital, Sao Paulo Medical School, Sao Paulo University, Av. Dr. Eneas de Carvalho Aguiar 255, 7 andar, sala 7037, Sao Paulo, SP 05403-000, Brazil
* Corresponding author. Hospital das Clínicas, Faculdade de Medicina da Universidade de São Paulo, Disciplina de Endocrinologia e Metabologia, Av. Dr. Enéas de CarvalhoAguiar, 155, 2° andar, bloco 6, São Paulo 05403-900, Brasil
E-mail addresses: anacl@usp.br; leticia.silveira@hc.fm.usp.br

Endocrinol Metab Clin N Am 46 (2017) 283–303
http://dx.doi.org/10.1016/j.ecl.2017.01.010
0889-8529/17/© 2017 Elsevier Inc. All rights reserved.

the reproductive system of mammals.[1] Congenital IHH is a rare condition with male pre-dominance, with a prevalence of 3 to 5 males to one female.[2,3] This condition is charac-terized by absent or incomplete pubertal development and the diagnosis of hypogonadism is typically made during the second or third decades of life, when the affected individuals present with pubertal delay, primary amenorrhea, or infertility. In some cases, the suspected diagnosis can be considered in childhood owing to the pres-ence of micropenis and/or cryptorchidism, especially when there is a positive family his-tory of hypogonadism. Biochemically, the diagnosis is confirmed by the finding of low serum levels of sex steroids associated with low or inappropriately normal luteinizing hor-mone and follicle-stimulating hormone serum levels. The remaining pituitary function is normal without anatomic abnormalities of the hypothalamic–pituitary–gonadal axis.[1,2] Around 50% to 60% of the affected individuals exhibit olfaction dysfunction (anosmia or hyposmia) in association with IHH, defining Kallmann syndrome. The olfaction defects occur owing to combined abnormal embryonic migration of GnRH neurons and olfactory fibers from their origin in the olfactory placode to the forebrain.[3–5] These patients usually present with hypoplasia or aplasia of the olfactory tract/bulbs associated to GnRH defi-ciency.[6] Currently, it is known that the clinical manifestations of congenital IHH may be heterogeneous. The same family may present with cases of normosmic IHH, Kallmann syndrome, pubertal delay, or isolated abnormalities, such as isolated anosmia or cranio-facial malformations.[7] Developmental anomalies such as cleft lip or palate, dental agen-esis, ear anomalies, congenital hearing impairment, renal agenesis, bimanual synkinesis, or skeletal anomalies may be associated with the Kallmann syndrome and some genetic mutations are associated more frequently with some of these defects.[8]

Congenital IHH is genetically heterogeneous, with both sporadic and familial cases. The new techniques of parallel sequencing in large scale have enabled the study of various genes simultaneously (gene panels) or even of the whole exoma, increasing the knowledge of the molecular bases of congenital IHH. The advent of these new tech-niques allowed an increase in the molecular diagnosis of patients congenital IHH from 30% to approximately 50% of cases.[8,9] A growing list of genes has been implicated in the molecular pathogenesis of the congenital IHH, highlighting the heterogeneity and complexity of the genetic basis of this condition. These genes encode neuropeptides and proteins involved in the development and migration of GnRH neurons, or in the con-trol of different stages of GnRH function (**Table 1**). The genetic causes of congenital IHH are reviewed here and have been categorized according to the stage of development of the gonadotrophic axis in which they participate (**Fig. 1**).

GENES IMPLICATED WITH DEVELOPMENT AND MIGRATION OF GONADOTROPIN-RELEASING HORMONE NEURONS

The development of GnRH neurons is unusual, because they originate outside the central nervous system in the olfactory placode and then migrate in close association with the olfactory fibers into the brain during embryonic development to their ultimate destination in the hypothalamus. This route provides a developmental link between the central control of reproduction and the sense of smell, which are both affected in Kall-mann syndrome. Several genes associated to congenital IHH affect the fate and migration of GnRH neurons, being implicated in the pathogenesis of both Kallmann syndrome and normosmic IHH (**Fig. 2**).

KAL1 or ANOS1

The *KAL1* gene, located at Xp22.31, was identified by a positional cloning strategy in 1991.[10] It encodes the glycoprotein anosmin-1, an extracellular 680 amino acid

Table 1
Genes implicated in congenital IHH

Gene	Chromosomal Location	IHH Phenotype	Clinical Features Associated	Syndromes Associated	Inheritance Pattern	Prevalence (%)
KAL1 (ANOS1)	Xp22.31	KS	Bimanual synkinesia Renal agenesis		X-linked	5
IL17RD	3p14.3	KS	Congenital hearing impairment		Autosomal recessive	3
SOX10	22q13.1	KS	Congenital hearing impairment	Waardenburg syndrome	Described in heterozygous state	2
FEZF1	7q31.32	KS			Autosomal recessive	Rare
CCDC141	2q31.2	KS			Autosomal recessive (?)	Rare
SEMA3A	7q21.11	KS			Autosomal dominant	Rare
SEMA7A	15q24.1	KS nIHH			Autosomal dominant	Rare
FGFR1	8p11.23	KS nIHH	Cleft lip and/or palate Septooptic dysplasia Skeletal anomalies Bimanual synkinesia Hand/foot malformation Combined pituitary hormone deficiency	Hartsfield syndrome	Autosomal dominant	10
FGF8	10q24.32	KS nIHH	Cleft lip and/or palate Skeletal anomalies Bimanual synkinesia Combined pituitary hormone deficiency		Autosomal dominant	<2
FGF17	8p21.3	KS nIHH		Dandy-Walker syndrome	Autosomal dominant (?)	Rare

(continued on next page)

Table 1
(continued)

Gene	Chromosomal Location	IHH Phenotype	Clinical Features Associated	Syndromes Associated	Inheritance Pattern	Prevalence (%)
HS6ST1	2q14.3	KS nIHH	Cleft lip and/or palate Skeletal anomalies		Autosomal dominant (?)	Rare
CHD7	8q12.2	KS nIHH	Congenital hearing impairment Semicircular canal hypoplasia	CHARGE syndrome	Autosomal dominant (?)	6
PROK2	3p13	KS nIHH			Autosomal recessive	3–6
PROKR2	20p12.3	KS nIHH	Combined pituitary hormone deficiency	Morning Glory syndrome	Autosomal recessive	3–6
WDR11	10q26.12	KS nIHH	Combined pituitary hormone deficiency		Autosomal dominant	Rare
NELF (NSMF)	9q34.3	KS nIHH			Autosomal dominant (?)	Rare
AXL	19q13.2	KS nIHH			Autosomal dominant (?)	NR
IGSF10	3q24	KS nIHH			Autosomal dominant (?)	Rare
GNRH1	8p21.2	nIHH			Autosomal recessive	Rare
KISS1	1q32.1	nIHH			Autosomal recessive	2
KISS1R (GPR54)	19p13.3	nIHH			Autosomal recessive	2
TAC3	12q3	nIHH			Autosomal recessive	Rare
TACR3	4q24	nIHH			Autosomal recessive	Rare

GNRHR	4q13.2	nIHH			Autosomal recessive	6–16
LEP	7q32.1	nIHH	Early onset of morbid obesity		Autosomal recessive	<2
LEPR	1p31.3	nIHH	Early onset of morbid obesity		Autosomal recessive	<2
PCSK1	5q15	nIHH	Early onset of morbid obesity		Autosomal recessive	<2
OTUD4	4q31.21	nIHH	Cerebellar ataxia	Gordon Holmes syndrome	Autosomal recessive	Rare
RNF216	7p22.1	nIHH	Cerebelar ataxia	Gordon Holmes syndrome	Autosomal recessive	Rare
PNPLA6	19p13.2	nIHH	Cerebelar ataxia	Gordon Holmes syndrome	Autosomal recessive	Rare
DMXL2	15q21.2	nIHH	Polyendocrine deficiencies and polyneuropathies		Autosomal recessive	Rare
NR0B1 (DAX1)	Xp21.2	nIHH	Adrenal hypoplasia		X-linked	Rare
HESX1	3p14.3	KS	Septooptic dysplasia Combined pituitary hormone deficiency		Autosomal dominant (?)	Rare

Abbreviations: CHARGE syndrome, coloboma, heart defects, choanal atresia, retarded growth and development, genital hypoplasia, ear anomalies and deafness; IHH, isolated hypogonadotropic hypogonadism; KS, Kallmann syndrome; nIHH, normosmic isolated hypogonadotropic hypogonadism.

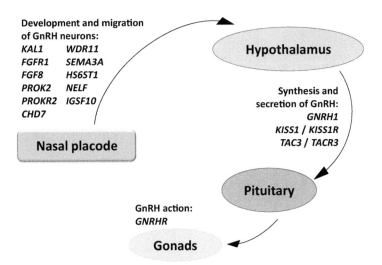

Fig. 1. Genes implicated in the embryonic development and migration of gonadotropin-releasing hormone (GnRH) secreting-neurons as well as in the synthesis, secretion, and action of the hypothalamic GnRH.

protein composed by a cysteine-rich region, a whey acidic protein domain, 4 fibronectinlike type III repeats, and several predicted heparin sulfate binding regions.[11] Anosmin-1 is involved in fibroblast growth factor (FGF) signaling, playing different cell functions, including cell adhesion, neurite/axonal elongation and fasciculation, and epithelial morphogenesis as well as in the migratory activity of GnRH neurons.[12] During the development, anosmin-1 is expressed transiently in the basement membranes of the developing olfactory bulb, retina, and kidney, being essential for axonal

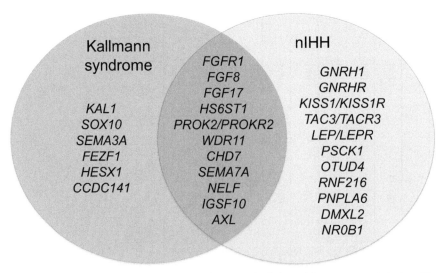

Fig. 2. Genes associated with Kallmann syndrome only (*left circle*) or normosmic isolated hypogonadotropic hypogonadism (nIHH) only (*right circle*) or both conditions (intersection).

guidance and migration of olfactory and GnRH neurons from the nasal placode to their final location in the brain.[11]

Mutations in *KAL1* are reported to be present in approximately 5% to 10% of all Kallmann syndrome patients and 15% to 50% of the familial cases with an X-linked pattern of inheritance.[5,13–16] Patients with *KAL1* mutations usually exhibit an almost uniformly severe and highly penetrant reproductive phenotype.[16] Most patients with X-linked Kallmann syndrome have micropenis and bilaterally undescended testes at birth, reflecting severe congenital GnRH and gonadotropin insufficiency.[16] Other anomalies frequently associated with X-linked Kallmann syndrome include high arched palate, cleft lip and/or palate, short metacarpals, unilateral renal agenesis, sensorineural hearing loss, bimanual synkinesia, and oculomotor abnormalities.

Fibroblast Growth Factors Family and Modulators

FGFs and their cell surface receptors comprise a large and complex family of signaling molecules that have been shown to play crucial roles in multiple aspects of vertebrate and invertebrate embryonic development, angiogenesis, wound healing, and tissue homeostasis.[17] In the presence of heparin sulfate glycosamino glycans, FGFs bind with high affinity to the receptor.

FGF receptor 1 (FGFR1) signaling is required in normal GnRH neuronal migration, differentiation, or survival within the hypothalamus, and also plays an essential role in the morphogenesis of the telencephalon, in particular of the olfactory bulbs.[17] *FGFR1* expression has been detected in the nasal placode, developing olfactory bulbs and the GnRH migratory pathways, as well as the hypothalamic GnRH neurons and their projections.[17]

FGFR1 was firstly associated with congenital IHH, in 2003, when Dodé and colleagues[18] reported the association of loss-of-function mutations in *FGFR1* with an autosomal-dominant form of Kallmann syndrome. *FGFR1* mutations may cause isolated defects in GnRH neuronal migration without necessarily affecting olfactory bulbs development and, because of that, *FGFR1* defects have been associated with both Kallmann syndrome and normosmic IHH.[17,19] Currently, *FGFR1* mutations are the second most common known molecular cause of Kallmann syndrome. *FGFR1* mutations are associated with marked phenotypic variability both within and among families and apparent incomplete penetrance.[20]

FGF8 is considered as a key ligand of the FGFR1 in the ontogenesis of GnRH neurons.[7,21] In 2008, Falardeau and colleagues[22] reported 6 missense mutations in *FGF8* in congenital IHH probands with variable olfactory phenotypes and different degrees of GnRH deficiency, including the rare adult-onset form of IHH. Like FGFR1, FGF8 mutations cause autosomal-dominant congenital IHH.[23] Other malformations most commonly associated with mutations of the FGF system include cleft lip-palate, dental agenesis, and bone defects, such as syndactyly and hand/foot malformation.[24,25]

More recently, Miraoui and colleagues[9] investigated genes belonging to the *FGF8* subfamily and identified *FGF17* heterozygous mutations in one normosmic IHH and 2 Kallmann syndrome patients. *FGF17* has emerged as the second-most critical FGFR1 ligand for GnRH neuron ontogeny and has a strong sequence identity with *FGF8*.[9] In the same study, *IL17RD* mutations, either in homozygous or heterozygous state, were identified in 8 Kallmann syndrome patients, 6 of them with hearing loss. The *IL17RD* gene encodes a membrane protein belonging to the interleukin-17 receptor (*IL-17R*) protein family. It is part of a group of modulators of FGF signaling, known as "similar expression to FGFs" (SEF). SEF seems to play critical roles in proliferation, migration, and angiogenesis, and interacts with *FGFR1* in transfected human embryonic kidney cells.[26] The localization patterns of Il17rd in the nasal region of mouse embryos suggested that *IL17RD* might have a role in the early stages of GnRH neuron fate specification.[9]

HS6ST1 encodes the heparan sulfate 6-O-sulfotransferase enzyme, an important component of *FGFR1* signaling. Heparan 6-O-sulfation is required for anosmin-1 and *FGFR1* functions. FGF8 and heparan sulfate bind to *FGFR1*, forming a complex and leading to activation of downstream signaling pathways. Interestingly, anosmin-1 acts as a modulatory co-ligand with FGF8 to activate the FGFR1 in a heparan sulfate-dependent manner.[27,28] Tornberg and colleagues[27] identified 7 variants in the *HS6ST1* gene in congenital IHH patients either with normal olfaction or variable degrees of olfactory dysfunction.

Some of the variants in *FGF17*, *IL17RD*, and *HS6ST1* were identified in combination with additional variants in other known IHH-associated genes, such as *FGFR1*, *KISS1R*, and *NELF*. Mutations in these genes might act synergistically in the pathogenesis of IHH, suggesting that one allelic defect in *FGF17*, *IL17RD*, or *HS6ST1* is most likely not sufficient cause the phenotype.[9,27]

Nasal Embryonic Luteinizing Hormone-Releasing Hormone Factor

Nasal embryonic luteinizing hormone-releasing hormone factor (*NELF*), also known as *NSMF*, is expressed in the olfactory sensory cells and GnRH cells during embryonic development. It serves as a common guidance molecule for the olfactory axon and GnRH neurons across the nasal region.[29] Monoallelic and biallelic mutations were identified in *NELF* in normosmic IHH and Kallmann syndrome patients, some of them in association with other IHH genes, including *FGFR1*, *HS6ST1*, *KAL1*, and *TACR3*.[30,31] These findings suggest that *NELF* is associated with normosmic IHH and Kallmann syndrome, either singly or in combination with a mutation in another gene.[7,27,31]

Prokineticin 2 and Prokineticin Receptor 2

Prokineticins are cysteine-rich secreted proteins that were originally identified as potent agents mediating gut motility in the digestive system, but were later shown to promote diverse biological functions, including normal development of the olfactory bulb and sexual maturation.[32]

Mutations in *PROKR2*, a G-protein–coupled receptor, and its ligand (PROK2) were first described by Dodé and colleagues,[33] who studied a cohort of 192 patients with Kallmann syndrome. Ten *PROKR2* and 4 *PROK2* defects were identified in this study. Later, Abreu and colleagues[34] studied a cohort of 107 Brazilian patients with congenital IHH. The identification of healthy patients harboring heterozygous mutations in these genes indicated that *PROKR2* haploinsufficiency is not sufficient to cause Kallmann syndrome or normosmic IHH. However, the frequent finding of heterozygous mutations in *PROKR2* in patients with congenital IHH has raised the question of a possible digenic mode of inheritance in these patients.[35] Mutations in *PROK2/PROKR2* are estimated to account for 5% to 10% of all Kallmann syndrome cases.[20] Because patients who carry mutations in *PROKR2* or *PROK2* have variable degrees of olfactory and reproductive dysfunction, mutations in *PROK2* and *PROKR2* should be considered in all GnRH-deficient subjects with or without anosmia.[34]

WDR11

The *WDR11* gene encodes a highly conserved protein throughout vertebrate evolution that is expressed in the developing olfactory and GnRH migratory pathway.[36] Kim and colleagues[37] screened 201 normosmic and hyposmic/anosmic patients with congenital IHH for mutations in *WDR11* and identified 5 different heterozygous missense mutations in 6 unrelated probands, including 5 normosmic patients and 1 anosmic patient. Because all *WDR11* mutations have been described in the heterozygous state, the inheritance pattern is most likely autosomal dominant.

Chromodomain-Helicase DNA-Binding Protein 7

CHARGE syndrome (OMIM #214800), is a multisystem disorder classically characterized by a variety of congenital anomalies including coloboma, heart defects, choanal atresia, retarded growth and development, genital hypoplasia, ear anomalies, and deafness. Notably, IHH and anosmia are consistent findings in this syndrome, suggesting that the same embryonic migration process could be disturbed in the Kallmann and CHARGE syndromes.

Dominant mutations in the chromodomain-helicase DNA-binding protein 7 (CHD-7) cause CHARGE syndrome (60%–70% of cases). Kim and colleagues[38] studied 197 patients with Kallmann syndrome or normosmic IHH without other features of the CHARGE phenotype. Several heterozygous mutations were identified in these patients, indicating that congenital IHH represents a milder allelic variant of CHARGE syndrome.[38] Later studies reported *CHD7* mutations in patients who had Kallmann syndrome and additional features of CHARGE syndrome.[39] These finding suggested that *CHD7* analysis is especially recommended in Kallmann syndrome patients who have at least 2 of the following features: ocular coloboma, choanal atresia/stenosis, characteristic external ear anomaly, cranial nerve dysfunction (facial palsy, sensorineural hearing loss, or hypoplastic cranial nerves on imaging), or balance disturbance. In addition, the *CHD7*-positive patient should also be screened for additional CHARGE features.[40] Currently, mutations in *CHD7* are reported to be present in approximately 7% of patients with Kallmann syndrome; however, when IHH is associated with hearing loss, *CHD7* mutations could be identified in approximately 40% of patients.[8]

Semaphorins 7A and 3A

Semaphorins are a class of secreted and membrane proteins that act as axonal growth cone guidance molecules. Sema3A and Sema7A-mutant mice have a reduced number of GnRH neurons in their brains. Sema3A is essential for the patterning of vomeronasal axons, whereas in Sema7A mutants, the olfactory system seems to remain unaffected.[41–43] Heterozygous loss-of-function mutations have been identified in *SEMA3A* in 28 patients with Kallmann syndrome, some of them in combination with mutations in other IHH genes.[43–45] Posteriorly, *SEMA7A* mutations were reported in 1 Kallmann and 1 normosmic IHH patient, both with previously identified mutations in other IHH genes.[43] These results suggest that *SEMA3A* and *SEMA7A* play a role in the IHH pathogenesis, but up to now it is not completely clear if single variants in this system, especially in *SEMA7A*, are sufficient to cause the disorder.[43–45]

Sex determining region Y-Box 10

Sex determining region Y-Box 10 (*SOX10*) belongs to the SOX transcription factor family, whose members are involved in several developmental and cellular processes.[46] Mutations in *SOX10* are a well-known cause of Waardenburg syndrome, characterized by deafness, skin/hair/iris hypopigmentation, Hirschsprung disease, and neurologic defects.[47] Study of *SOX10*-null mutant mice revealed a developmental role of *SOX10* in olfactory unsheathing glial cells. These mice showed an almost complete absence of these cells along the olfactory nerve pathway, as well as defasciculation and misrouting of the nerve fibers, impaired migration of GnRH cells, and disorganization of the olfactory nerve layer of the olfactory bulbs.[47] In addition, a high frequency of olfactory bulb agenesis was identified recently in patients with Waardenburg syndrome, raising the hypothesis that SOX10 mutations might be involved in the Kallmann syndrome pathogenesis. Indeed, SOX10 mutations were identified in 8 individuals with Kallmann syndrome, 7 of them with hearing loss, suggesting that SOX10 should be screened in patients with Kallmann syndrome and deafness.[47,48]

FEZ family zinc finger 1 and CCDC141

FEZ family zinc finger 1 (FEZF1) encodes a transcriptional repressor selectively expressed during embryogenesis in the olfactory epithelium, amygdala, and hypothalamus.[49,50] In mice, the Fezf1 product enables axons of olfactory receptor neurons and GnRH neurons to enter the central nervous system. Fezf1-deficient mice have impaired axonal projection of pioneer olfactory receptor neurons, which are not able to cross the cribriform plate toward the olfactory bulb.[51,52] Kotan and colleagues[50] screened a cohort of 30 Kallmann syndrome patients using candidate gene screening, autozygosity mapping, and whole-exome sequencing, in the search for new causative genes. Homozygous loss-of-function mutations were identified in FEZF1 in 2 independent consanguineous families, each with 2 affected siblings. The inheritance pattern in both families was consistent with an autosomal-recessive condition.[50] Curiously, in one of these families, a nonsense homozygous mutation in the CCDC141 gene was also found in the same siblings harboring a missense FEZF1 homozygous mutation, and the parents and unaffected siblings were all heterozygous. CCDC141 encodes the coiled-coil domain containing protein 141, a cytoskeletal associated protein. The CCDC141 gene product has been implicated in cortical neuronal migration; however, its function is not well-known.[53] Kotan and colleagues[50] demonstrated that Ccdc141 is expressed in GnRH neurons and olfactory fibers in mice and that knockdown of Ccdc141 reduces GnRH neuronal migration. These findings corroborate the hypothesis that mutations in this gene might cause additional detrimental effects in patients with Kallmann syndrome already harboring FEZF1 defects.[50]

AXL

AXL is a receptor tyrosine kinase described in 1991.[54] The Tyro3, Axl, and Mer (TAM) family of receptor tyrosine kinases are differentially expressed in GnRH neuronal cells. Axl/Tyro3-null mice have delayed first estrus and abnormal cyclicity owing to developmental defects in GnRH neuron migration and survival.[54] Three AXL mutations were recently identified in 2 Kallmann syndrome and 2 normosmic IHH subjects.[55]

Immunoglobulin Superfamily Member 10

Using exome and candidate gene sequencing, Howard and colleagues[56] recently identified rare mutations in the IGSF10 gene in 6 families with self-limited delayed puberty. Strong expression of IGSF10 was demonstrated in embryonic nasal mesenchyme during GnRH neuronal migration to the hypothalamus, suggesting a potential role of the immunoglobulin superfamily member 10 (IGSF10), in the regulation of GnRH neuronal migration. In addition, IGSF10 knockdown caused a reduced migration of immature GnRH neurons in vitro, and impaired the migration and extension of GnRH neurons in a zebrafish model.[56] Notably, rare predicted damaging variants in IGSF10 gene were also identified in few patients with functional and congenital IHH patients. However, the definitive role of this gene in the pathogenesis of congenital IHH remains to be determined.[56]

GENES IMPLICATED WITH GONADOTROPIN-RELEASING HORMONE SYNTHESIS AND SECRETION

Gonadotropin-Releasing Hormone 1

The human *GNRH1* gene encodes the preprohormone that is ultimately processed to produce GnRH decapeptide.[57] Although it may be considered the most obvious candidate gene for congenital IHH, *GNRH1* mutations are a very rare cause of normosmic IHH. Despite a large number of individuals screened, only 3 homozygous *GNRH1* mutations were described in patients with normosmic IHH, in an autosomal-recessive mode of inheritance.[58–60] In addition, one heterozygous *GNRH1* (p.R31C) mutation that affects the conserved GnRH decapeptide sequence was identified in 9 normosmic IHH subjects from 4 unrelated families, giving evidence for a putative "hot spot."[59,61] This mode is in contrast with the autosomic-recessive mode of inheritance observed for the other GnRH1 mutations. In vitro studies showed a reduction of the mutant decapeptide capacity to bind GnRH receptor; however, a dominant negative effect was not demonstrated.[61] An effect of haploinsufficiency has been suggested for this variant, leading to partial hypogonadism.[60] Nevertheless, the role of this heterozygous p.R31C mutation is not clear and raises a discussion on the pathogenic mechanism underlying GnRH mutations.

Kisspeptin 1 and Kisspeptin 1 Receptor

Kisspeptin, encoded by the *KISS1* gene, is the most potent known stimulator of GnRH-dependent luteinizing hormone secretion. Kisspeptin acts exclusively through its cognate receptor, *KISS1R*, a heptahelical G-protein–coupled receptor, expressed in the surface of the GnRH secreting neurons. In the central nervous system, kisspeptin expression is highest in the arcuate and anteroventralperiventricular nuclei, known to send projections to the medial preoptic area, where GnRH cell bodies are mainly located. The kisspeptin/KISS1R system is currently recognized as the gatekeeper of the reproductive function.[62–64]

Loss-of-function mutations of *KISS1R* were first reported in patients with congenital IHH belonging to large consanguineous families by 2 independent researcher groups in 2003.[62,63] Since then, several different loss-of-function mutations have been described in the *KISS1R* gene in patients with partial or complete normosmic IHH.[65] Family segregation analyses of these patients showed that individuals with heterozygous alterations in *KISS1R* had a normal pubertal development, confirming a model of autosomal-recessive inheritance for this disease. *KISS1R* mutations are responsible for about 5% of cases of normosmic IHH.[20,65] Patients with mutations in the gene *KISS1R* have no olfactory changes or other associated clinical conditions.

KISS1 mutations were rarely associated with normosmic IHH. In 2012, Topaloglu and colleagues[66] described the first homozygous mutation in *KISS1* associated with IHH.

Tachykinin 3 and Tachykinin 3 receptor

A genome-wide single nucleotide polymorphism analysis performed in 9 consanguineous Turkish families with multiple members affected by normosmic IHH led to the identification of inactivating mutations in the genes *TAC3* and *TACR3* in 4 unrelated families.[67] The *TAC3* encodes neurokinin-B, a member of the substance P–related tachykinin family, whereas *TACR3* encodes neurokinin B receptor, a member of the rhodopsin family of G-protein–coupled receptors.[67] It is currently known that mutations in the complex *TAC3/TACR3* are a relatively common cause of normosmic IHH, occurring in more than 5% of affected individuals.[68]

Gonadotropin-Releasing Hormone Receptor

The GnRH receptor (encoded by the *GNRHR* gene) belongs to the rhodopsin family of G-protein–coupled receptors, composed of 7 helical transmembrane domains, an extracellular amino-terminal domain, characterized by the absence of a cytoplasmic domain intracellular carboxy-terminal present in other receptors of this family.[20] The GnRH receptor is expressed on the surface of gonadotrophes. Upon ligand binding, activation of the GnRH receptor increases calcium mobilization and stimulates influx of extracellular calcium activates phospholipase C, increasing inositol triphosphate and resulting in mobilization of intracellular calcium, stimulating the synthesis and release of luteinizing hormone and follicle-stimulating hormone.[69]

Inactivating mutations in the *GNRHR* gene were the first identified genetic causes of normosmic IHH.[70] Since the first description in 1997 by de Roux and colleagues,[70] more than 20 different mutations in homozygous or compound heterozygous, were reported in cases of sporadic or familial normosmic IHH, with no other associated malformations, and always with an autosomal-recessive inheritance.[71,72] *GNRHR* mutations have been shown to be responsible for significant proportion cases of normosmic IHH, with a prevalence of approximately 17% in sporadic cases and 40% in familial cases with the autosomal-recessive pattern of inheritance.[71–73]

GNRHR mutations have been associated with a broad phenotypic reproductive spectrum, varying from partial to complete GnRH resistance.[72,74,75] Indeed, a good genotype–phenotype correlation has been observed, considering that individuals homozygous for complete loss-of-function *GNRHR* mutations in general present with a phenotype of complete IHH and patients carrying partially inactivating mutations usually have partial IHH, with reports of reversal of the hypogonadism and milder cases, as the so-called fertile eunuch syndrome.[72,75]

HYPOGONADOTROPIC HYPOGONADISM ASSOCIATED WITH OTHER SYNDROMES
Leptin, Leptin Receptor, and PCSK1

The early onset of severe obesity associated with IHH may suggest loss-of-function mutations in the *LEP*, *LEPR*, or *PCSK1* genes. Leptin is a fat-derived hormone that regulates body weight by inhibiting food intake and stimulating energy expenditure. Leptin acts through the leptin receptor, a single transmembrane domain peptide expressed on human pituitary cells, as well as in many different sites of the central nervous system (choroid plexus, and the arcuate, ventromedial, dorsomedial and paraventricular nuclei).[76]

The importance of leptin in the reproductive axis was suggested because of the observation that leptin-deficient (*ob/ob*) or leptin-resistant (*db/db*) mice also presented with failure of pubertal development.[77] Furthermore, exogenous administration of leptin accelerated puberty in mice and normalized reproductive deficiencies in leptin-deficient (*ob/ob*) mice, suggesting that leptin may be a link between body fat and reproductive capability.[77] Accordingly, loss of body fat owing to starvation or excessive exercise is known to suppress reproduction and results in amenorrhea and infertility.[78–80]

Inactivating mutations in *LEP* or the gene encoding its receptor, *LEPR*, have been found in patients with severe obesity and IHH. These inactivating mutations account for less than 5% of normosmic IHH and have an autosomal-recessive pattern of transmission.[81]

Exactly how the effects of leptin are transmitted to GnRH neurons is unknown. Experimental data suggest that kisspeptin neurons are sensitive to changes in leptin concentrations and metabolic conditions, yet they do not express functional leptin receptor, which indicates the mode of action is indirect.[82,83] In summary, in humans, leptin and its receptor has a permissive role in the control of reproduction, being necessary but not sufficient for the onset of puberty and maintenance of fertility.[84]

The *PCSK1* gene encoded the proprotein convertase-1, a neuroendocrine convertase 1 (NEC1) that processes large precursor proteins into mature bioactive products.[85] Proprotein convertase-1 cleaves proopiomelanocortin (POMC) and acts in combination with proprotein convertase-2 to process proinsulin and proglucagon in pancreatic islets.[85] The first report of a patient with congenital NEC1 deficiency associated with obesity and IHH was published in 1995.[86] Mutations in this gene have been described in homozygous or compound heterozygous state, suggesting a pattern of autosomal recessive inheritance. The clinical characteristics generally include obesity, abnormal glucose homeostasis, and IHH.[86–88]

OTUD4/RNF216/PNPLA6

Gordon Holmes syndrome is characterized by cerebellar ataxia/atrophy and normosmic IHH.[89,90] Using whole-exome sequencing, digenic homozygous mutations in the *RNF216* and *OTUD4* genes were recently identified in a consanguineous family whose members were affected by ataxia and IHH.[91] Additional screening, by targeted sequencing of candidate genes in similarly affected patients, identified compound heterozygous truncating mutations in *RNF216* in an unrelated patient and single heterozygous deleterious mutations in 4 other patients. All patients had progressive ataxia and dementia. Neuronal loss was observed in cerebellar pathways and the hippocampus and defects were detected at the hypothalamic and pituitary levels of the reproductive endocrine axis.[91] Both *RNF216* and *OTUD4* encode proteins that regulate ubiquitination, indicating that abnormalities in this fundamental cellular process can have pathologic effects on pituitary components of the reproductive endocrine cascade.[91] Mutations affecting *RNF216* and *OTUD4* can synergize to cause neurologic syndrome associated with congenital IHH.[91]

Investigating the genetic causes of Boucher-Neuhauser and Gordon Holmes syndromes by exome sequencing approach, it was demonstrated that both syndromes were caused by recessive *PNPLA6* mutations.[92] It has been suggested that the deficiency of *PNPLA6* may cause a delayed neurodegeneration and a reproductive failure is owing to impaired gonadotropin release.[90]

DMXL2

A homozygous in-frame deletion of 15 nucleotides in *DMXL2* gene was identified in 3 brothers with a very complex neurologic endocrine syndrome characterized by gonadotropic axis deficiency, central hypothyroidism, peripheral demyelinating sensorimotor polyneuropathy, mental retardation, and profound hypoglycemia progressing to nonautoimmune insulin-dependent diabetes mellitus.[93] The mutated cex-hibited lower *DMXL2* mRNA expression levels in peripheral blood. Similarly, low levels of Dmxl2 expression in neuronal cells of mice lead to a partial gonadotropic axis deficiency, resulting in a very low fertility, owing to a loss of GnRH neurons in the hypothalamus, suggesting a new mechanism of GnRH deficiency.[93]

NR0B1

NR0B1 (also know as *DAX1*) is an orphan member of the nuclear receptor superfamily that functions in the proper formation of the adult adrenal gland.[94] The *NR0B1* gene product is a transcription factor expressed in the adrenal cortex, gonads, hypothalamus, and pituitary gonadotropes.[95] *DAX1* mutations cause congenital adrenal hypoplasia associated with IHH. The expression of DAX1 in the first stages of gonadal and adrenal differentiation and in the developing hypothalamus provided a basis for adrenal insufficiency and IHH in affected males, and was consistent with a role for *DAX1* in gonadal sex function.[96] More than 60 mutations in the *NR0B1* gene have been described in patients with congenital adrenal hypoplasia and most of these mutations are frameshift or nonsense mutations located throughout the gene, leading to truncation of the carboxy-terminal region and missense mutations are less common.[97] The pathogenesis of HH in *NR0B1* mutation is complex and seems to involve combined hypothalamic and pituitary defect.

Homeobox Gene Expressed in Embryonic Stem Cells 1

Homeobox gene expressed in embryonic stem cells 1 (HESX1) is a developmental gene identified in mouse that encodes an embryologic transcription repressor important for organ commitment and cell differentiation and proliferation.[98,99] HESX1 defects have been associated with the phenotype of septooptic dysplasia, isolated growth hormone deficiency and combined pituitary hormone deficiency in humans.[99–101]

Newbern and colleagues[101] screened 217 individuals with congenital IHH, including normosmic IHH and Kallmann syndrome, and identified heterozygous missense mutations in 3 Kallmann syndrome patients. It was hypothesized that Kallmann syndrome might represent a milder phenotypic manifestation of HESX1 mutations in these cases.[101]

REVERSAL OF HYPOGONADISM

Congenital IHH has been traditionally considered a lifelong and permanent condition. However, anecdotal reports of spontaneous recovery of the reproductive function after testosterone therapy have been described for many years.[102,103] Currently, the prevalence of IHH reversal is observed in 10% to 15%, occurring in both males and females.[104] Reversal of congenital IHH has been reported in patients with normosmic IHH and Kallmann syndrome, but is more common in patients with a phenotype of partial IHH.[4,5,68,72] Reversal should be suspected if testicular volume increases during testosterone administration or in cases of spontaneous fertility in IHH patients. A brief discontinuation of hormonal therapy to assess reversibility is indicated in these cases.[4] Nevertheless, the reversibility may not always be lifelong, and relapse of the hypogonadism has been observed in up to 5% of cases.[5] Interestingly, IHH reversal has been reported in several patients with confirmed pathogenic mutations in IHH genes, occurring more commonly in association with *GNRHR, FGFR1, TAC3/TACR3, CHD7,* and *PROKR2.* These observations indicate that the effects of a genetic defect can be overcome.[3] The triggers leading to reversal of IHH are not well-understood. Potential mechanisms involve the upregulation of genes involved in the regulation of GnRH axis or plasticity of the GnRH-producing neurons in adulthood in response to sexual steroids administration.[4,5] Interestingly, hypothalamic progenitor cells in rat can give rise to GnRH neurons, suggesting that postnatal genesis of GnRH neurons can occur in certain circumstances.[3,105]

OLIGOGENIC INHERITANCE

There are several disorders that were thought initially to be monogenic, but have subsequently proven to be caused by more than one gene defect.[7] Over the years, the traditional Mendelian view of congenital IHH as a monogenic disorder has been revised after the identification of oligogenic forms of congenital IHH. Mutations in more than 1 gene have been reported in several cases in normosmic IHH/Kallmann syndrome, involving different combinations of genes.[7,9,30,33,106,107] The genes more frequently associated to digenic inheritance include *FGFR1, FGF8, KAL1, PROKR2, PROK2, GNRHR, KISS1R*, and *NELF*.[7] In some of these cases, the segregation pattern of these digenic/oligogenic mutations in the pedigree can partially account for the phenotypic variability among individual family members.[13] Currently, oligogenic inheritance account for 10% to 20% of congenital IHH cases.[13,108]

SUMMARY

Congenital IHH is a rare disease with an uncovered complex model of genetics (monogeniticy and oligogenicity) that might apply to a large proportion of patients. At present, more than 25 different genes have been implicated in congenital IHH, which accounts for approximately 50% of cases.[8,9] The greater accessibility of new genetic sequencing methods probably will increase the percentage of patients with defined molecular diagnosis through the use of gene panels and new genes not yet described could be associated with congenital IHH using the exomic sequencing techniques.

REFERENCES

1. Silveira LF, Latronico AC. Approach to the patient with hypogonadotropic hypogonadism. J Clin Endocrinol Metab 2013;98(5):1781–8.
2. Seminara SB, Hayes FJ, Crowley WF Jr. Gonadotropin-releasing hormone deficiency in the human (idiopathic hypogonadotropic hypogonadism and Kallmanns syndrome): pathophysiological and genetic considerations. Endocr Rev 1998;19(5):521–39.
3. Mitchell AL, Dwyer A, Pitteloud N, et al. Genetic basis and variable phenotypic expression of Kallmann syndrome: towards a unifying theory. Trends Endocrinol Metab 2011;22(7):249–58.
4. Raivio T, Falardeau J, Dwyer A, et al. Reversal of idiopathic hypogonadotropic hypogonadism. N Engl J Med 2007;357(9):863–73.
5. Sidhoum VF, Chan YM, Lippincott MF, et al. Reversal and relapse of hypogonadotropic hypogonadism: resilience and fragility of the reproductive neuroendocrine system. J Clin Endocrinol Metab 2014;99(3):861–70.
6. Quinton R, Duke VM, De Zoysa PA, et al. The neuroradiology of Kalman's syndrome: a genotypic and phenotypic analysis. J Clin Endocrinol Metab 1996; 81(8):3010–7.
7. Pitteloud N, Quinton R, Pearce S, et al. Digenic mutations account for variable phenotypes in idiopathic hypogonadotropic hypogonadism. J Clin Invest 2007;117(2):457–63.
8. Boehm U, Bouloux PM, Dattani MT, et al. Expert consensus document: European consensus statement on congenital hypogonadotropic hypogonadism-pathogenesis, diagnosis and treatment. Nat Rev Endocrinol 2015;11(9):547–64.
9. Miraoui H, Dwyer AA, Sykiotis GP, et al. Mutations in FGF17, IL17RD, DUSP6, SPRY4, and FLRT3 are identified in individuals with congenital hypogonadotropic hypogonadism. Am J Hum Genet 2013;92(5):725–43.
10. Franco B, Guioli S, Pragliola A, et al. A gene deleted in Kallmann's syndrome shares homology with neural cell adhesion and axonal path-finding molecules. Nature 1991;353(6344):529–36.
11. Legouis R, Hardelin JP, Levilliers J, et al. The candidate gene for the x-linked Kallmann syndrome encodes a protein related to adhesion molecules. Cell 1991;67(2):423–35.

12. Hardelin J-P, Levilliers J, del Castillo I, et al. X chromosome-linked Kallmann syndrome: stop mutations validate the candidate gene. Proc Natl Acad Sci U S A 1992;89(17):8190–4.
13. Sykiotis GP, Plummer L, Hughes VA, et al. Oligogenic basis of isolated gonadotropin-releasing hormone deficiency. Proc Natl Acad Sci U S A 2010; 107(34):15140–4.
14. Kauffman AS, Smith JT. Kisspeptin signaling in reproductive biology. New York: Springer; 2013.
15. Dwyer AA, Sykiotis GP, Hayes FJ, et al. Trial of recombinant follicle-stimulating hormone pretreatment for gnrh-induced fertility in patients with congenital hypogonadotropic hypogonadism. J Clin Endocrinol Metab 2013;98(11):E1790–5.
16. Oliveira LM, Seminara SB, Beranova M, et al. The importance of autosomal genes in Kallmann syndrome: genotype-phenotype correlations and neuroendocrine characteristics 1. The J Clin Endocrinol Metab 2001;86(4):1532–8.
17. Kim SH, Hu Y, Cadman S, et al. Diversity in fibroblast growth factor receptor 1 regulation: learning from the investigation of Kallmann syndrome. J Neuroendocrinol 2008;20(2):141–63.
18. Dodé C, Levilliers J, Dupont JM, et al. Loss-of-function mutations in FGFR1 cause autosomal dominant Kallmann syndrome. Nat Genet 2003;33(4):463–5.
19. Xu N, Qin Y, Reindollar RH, et al. A mutation in the fibroblast growth factor receptor 1 gene causes fully penetrant normosmic isolated hypogonadotropic hypogonadism. J Clin Endocrinol Metab 2007;92(3):1155–8.
20. Bianco SD, Kaiser UB. The genetic and molecular basis of idiopathic hypogonadotropic hypogonadism. Nat Rev Endocrinol 2009;5(10):569–76.
21. Olsen SK, Li JY, Bromleigh C, et al. Structural basis by which alternative splicing modulates the organizer activity of FGF8 in the brain. Genes Dev 2006;20(2): 185–98.
22. Falardeau J, Chung WC, Beenken A, et al. Decreased FGF8 signaling causes deficiency of gonadotropin-releasing hormone in humans and mice. J Clin Invest 2008;118(8):2822–31.
23. Trarbach EB, Abreu AP, Silveira LF, et al. Nonsense mutations in FGF8 gene causing different degrees of human gonadotropin-releasing deficiency. J Clin Endocrinol Metab 2010;95(7):3491–6.
24. Costa-Barbosa FA, Balasubramanian R, Keefe KW, et al. Prioritizing genetic testing in patients with Kallmann syndrome using clinical phenotypes. J Clin Endocrinol Metab 2013;98(5):E943–53.
25. Villanueva C, Jacobson-Dickman E, Xu C, et al. Congenital hypogonadotropic hypogonadism with split hand/foot malformation: a clinical entity with a high frequency of FGFR1 mutations. Genet Med 2015;17(8):651–9.
26. Yang RB, Ng CK, Wasserman SM, et al. A novel interleukin-17 receptor-like protein identified in human umbilical vein endothelial cells antagonizes basic fibroblast growth factor-induced signaling. J Biol Chem 2003;278(35):33232–8.
27. Tornberg J, Sykiotis GP, Keefe K, et al. Heparan sulfate 6-o-sulfotransferase 1, a gene involved in extracellular sugar modifications, is mutated in patients with idiopathic hypogonadotrophic hypogonadism. Proc Natl Acad Sci 2011; 108(28):11524–9.
28. Hu Y, Bouloux P-M. Novel insights in FGFR1 regulation: lessons from Kallmann syndrome. Trends Endocrinol Metab 2010;21(6):385–93.
29. Kramer PR, Wray S. Novel gene expressed in nasal region influences outgrowth of olfactory axons and migration of luteinizing hormone-releasing hormone (LHRH) neurons. Genes Dev 2000;14(14):1824–34.

30. Miura K, Acierno JS, Seminara SB. Characterization of the human nasal embryonic LHRH factor gene, NELF, and a mutation screening among 65 patients with idiopathic hypogonadotropic hypogonadism (IHH). J Hum Genet 2004;49(5): 265–8.

31. Xu N, Kim H-G, Bhagavath B, et al. Nasal embryonic LHRH factor (NELF) mutations in patients with normosmic hypogonadotropic hypogonadism and Kallmann syndrome. Fertil Steril 2011;95(5):1613–20.

32. Li JD, Hu WP, Boehmer L, et al. Attenuated circadian rhythms in mice lacking the prokineticin 2 gene. J Neurosci 2006;26(45):11615–23.

33. Dodé C, Teixeira L, Levilliers J, et al. Kallmann syndrome: mutations in the genes encoding prokineticin-2 and prokineticin receptor-2. PLoS Genet 2006;2(10): e175.

34. Abreu AP, Trarbach EB, de Castro M, et al. Loss-of-function mutations in the genes encoding prokineticin-2 or prokineticin receptor-2 cause autosomal recessive Kallmann syndrome. J Clin Endocrinol Metab 2008;93(10):4113–8.

35. Matsumoto S-I, Yamazaki C, Masumoto K-H, et al. Abnormal development of the olfactory bulb and reproductive system in mice lacking prokineticin receptor PKR2. Proc Natl Acad Sci U S A 2006;103(11):4140–5.

36. Valdes-Socin H, Almanza MR, Fernández-Ladreda MT, et al. Reproduction, smell, and neurodevelopmental disorders: genetic defects in different hypogonadotropic hypogonadal syndromes. Neurological and Psychiatric Disorders in Endocrine Diseases 2015;29.

37. Kim HG, Ahn JW, Kurth I, et al. WDR11, a WD protein that interacts with transcription factor EMX1, is mutated in idiopathic hypogonadotropic hypogonadism and Kallmann syndrome. Am J Hum Genet 2010;87(4):465–79.

38. Kim HG, Kurth I, Lan F, et al. Mutations in CHD7, encoding a chromatin-remodeling protein, cause idiopathic hypogonadotropic hypogonadism and Kallmann syndrome. Am J Hum Genet 2008;83(4):511–9.

39. Jongmans MC, Admiraal RJ, van der Donk KP, et al. CHARGE syndrome: the phenotypic spectrum of mutations in the CHD7 gene. J Med Genet 2006; 43(4):306–14.

40. Bergman JE, de Ronde W, Jongmans MC, et al. The results of CHD7 analysis in clinically well-characterized patients with Kallmann syndrome. J Clin Endocrinol Metab 2012;97(5):E858–62.

41. Cariboni A, Davidson K, Rakic S, et al. Defective gonadotropin-releasing hormone neuron migration in mice lacking SEMA3A signalling through NRP1 and NRP2: implications for the aetiology of hypogonadotropic hypogonadism. Hum Mol Genet 2011;20(2):336–44.

42. Messina A, Ferraris N, Wray S, et al. Dysregulation of semaphorin7a/β1-integrin signaling leads to defective gnrh-1 cell migration, abnormal gonadal development and altered fertility. Hum Mol Genet 2011;20(24):4759–74.

43. Känsäkoski J, Fagerholm R, Laitinen EM, et al. Mutation screening of SEMA3A and SEMA7A in patients with congenital hypogonadotropic hypogonadism. Pediatr Res 2014;75(5):641–4.

44. Young J, Metay C, Bouligand J, et al. SEMA3A deletion in a family with Kallmann syndrome validates the role of semaphorin 3A in human puberty and olfactory system development. Hum Reprod 2012;27(5):1460–5.

45. Hanchate NK, Giacobini P, Lhuillier P, et al. SEMA3A, a gene involved in axonal pathfinding, is mutated in patients with Kallmann syndrome. PLoS Genet 2012; 8(8):e1002896.

46. Elmaleh-Bergès M, Baumann C, Noël-Pétroff N, et al. Spectrum of temporal bone abnormalities in patients with Waardenburg syndrome and SOX10 mutations. AJNR Am J Neuroradiol 2013;34(6):1257–63.

47. Pingault V, Bodereau V, Baral V, et al. Loss-of-function mutations in SOX10 cause Kallmann syndrome with deafness. Am J Hum Genet 2013;92(5):707–24.

48. Vaaralahti K, Tommiska J, Tillmann V, et al. De novo SOX10 nonsense mutation in a patient with Kallmann syndrome and hearing loss. Pediatr Res 2014;76(1): 115–6.

49. Eckler MJ, McKenna WL, Taghvaei S, et al. Fezf1 and fezf2 are required for olfactory development and sensory neuron identity. J Comp Neurol 2011;519(10): 1829–46.

50. Kotan LD, Hutchins BI, Ozkan Y, et al. Mutations in FEZF1 cause Kallmann syndrome. Am J Hum Genet 2014;95(3):326–31.

51. Hirata T, Nakazawa M, Yoshihara S, et al. Zinc-finger gene fez in the olfactory sensory neurons regulates development of the olfactory bulb non-cell-autonomously. Development 2006;133(8):1433–43.

52. Murata K, Tamogami S, Itou M, et al. Identification of an olfactory signal molecule that activates the central regulator of reproduction in goats. Curr Biol 2014;24(6):681–6.

53. Fukuda T, Sugita S, Inatome R, et al. CAMDI, a novel disrupted in schizophrenia 1 (DISC1)-binding protein, is required for radial migration. J Biol Chem 2010; 285(52):40554–61.

54. O'Bryan JP, Frye RA, Cogswell PC, et al. Axl, a transforming gene isolated from primary human myeloid leukemia cells, encodes a novel receptor tyrosine kinase. Mol Cell Biol 1991;11(10):5016–31.

55. Salian-Mehta S, Xu M, Knox AJ, et al. Functional consequences of AXL sequence variants in hypogonadotropic hypogonadism. The J Clin Endocrinol Metab 2014;99(4):1452–60.

56. Howard SR, Guasti L, Ruiz-Babot G, et al. IGSF10 mutations dysregulate gonadotropin-releasing hormone neuronal migration resulting in delayed puberty. EMBO Mol Med 2016;8(6):626–42.

57. Mason AJ, Hayflick JS, Zoeller RT, et al. A deletion truncating the gonadotropin-releasing hormone gene is responsible for hypogonadism in the hpg mouse. Science 1986;234(4782):1366–71.

58. Bouligand J, Ghervan C, Tello JA, et al. Isolated familial hypogonadotropic hypogonadism and a GNRH1 mutation. N Engl J Med 2009;360(26):2742–8.

59. Chan Y-M, de Guillebon A, Lang-Muritano M, et al. GNRH1 mutations in patients with idiopathic hypogonadotropic hypogonadism. Proc Natl Acad Sci U S A 2009;106(28):11703–8.

60. Mengen E, Tunc S, Kotan LD, et al. Complete idiopathic hypogonadotropic hypogonadism due to homozygous GNRH1 mutations in the mutational hot spots in the region encoding the decapeptide. Horm Res Paediatr 2016;85(2):107–11.

61. Maione L, Albarel F, Bouchard P, et al. R31C GNRH1 mutation and congenital hypogonadotropic hypogonadism. PLoS One 2013;8(7):e69616.

62. Seminara SB, Messager S, Chatzidaki EE, et al. The GPR54 gene as a regulator of puberty. N Engl J Med 2003;349(17):1614–27.

63. de Roux N, Genin E, Carel J-C, et al. Hypogonadotropic hypogonadism due to loss of function of the kiss1-derived peptide receptor GPR54. Proc Natl Acad Sci 2003;100(19):10972–6.

64. Navarro VM, Castellano JM, García-Galiano D, et al. Neuroendocrine factors in the initiation of puberty: the emergent role of kisspeptin. Rev Endocr Metab Disord 2007;8(1):11–20.

65. Tusset C, Trarbach B, Silveira LFG, et al. Aspectos clínicos e moleculares do hipogonadismohipogonadotrófico isolado congênito. Arq Bras Endocrinol Metabol 2011;55(8):501–11.

66. Topaloglu AK, Tello JA, Kotan LD, et al. Inactivating KISS1 mutation and hypogonadotropic hypogonadism. N Engl J Med 2012;366(7):629–35.

67. Topaloglu AK, Reimann F, Guclu M, et al. TAC3 and TACR3 mutations in familial hypogonadotropic hypogonadism reveal a key role for neurokinin B in the central control of reproduction. Nat Genet 2009;41(3):354–8.

68. Gianetti E, Tusset C, Noel SD, et al. TAC3/TACR3 mutations reveal preferential activation of gonadotropin-releasing hormone release by neurokinin B in neonatal life followed by reversal in adulthood. J Clin Endocrinol Metab 2010; 95(6):2857–67.

69. Kakar SS, Musgrove LC, Devor DC, et al. Cloning, sequencing, and expression of human gonadotropin releasing hormone (gnrh) receptor. Biochem Biophys Res Commun 1992;189(1):289–95.

70. de Roux N, Young J, Misrahi M, et al. A family with hypogonadotropic hypogonadism and mutations in the gonadotropin-releasing hormone receptor. N Engl J Med 1997;337(22):1597–603.

71. Chevrier L, Guimiot F, de Roux N. GnRH receptor mutations in isolated gonadotropic deficiency. Mol Cell Endocrinol 2011;346(1–2):21–8.

72. Beneduzzi D, Trarbach EB, Min L, et al. Role of gonadotropin-releasing hormone receptor mutations in patients with a wide spectrum of pubertal delay. Fertil Steril 2014;102(3):838–46.

73. Beranova M, Oliveira LMB, Bedecarrats GY, et al. Prevalence, phenotypic spectrum, and modes of inheritance of gonadotropin-releasing hormone receptor mutations in idiopathic hypogonadotropic hypogonadism 1. The J Clin Endocrinol Metab 2001;86(4):1580–8.

74. Seminara SB, Beranova M, Oliveira LM, et al. Successful use of pulsatile gonadotropin-releasing hormone (gnrh) for ovulation induction and pregnancy in a patient with gnrh receptor mutations 1. The J Clin Endocrinol Metab 2000;85(2):556–62.

75. Pitteloud N, Boepple PA, DeCruz S, et al. The fertile eunuch variant of idiopathic hypogonadotropic hypogonadism: spontaneous reversal associated with a homozygous mutation in the gonadotropin-releasing hormone receptor 1. The J Clin Endocrinol Metab 2001;86(6):2470–5.

76. Wauters M, Considine RV, Van Gaal LF. Human leptin: from an adipocyte hormone to an endocrine mediator. Eur J Endocrinol 2000;143(3):293–311.

77. Chehab FF, Lim ME, Lu R. Correction of the sterility defect in homozygous obese female mice by treatment with the human recombinant leptin. Nat Genet 1996; 12(3):318–20.

78. Licinio J. Leptin in anorexia nervosa and amenorrhea. Mol Psychiatry 1997;2(4): 267–9.

79. Hill JW, Elmquist JK, Elias CF. Hypothalamic pathways linking energy balance and reproduction. Am J Physiol Endocrinol Metab 2008;294(5):E827–32.

80. Clément K, Vaisse C, Lahlou N, et al. A mutation in the human leptin receptor gene causes obesity and pituitary dysfunction. Nature 1998;392(6674): 398–401.

81. Strobel A, Issad T, Camoin L, et al. A leptin missense mutation associated with hypogonadism and morbid obesity. Nat Genet 1998;18(3):213–5.
82. Quennell JH, Mulligan AC, Tups A, et al. Leptin indirectly regulates gonadotropin-releasing hormone neuronal function. Endocrinology 2009; 150(6):2805–12.
83. Bellefontaine N, Chachlaki K, Parkash J, et al. Leptin-dependent neuronal NO signaling in the preoptic hypothalamus facilitates reproduction. J Clin Invest 2014;124(6):2550–9.
84. Tena-Sempere M. KiSS-1 and reproduction: focus on its role in the metabolic regulation of fertility. Neuroendocrinology 2006;83(5–6):275–81.
85. Jansen E, Ayoubi TA, Meulemans SM, et al. Neuroendocrine-specific expression of the human prohormone convertase 1 gene hormonal regulation of transcription through distinct camp response elements. J Biol Chem 1995;270(25): 15391–7.
86. O'Rahilly S, Gray H, Humphreys PJ, et al. Impaired processing of prohormones associated with abnormalities of glucose homeostasis and adrenal function. N Engl J Med 1995;333(21):1386–91.
87. Farooqi IS, Volders K, Stanhope R, et al. Hyperphagia and early-onset obesity due to a novel homozygous missense mutation in prohormone convertase 1/3. J Clin Endocrinol Metab 2007;92(9):3369–73.
88. Farooqi IS, O'Rahilly S. Mutations in ligands and receptors of the leptin-melanocortin pathway that lead to obesity. Nat Clin Pract Endocrinol Metab 2008;4(10):569–77.
89. Balasubramanian R, Crowley WF. Isolated gnrh deficiency: a disease model serving as a unique prism into the systems biology of the gnrh neuronal network. Mol Cell Endocrinol 2011;346(1–2):4–12.
90. Topaloglu AK, Lomniczi A, Kretzschmar D, et al. Loss-of-function mutations in PNPLA6 encoding neuropathy target esterase underlie pubertal failure and neurological deficits in Gordon Holmes syndrome. J Clin Endocrinol Metab 2014;99(10):E2067–75.
91. Margolin DH, Kousi M, Chan YM, et al. Ataxia, dementia, and hypogonadotropism caused by disordered ubiquitination. N Engl J Med 2013;368(21): 1992–2003.
92. Synofzik M, Gonzalez MA, Lourenco CM, et al. PNPLA6 mutations cause Boucher-Neuhauser and Gordon Holmes syndromes as part of a broad neurodegenerative spectrum. Brain 2014;137(Pt 1):69–77.
93. Tata B, Huijbregts L, Jacquier S, et al. Haploinsufficiency of dmxl2, encoding a synaptic protein, causes infertility associated with a loss of gnrh neurons in mouse. PLoS Biol 2014;12(9):e1001952.
94. Niakan KK, McCabe ER. DAX1 origin, function, and novel role. Mol Genet Metab 2005;86(1–2):70–83.
95. Silveira LF, MacColl GS, Bouloux PM. Hypogonadotropic hypogonadism. Semin Reprod Med 2002;20(4):327–38.
96. Swain A, Zanaria E, Hacker A, et al. Mouse dax1 expression is consistent with a role in sex determination as well as in adrenal and hypothalamus function. Nat Genet 1996;12(4):404–9.
97. Achermann JC, Jameson JL. Advances in the molecular genetics of hypogonadotropic hypogonadism. J Pediatr Endocrinol Metab 2001;14(1):3–15.
98. Hermesz E, Mackem S, Mahon KA. Rpx: a novel anterior-restricted homeobox gene progressively activated in the prechordal plate, anterior neural plate and Rathke's pouch of the mouse embryo. Development 1996;122(1):41–52.

99. Dattani MT, Martinez-Barbera J-P, Thomas PQ, et al. Mutations in the homeobox gene HESX1/hesx1 associated with septo-optic dysplasia in human and mouse. Nat Genet 1998;19(2):125–33.
100. Carvalho LR, Woods KS, Mendonca BB, et al. A homozygous mutation in HESX1 is associated with evolving hypopituitarism due to impaired repressor-corepressor interaction. J Clin Invest 2003;112(8):1192–201.
101. Newbern K, Natrajan N, Kim HG, et al. Identification of HESX1 mutations in Kallmann syndrome. Fertil Steril 2013;99(7):1831–7.
102. Rezvani I, DiGeorge A, Rutano J, et al. Delayed puberty and anosmia; coincidence or Kallmann variant? Pediatr Res 1975;9:224.
103. Bauman A. Markedly delayed puberty or Kallmann's syndrome variant. J Androl 1986;7(4):224–7.
104. Dwyer AA, Raivio T, Pitteloud N. Management of endocrine disease: reversible hypogonadotropic hypogonadism. Eur J Endocrinol 2016;174(6):R267–74.
105. Salvi R, Arsenijevic Y, Giacomini M, et al. The fetal hypothalamus has the potential to generate cells with a gonadotropin releasing hormone (gnrh) phenotype. PLoS One 2009;4(2):e4392.
106. Cole LW, Sidis Y, Zhang C, et al. Mutations in prokineticin 2 and prokineticin receptor 2 genes in human gonadotrophin-releasing hormone deficiency: molecular genetics and clinical spectrum. J Clin Endocrinol Metab 2008;93(9):3551–9.
107. Canto P, Munguia P, Söderlund D, et al. Genetic analysis in patients with Kallmann syndrome: coexistence of mutations in prokineticin receptor 2 and KAL1. J Androl 2009;30(1):41–5.
108. Quaynor SD, Kim HG, Cappello EM, et al. The prevalence of digenic mutations in patients with normosmic hypogonadotropic hypogonadism and Kallmann syndrome. Fertil Steril 2011;96(6):1424–30.e6.

Genetics of Diabetes Insipidus

Marie Helene Schernthaner-Reiter, MD, PhD, MSci[a,b,*],
Constantine A. Stratakis, MD, D(med)Sci[b], Anton Luger, MD[a]

KEYWORDS

- Familial neurohypophyseal diabetes insipidus
- Familial nephrogenic diabetes insipidus • Arginine vasopressin
- Arginine vasopressin receptor type 2 • Aquaporin 2 • Wolfram syndrome

KEY POINTS

- Familial neurohypophyseal diabetes insipidus is most commonly caused by autosomal dominant *arginine vasopressin (AVP)* mutations; it demonstrates a gradual onset during infancy or early childhood and is treated by 1-desamino-8-D-arginine vasopressin (dDAVP).
- Familial nephrogenic diabetes insipidus is most often caused by X-linked mutations in the *arginine vasopressin receptor type 2 (AVPR2)* and hence affects mainly boys and men; it is characterized by onset in early infancy and standard treatment consists of thiazide diuretics and indomethacin.
- Alternative treatments of familial nephrogenic diabetes insipidus, including stabilization of AVPR2 by molecular chaperones and stimulation of AVPR2-independent aquaporin (AQP) 2 cell surface translocation, are currently under investigation.

INTRODUCTION

Diabetes insipidus is a disease characterized by polyuria and polydipsia. It may be caused by inadequate posterior pituitary arginine vasopressin (AVP) production (neurohypophyseal diabetes insipidus or central diabetes insipidus), renal vasopressin signaling defects (nephrogenic diabetes insipidus), or increased AVP degradation by placental vasopressinase in pregnancy (gestational diabetes insipidus), and it may occasionally be due to secondary suppression of AVP production after excessive fluid intake (primary polydipsia).

Disclosures: The authors have nothing to disclose.
[a] Clinical Division of Endocrinology and Metabolism, Department of Internal Medicine III, Medical University of Vienna, Waehringer Guertel 18-20, Vienna 1090, Austria; [b] Section on Endocrinology and Genetics, *Eunice Kennedy Shriver* National Institute of Child Health and Human Development, National Institutes of Health, 31 Center Drive, Bethesda, MD 20892, USA
* Corresponding author.
E-mail address: helene@schernthaner.eu

Endocrinol Metab Clin N Am 46 (2017) 305–334
http://dx.doi.org/10.1016/j.ecl.2017.01.002
0889-8529/17/© 2017 Elsevier Inc. All rights reserved.

endo.theclinics.com

The complete loss of AVP function leads to a daily urine production of approximately 12 L, resulting in an average urination frequency of once per hour over 24 hours.[1] Acquired forms are most often caused by hypothalamic or pituitary injury, often through adenomas, craniopharyngiomas, other infiltrating or metastatic disease, trauma, ischemia, or autoimmune disorders.

This article reviews the genetic causes of central diabetes insipidus and nephrogenic diabetes insipidus in the context of its pathogenic mechanisms, diagnosis, and treatments.

THE POSTERIOR PITUITARY-DISTAL TUBULE AXIS: ARGININE VASOPRESSIN PRODUCTION, RELEASE, AND MECHANISMS OF ACTION

The gene product of *AVP* is a larger precursor peptide (prepro-AVP), consisting of a signal peptide, the AVP moiety, neurophysin II (NPII), and the glycopeptide copeptin (**Fig. 1**).[2,3] Prepro-AVP is produced by the magnocellular neurons of the supraoptic and paraventricular hypothalamic nuclei. These vasopressinergic neurons project from the hypothalamus through the diaphragma sellae and form the posterior pituitary gland.[4] Cotranslationally, prepro-AVP is targeted to the endoplasmic reticulum (ER) by its signal peptide, where pro-AVP is created by removal of the signal peptide, the glycosylation of copeptin, folding, and formation of 8 disulfide bonds. Pro-AVP is then further glycosylated in the Golgi apparatus and packaged into dense core granules. In these, proteolytic cleavage into AVP, its carrier protein NPII, and the glycoprotein copeptin occurs by prohormone convertases during axonal transport into the posterior pituitary, where all 3 peptides are stored within neurosecretory vesicles, which are released after neuronal stimulation by calcium-mediated exocytosis.[5–8] Release of AVP is regulated by the osmotic pressure of the plasma and interstitium, which can be sensed by osmoregulatory hypothalamic neurons as well as by circulating blood volume, sensed by carotid, aortic, and atrial baroreceptors, or nausea.[9–12]

After release into the circulation, AVP binds to its receptor, AVPR2, which is expressed on the basolateral surface of the epithelial cells of the renal collecting duct (**Fig. 2**).[13,14] AVPR2 is a 7 membrane–spanning, G protein–coupled receptor; after AVP binding, AVPR2 releases $G_s\alpha$, which activates the adenylyl cyclase, causing cyclic adenosine monophosphate (cAMP) release and thereby cAMP-dependent protein kinase (PKA) activation. The PKA phosphorylates AQP2 at a C-terminal residue, which stimulates the insertion of subapical storage vesicles containing AQP2 oligomers into the cell membrane (see **Fig. 2**).[15–17] Thereby, water can diffuse into the principal cells of the collecting duct and exit into the interstitium through the constitutively expressed AQP3 and AQP4 on the basolateral side, which reduces urinary water loss by reducing urine volume and increasing urine osmolality.[18–20] The importance of renal PKA signaling in the pathogenesis of nephrogenic diabetes insipidus is underlined by the finding that mice expressing a dominant-negative PKA regulatory subunit display a diabetes insipidus phenotype.[21] In addition, AVP stimulates sodium reabsorption in the collecting duct via the epithelial sodium channel,[22,23] and it increases urea transport by regulating the urea transporter A1.[24,25] In the longer term, AVP-dependent PKA signaling also leads to an up-regulation of *AQP2* transcription via stimulation of the cAMP response element binding protein, which is also activated by the PKA.[26]

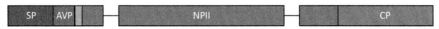

Fig. 1. The structure of the AVP gene in terms of components of the AVP peptide (prepro-AVP), including the N-terminal signal peptide (SP), the AVP moiety, the NPII moiety, and the C-terminal copeptin.

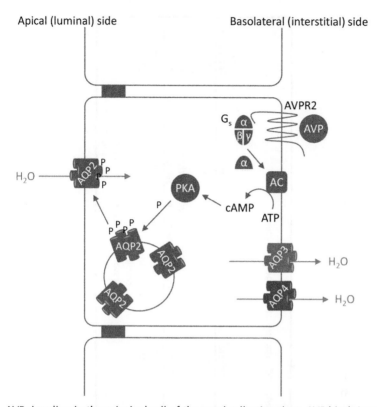

Fig. 2. AVP signaling in the principal cell of the renal collecting duct. AVP binds its receptor AVPR2 on the interstitial side; this activates $G_s\alpha$, which in turn activates the adenylyl cyclase, leading to increasing intracellular cAMP levels. This is followed by an activation of the PKA, which phosphorylates AQP2, thereby stimulating the translocation of subapical AQP2-containing vesicles to the apical cell membrane. Water can thereby enter the apical side of the collecting duct and leave the cell into the interstitium via basolateral AQP3 and AQP4 channels.

During maximal activation of the posterior pituitary-distal tubule axis, urine osmolality can increase up to approximately 1200 mOsm/L and urine flow can decrease down to 0.5 mL/min, whereas a complete absence of vasopressin stimulation, such as during complete diabetes insipidus, leaves the collecting ducts impermeable to water, hence leading to urine excretion rates of up to 20 mL/min and urine concentrations as low as 50 mOsm/L.[27]

DIAGNOSIS

Diagnostically, a fluid deprivation test in conjunction with dDAVP administration is most commonly used to establish diabetes insipidus and to distinguish between nephrogenic or gestational forms versus neurohypophyseal forms. In severe forms of diabetes insipidus, fluid deprivation fails to adequately stimulate urine concentration to values greater than 300 mOsm/L; dDAVP administration rescues urine concentration in central diabetes insipidus and gestational diabetes insipidus but has no or little effect on nephrogenic diabetes insipidus (**Table 1**).[1,28,29] The interpretation of those tests becomes more difficult in partial neurohypophyseal or nephrogenic forms, in

Table 1
Different types of familial diabetes insipidus, their diagnosis and treatment, and summary of their genetic causes

Type of Diabetes Insipidus	Diagnosis		Standard Treatment	Affected Gene	Inheritance	Onset	Known Mutations
	Fluid Deprivation	dDAVP Stimulation					
Neurohypophyseal	No response	Increase of urine osmolality	dDAVP	AVP	Autosomal dominant	1–6 y	73
					Autosomal recessive	Early infancy	3
				WFS1	Autosomal recessive	Second/third decade	>170
Nephrogenic	No response	No response	Thiazide, indomethacin	AVPR2	X-linked	Early infancy	>200
				AQP2	Autosomal dominant	Early infancy	52
					Autosomal recessive	Infancy, early childhood	11

which urine concentration during fluid deprivation is often still conserved. Further-more, in partial nephrogenic diabetes insipidus, where there may be some response to fluid deprivation, differential diagnosis versus primary polydipsia is often difficult to establish because primary polydipsia often also leads to somewhat submaximal urine concentration by adaptation to a large fluid intake.[1,28,29]

The infusion of hypertonic saline to raise serum sodium levels is also sometimes used and should lead to maximal stimulation of pituitary AVP secretion and hence urine concentration, analogous to water deprivation, in complete diabetes insipidus.[29]

On MRI of the sella, central diabetes insipidus is usually characterized by the absence of the characteristic posterior pituitary bright spot in T1-weighted imaging, whereas the bright spot is thought to be preserved in nephrogenic DI; however, this is relatively unspecific, because an absent bright spot is often also noted in nephro-genic diabetes insipidus, possibly due to the depletion of intracellular AVP stores in the vasopressinergic neurons. On the other hand, a bright spot should always be visible in primary polydipsia.[30–32]

Although the measurement of serum AVP levels is theoretically a good option to identify complete central diabetes insipidus (where even maximal stimulation by water deprivation is not able to elicit an adequate increase in AVP levels) and nephrogenic diabetes insipidus (where AVP levels are compensatorily up-regulated), practically serum AVP is difficult to measure accurately due to its preanalytic instability and the lack of reliable assays. Copeptin, however, the C-terminal part of prepro-AVP, can be detected in serum and is much more stable than AVP. The measurement of copep-tin as a surrogate parameter for AVP levels in the diagnosis of diabetes insipidus is currently being developed.[33] Measurement of urinary AQP2 levels have been sug-gested in the diagnosis of central diabetes insipidus.[34]

FAMILIAL NEUROHYPOPHYSEAL DIABETES INSIPIDUS

Familial neurohypophyseal diabetes insipidus (OMIM#125700) may be caused by mu-tations in the AVP (OMIM*192340) gene as well as in rarer cases by mutations in the WFS1 gene. Cases of X-linked central diabetes insipidus have been described in the literature, but no genetic cause has been identified yet.

Familial neurohypophyseal diabetes insipidus usually manifests at an age of several months to several years (typically between 1 and 6 years of age), with a gradual onset due to the progressive destruction of vasopressinergic neurons[35,36]; in early stages of disease development, patients may display partial AVP deficiency that can be over-come by fluid deprivation or other stimuli for AVP secretion, such as nausea or postural hypotension.[35,36] In addition, there is a wide spectrum of disease manifestations, where even the same mutation can lead to heterogeneous clinical presentations in different family members.[37,38] In the autosomal recessive forms of familial neurohypophyseal diabetes insipidus, age of manifestation was lower than in the dominant mutations (me-dians: 2 months vs 2 years, respectively).[39] A decrease of symptoms with age can often be observed; the mechanism for this phenomenon is not entirely clear but could relate to an age-dependent decrease in glomerular filtration rates.[40–42] Although polyuria and polydipsia are usually the earliest symptoms, those may be difficult to recognize in in-fants. Affected children, however, often also present with failure to thrive; in these cases, catch-up growth is usually observed once dDAVP therapy is initiated.[42,43] Diag-nostically, AVP is generally low/absent and the lack of a posterior pituitary bright spot on MRI may be observed[30,44,45]; a fluid deprivation test results in a complete absence of urine concentration as well as AVP stimulation, whereas a complete rescue of urine osmolality after dDAVP, or desmopressin, administration is expected.

Treatment of familial neurohypophyseal diabetes insipidus is performed with the AVPR2-selective AVP analog dDAVP, which leads to a cessation of polyuria, hence also normalizing polydipsia and thirst.[46]

Arginine Vasopressin Mutations Causing Familial Neurohypophyseal Diabetes Insipidus

Most frequently, familial neurohypophyseal diabetes insipidus is caused by mutations in the *AVP* gene, also referred to as *AVP-NPII*, leading to absence or deficiency of AVP.[47] A large majority of familial neurohypophyseal diabetes insipidus–causing *AVP* mutations are inherited in an autosomal dominant fashion; 3 *AVP* mutations leading to a recessive transmission have been described in 5 kindreds (discussed later).

Autosomal dominant familial neurohypophyseal diabetes insipidus due to arginine vasopressin mutations

AVP is located on chromosome 20p13 and consists of 3 exons. A 19 amino acid signal sequence, which is responsible for ER targeting of prepro-AVP, is followed by the 9 amino acid AVP moiety on exon 1. It is followed by NPII, which is encoded on exons 1, 2, and 3 (93 amino acids). Finally, NPII is followed by copeptin, encoded on exon 3 (39 amino acids) (see **Fig. 1**).[48]

Most autosomal dominantly inherited cases of neurohypophyseal diabetes insipidus are due to *AVP* mutations located in the *NPII* moiety or the signal peptide whereas a few mutations are located directly in the *AVP* moiety; currently, 72 disease-causing mutations have been identified (**Table 2**). Most mutations are missense or nonsense mutations; however, small deletions, indels, and 1 splice site mutation have also been described. The mutations are largely predicted to interfere with processing or folding of the AVP precursors.[29,42] No clear genotype-phenotype correlation has been observed, with the exception of the c.55G>A (p.Ala19Thr) mutation, which leads to impaired cleavage of the signal peptide and to a later onset of disease.[41,49]

Mechanistically, autosomal dominant neurohypophyseal diabetes insipidus–causing AVP mutants are expressed but retained in the ER, where they are thought to accumulate and lead to cell death of vasopressinergic neurons. Some mutants were demonstrated to form densely packed aggregates with a fibrillar structure,[42,50] ultimately leading to autophagic cell death and loss of vasopressinergic neurons.[51–53] In mice, progression of polyuria was paralleled by the formation of inclusion bodies in vasopressinergic neurons.[54] This hypothesis is consistent with autopsy studies, which showed a loss of AVP-secreting cells in patients with familial neurohypophyseal diabetes insipidus.[55,56] Furthermore, the mutant prohormones can act in a dominant-negative fashion by heterodimerizing with wild-type pro-AVP, thereby preventing its processing,[57] suggesting that this additional mechanism may also contribute to disease development. Murine studies showed that a reduction of AVP stimulation (by exogenous AVP administration or a low-sodium diet) may also delay neuronal cell death and thereby disease onset[58]; this could be useful in future therapeutic approaches.

Autosomal recessive familial neurohypophyseal diabetes insipidus due to arginine vasopressin mutations

Rarely, *AVP* mutations can lead to an autosomal recessive transmission of neurohypophyseal diabetes insipidus (**Table 3**). The c.77C>T mutation (p.Pro26Leu), located within the *AVP* moiety, inhibits AVP-AVPR2 binding, causing a reduction of the biological activity of AVP by approximately 30-fold; accordingly, the circulating

Table 2
AVP mutations, their locations, and corresponding references in autosomal dominant familial neurohypophyseal diabetes insipidus

Mutation				
cDNA Level	Protein Level	Mutation Type	Location	Reference
c.-3A>C	NR	Mutation in regulatory sequence	5′ UTR	[118]
c.1–33_4del	p.M1_T4del	37 bp deletion, alternative start site	Signal peptide	[119]
c.1A>G	p.M1_T4del	Missense, alternative start site	Signal peptide	[120]
c.3Gdel	p.M1_T4del	Small deletion, alternative start site	Signal peptide	[45,121]
c.3G>A	p.M1_T4del	Missense, alternative start site	Signal peptide	[120]
c.50C>T	p.S17F	Missense	Signal peptide	[121]
c.52_54delTCC	p.S18del	Small deletion	Signal peptide	[66]
c.55G>A	p.A19T	Missense	Signal peptide	[41]
c.56C>T	p.A19V	Missense	Signal peptide	[121]
c.61T>C	p.Y21H	Missense	AVP	[122]
c.62A>C	p.Y21S	Missense	AVP	[123]
c.64–66delTTC	p.F22del	Small deletion	AVP	[124]
c.123C>G	p.C41W	Missense	NPII	[125]
c.133G>C	p.G45R	Missense	NPII	[121]
c.133G>T	p.G45C	Missense	NPII	[126]
c.143G>T	p.G48V	Missense	NPII	[127]
c.151C>T	p.R51C	Missense	NPII	[121]
c.154T>C	p.C52R	Missense	NPII	[128]
c.160G>A	p.G54R	Missense	NPII	[129]
c.160G>C	p.G54R	Missense	NPII	[40]
c.161G>A	p.G54E	Missense	NPII	[130]
c.161G>T	p.G54V	Missense	NPII	[131]
c.164C>T	p.P55L	Missense	NPII	[132]
c.173G>T	p.C58F	Missense	NPII	[133]
c.175T>C	p.C59R	Missense	NPII	[73]
c.176G>A	p.C59Y	Missense	NPII	[134]
c.177_179delCGC	p.C59del/A60W	Small deletion	NPII	[135]
c.192_193delinsAA	p.C65S	Small indel, missense	NPII	[136]
c.194G>T	p.C65F	Missense	NPII	[137]
c.200T>C	p.V67A	Missense	NPII	[120]
c.207_209delGGC	p.A70del	Small deletion	NPII	[138]
c.218T>C	p.L73P	Missense	NPII	[139]
c.230_232delGAG	p.E78del	Small deletion	NPII	[140]
c.232G>A	p.E78K	Missense	NPII	[141]
c.233A>G	p.E78G	Missense	NPII	[121]
c.242T>C	p.L81P	Missense	NPII	[121]

(continued on next page)

Table 2
(continued)

cDNA Level	Protein Level	Mutation Type	Location	Reference
c.251C>T	p.P84L	Missense	NPII	[38]
c.260C>A	p.S87Y	Missense	NPII	[137]
c.260C>T	p.S87F	Missense	NPII	[142]
c.262G>A	p.G88S	Missense	NPII	[143]
c.262G>C	p.G88R	Missense	NPII	[121]
c.263G>T	p.G88V	Missense	NPII	[144]
c.274T>A	p.C92S	Missense	NPII	[137]
c.275G>A	p.C92Y	Missense	NPII	[142]
c.275G>C	p.C92S	Missense	NPII	[121]
c.276C>A	p.C92*	Nonsense	NPII	[121]
c.276C>G	p.C92W	Missense	NPII	[125]
c.277G>T	p.G93W	Missense	NPII	[145]
c.286G>T	p.G96C	Missense	NPII	[121]
c.287G>A	p.G96D	Missense	NPII	[120]
c.287G>T	p.G96V	Missense	NPII	[146]
c.289C>T	p.R97C	Missense	NPII	[147]
c.290G>C	p.R97P	Missense	NPII	[148]
c.292T>A	p.C98S	Missense	NPII	[149]
c.292T>G	p.C98G	Missense	NPII	[150]
c.293_294delinsCT	p.C98S	Missense	NPII	[137]
c.294C>A	p.C98*	Nonsense	NPII	[145]
c.295G>C	p.A99P	Missense	NPII	[35]
c.310T>G	p.C104G	Missense	NPII	[120]
c.311G>A	p.C104Y	Missense	NPII	[151]
c.311G>T	p.C104F	Missense	NPII	[152]
c.313T>C	p.C105R	Missense	NPII	[153]
c.314G>A	p.C105Y	Missense	NPII	[154]
c.322G>T	p.E108*	Nonsense	NPII	[155]
c.322+1delG	NR	Splice site mutation, intron 2 retention	NPII	[156]
c.330C>A	p.C110*	Nonsense	NPII	[121]
c.337G>T	p.E113*	Nonsense	NPII	[157]
c.342_343delinsGT	p.P114*	Small indel, nonsense	NPII	[121]
c.343G>T	p.E115*	Nonsense	NPII	[158]
c.346T>C	p.C116R	Missense	NPII	[159]
c.346T>G	p.C116G	Missense	NPII	[159]
c.348C>G	p.C116W	Missense	NPII	[120]
c.352G>T	p.E118*	Nonsense	NPII	[121]

Reference sequence NM_000490.
Abbreviations: NR, not reported; UTR, untranslated region.

Table 3
AVP mutations, their locations, and corresponding references in autosomal recessive familial neurohypophyseal diabetes insipidus

Mutation				
cDNA Level	Protein Level	Mutation Type	Location	Reference
c.77C>T	p.P26L	Missense	AVP	59,60
c.77C>T	p.P26L	Missense	AVP	39
c.121-2A>G	NR	Splice site mutation	NPII	
10,396 bp deletion	NR	Large deletion	NPII, copeptin, and regulatory sequences	61

Reference sequence NM_000490.
Abbreviation: NR, not reported.

levels of AVP p.Pro26Leu are compensatorily increased in affected patients. This mutation was detected in 2 apparently unrelated consanguineous families.[59,60] Clinically, this form manifests in early infancy or childhood and is characterized by the absence of the posterior pituitary bright spot and a good therapeutic response to dDAVP.

The same c.77C>T mutation was detected in a compound heterozygous boy with diabetes insipidus who additionally carried a novel *AVP* splice site mutation (c.121-2A>G); manifestation was in the first months of life, and treatment by dDAVP was successful. The functional consequences of the splice site mutation were not described, but the recessive transmission of the disease suggests the absence of translated prepro-AVP.[39]

A large 10-kb homozygous deletion encompassing almost the whole *AVP* gene as well as the intergenic region between oxytocin and *AVP* was detected in affected members of a consanguineous family. This led to disease manifestation in the first days of life, and symptoms responded well to dDAVP treatment.[61]

Neurohypophyseal Diabetes Insipidus Due to WFS1 Mutations

Wolfram syndrome is a rare autosomal recessive disorder that is characterized by central diabetes insipidus, diabetes mellitus, optic atrophy, and deafness (DIDMOAD, OMIM#222300).[62] It is largely caused by homozygous or compound heterozygous mutations in the *WFS1* gene (OMIM*606201) located on chromosome 4p, encoding wolframin.[63] Wolframin functions as an ER channel and regulates intracellular Ca^{2+} levels.[64] Although the disease is defined by the presence of diabetes mellitus and optic atrophy, approximately 70% of patients also present with central diabetes insipidus due to AVP deficiency.[62,65] A case of a patient with isolated familial neurohypophyseal diabetes insipidus on the basis of compound heterozygous *WFS1* mutations was recently described; even after extensive follow-up of 10 years, there was no evidence of optic atrophy or diabetes mellitus[66]; the investigators of another study hypothesized that a dosage effect of specific *WFS1* mutations with different tissue sensitivities to WFS1 deficiency may be responsible for partial phenotypes.[67] Clinically, diabetes insipidus in the context of Wolfram syndrome is characterized by late onset in the second or third decade of life.[62] In pancreatic beta cells, defective wolframin forms ER aggregates and causes ER stress, leading to cell death,[68] and there is histologic evidence of neuron loss in the supraoptic nucleus[69]; however, the mechanism by which defective wolframin leads to central diabetes insipidus is currently not known.

Proprotein Convertase Subtilisin/Kexin Type 1 and Fibroblast Growth Factor 8 — Potential Roles in Diabetes Insipidus

A recent study described a case of a patient with proprotein convertase subtilisin/kexin type 1 (PCSK1) deficiency due to compound heterozygous *PCSK1* mutations presenting with obesity, hypopituitarism, and central diabetes insipidus, which was treated with dDAVP; although the pathologic mechanism for diabetes insipidus in this patient is unclear, the investigators point out that PCSK1 and proprotein convertase subtilisin/kexin type 2 (PCSK2) are both involved in pro-AVP processing in mice, whereas PCSK1 is known to be involved in the processing of other hypothalamic prohormones.[70]

In a patient with holoprosencephaly and an absent corpus callosum, who presented in infancy with central diabetes insipidus and a deficient corticotrope axis, a homozygous fibroblast growth factor 8 (*FGF8*) mutation was identified, suggesting a role of FGF8 in pituitary and forebrain development.[71]

X-linked Familial Neurohypophyseal Diabetes Insipidus

There are some reports of X-linked neurohypophyseal diabetes insipidus, with no known genetic mutations. A report describes 4 male patients from 1 kindred with a young age of manifestation (<1 year), decreased basal and stimulated AVP, and remission on standard doses of dDAVP. No *AVP* gene mutations were detected; reduction or absence of the posterior pituitary bright spot in these patients could indicate posterior pituitary degeneration similar to autosomal dominant familial neurohypophyseal diabetes insipidus.[72,73]

NEPHROGENIC DIABETES INSIPIDUS

Genetic causes of nephrogenic diabetes insipidus are inactivating mutations of *AVPR2* (90% of congenital nephrogenic diabetes insipidus) and *AQP2* (10% of congenital nephrogenic diabetes insipidus) and a resulting insensitivity of the distal nephron to AVP, causing impaired water reabsorption.[1] Mutations in *AVPR2* (OMIM*300538) lead to X-linked nephrogenic diabetes insipidus (OMIM#304800); *AQP2* (OMIM*107777) mutations mostly cause autosomal recessive nephrogenic diabetes insipidus (OMIM#125800), with some cases of autosomal dominant nephrogenic diabetes insipidus. Almost all described cases of congenital nephrogenic diabetes insipidus can be attributed to mutations in 1 of those 2 genes.[1]

Standard treatment consists of symptomatic relief by reducing dietary sodium intake and ensuring replacement of urinary fluid losses, inhibition of tubular sodium reabsorption by thiazide diuretics, and the administration of a prostaglandin synthetase inhibitor, most often indomethacin.[1,29,74–76] Addition of the potassium-sparing diuretic amiloride further reduces urine volume when added to hydrochlorothiazide.[29,77] Generally, these treatments reduce urine volume by approximately 30% to 70%.[78]

Therapeutically, there is a spectrum of AVP resistance in these patients; although most patients do not respond to AVP, some mutations confer only partial AVP resistance that may be overcome by physiologic or supraphysiologic dDAVP doses.[43,79] Although this may not significantly alter symptoms during basal conditions and with free access to fluids, it can improve responses during episodes of dehydration.

Depending on the disease mechanism, novel targeted therapeutic strategies are currently being developed; they are described in detail later.

X-linked Nephrogenic Diabetes Insipidus

The incidence of X-linked nephrogenic diabetes insipidus was estimated to be approximately 450,000 in 8.8 million male live births (in the province of Quebec,

Canada).[1] AVPR2 is a 371 amino acid, 7 transmembrane–spanning protein belonging to the rhodopsin family, which is encoded on Xq28. Mutations in *AVPR2* are associated with X-linked nephrogenic diabetes insipidus, consequently a majority of patients are male.[80] Some female patients have been described; however, in most cases they exhibit a milder clinical phenotype of partial diabetes insipidus.[81] The variability in female clinical presentation is thought to be due to skewed X-chromosomal inactivation.[82,83] Some recurrent mutations have been identified, although most patients have individual mutations. More than 200 different *AVPR2* mutations have been described in more than 300 families.[84] Most mutations are missense mutations leading to the presence of misfolded AVPR2 retained in the ER.

AVPR2 is activated by the binding of AVP; this leads to the activation and release of $G_s\alpha$, which causes downstream apical translocation of AQP2 via PKA activation (see **Fig. 2** and discussed previously). Depending on their effect, 5 different classes of *AVPR2* mutations have been defined: (1) truncating mutations, promoter alterations, or splice site mutations, probably leading to nonsense-mediated decay and a lack of mRNA and protein expression; (2) missense mutation or indels without frameshift leading to fully translated proteins, which misfold and are retained in the ER, followed by proteasomal degradation; and finally, missense mutations or indels leading to fully translated and processed proteins (3) may fail to properly bind $G_s\alpha$, followed by reduced downstream PKA signaling after AVP binding, (4) may demonstrate reduced binding affinity for AVP by disturbances to the AVP binding pocket, or (5) may be misrouted to different cell organelles and be not or insufficiently expressed on the plasma membrane.[85] In cases of partial nephrogenic diabetes insipidus, often a combination of these effects is observed, where some AVPR2 is retained in the ER but the rest is expressed on the cell surface, where it may show defective AVP binding or defective coupling to PKA signaling.[85,86]

Although a large majority of AVPR2 mutations lead to complete diabetes insipidus, a few mutations were described that cause only a partial phenotype.[32,87–89] Described cases include mutations that lead to good AVPR2 cell surface expression but reduced AVP binding affinity.[88] Furthermore, in the case of splice site mutations, which often lead to nonsense-mediated decay, a small amount of correctly spliced transcript may compensate to some degree and also lead to a partial phenotype.[43]

Missense mutations, which cause different substitutions in the same residue, can have very different clinical consequences: AVPR2 p.Arg137His leads to nephrogenic diabetes insipidus whereas p.Arg137Cys and p.Arg137Leu cause constitutive AVPR2 activation and increased downstream cAMP signaling; this leads to the nephrogenic syndrome of inappropriate antidiuresis, which, analogous to the syndrome of inappropriate AVP secretion, is associated with hyponatremia and water retention.[90,91]

Onset of symptoms of X-linked nephrogenic diabetes insipidus (polyuria, increased thirst, and polydipsia and failure to thrive) is usually in early infancy.[92] Hyponatremia generally does not occur with free access to fluids but can become a problem during states of dehydration.[36]

Novel targeted therapeutic strategies are currently under development. Firstly, cell-permeable AVPR2 agonists or antagonists that could act as molecular chaperones are suggested to be able to prevent mutant AVPR2 misfolding and ER retention; this could lead to cell surface expression of the mutant receptors, which could then be activated by endogenous AVP. This strategy was tested in cell culture as well as in 1 small clinical trial.[93–96] The effects of this approach, however, have only been shown in few specific *AVPR2* missense mutations. Secondly, tubular AQP2 cell surface expression could be stimulated by receptors and signaling pathways other than AVPR2-PKA. In mouse and rat models for *AVPR2*-dependent nephrogenic diabetes insipidus, agonists of the prostaglandin EP2 and EP4 receptors were shown to increase AQP2 cell surface expression and ameliorate diabetes insipidus symptoms.[97,98] Secretin receptors agonists and phosphodiesterase inhibitors are also potential targets for the activation of alternative pathways to increase AQP2 surface expression.[99,100]

Aquaporin 2 Mutations in Nephrogenic Diabetes Insipidus

AQP2 encodes the water channel allowing AVP-stimulated water reabsorption from the renal distal tubule (discussed previously). AQP2 is a 271 amino acid protein, which is encoded on chromosome 12q13.[101] It consists of 6 transmembrane–spanning domains and a cytosolic C-terminus. Posttranslationally, AQP2 is folded and processed through the ER; it forms homotetramers, which are stored in subapical vesicles. Translocation and membrane expression of AQP2 from those vesicles after AVPR2 activation is achieved by C-terminal phosphorylation of AQP2 by the PKA at Ser256 (see **Fig. 2**).[16,102]

Homozygous or compound heterozygous loss-of-function mutations in *AQP2* lead to autosomal recessive nephrogenic diabetes insipidus[103,104]; some heterozygous *AQP2* mutations are described as leading to an autosomal dominant form (discussed later).

Autosomal recessive nephrogenic diabetes insipidus

Forty-seven families with 52 different mutations causing autosomal recessive nephrogenic diabetes insipidus have been described (**Table 4**). A majority of those are missense mutations located throughout the gene, which lead to AQP2 misfolding and retention in the ER, followed by proteasomal degradation. Even though molecular genetics show that at least some of those mutants form functional water channels, there is negligible cell surface expression leading to severe diabetes insipidus in most affected patients. Consequently, similarly to X-linked nephrogenic diabetes insipidus, the large majority of autosomal recessive nephrogenic diabetes insipidus leads to a complete phenotype. Some mutations, however, leading to some cell surface expression of AQP2 and partial responses to fluid deprivation and/or dDAVP have been described (see **Table 4**)[105–107]: the AQP2 p.Val168Met mutation allows a greater amount of cell surface expression of a partially functional channel; clinically the partial nephrogenic diabetes insipidus due to this mutation responded to dDAVP treatment by marginal increases in urine osmolality and decreased water intake.[106]

Two families with autosomal recessive nephrogenic diabetes insipidus and interesting compound heterozygous *AQP2* mutations were identified: the AQP2 p.Pro262-Leu mutation, whose location in the C-terminal tail is typical for autosomal dominant nephrogenic diabetes insipidus, fails to correctly localize to the cell surface only when coexpressed with another mutation causing ER retention (in these cases, p.Ala190Thr or p.Arg187Cys); however, when coexpressed with the wild type (such as in the healthy parent), the erroneous intracellular targeting is overridden by the wild-type protein and both correctly localize to the cell surface.[108]

Autosomal dominant nephrogenic diabetes insipidus

Currently, 11 mutations leading to autosomal dominant nephrogenic diabetes insipidus are known (**Table 5**). In the dominant form, mutations are located at the C-terminus of AQP2, which is important for intracellular trafficking and localization, in contrast to the recessive form where mutations are generally located between the first and last transmembrane domains (see **Table 5**). Some cases of autosomal dominant nephrogenic diabetes insipidus are due to missense mutations; all other mutations are small indels causing frameshifts and an extended C-terminal tail.

Table 4
Homozygous and compound heterozygous *AQP2* mutations, pathogenic mechanisms, and corresponding phenotypes in autosomal recessive nephrogenic diabetes insipidus

Mutation			Pathogenic Mechanism	Phenotype	Age at Onset	Urine Osmolality (mOsm/L)			Reference
cDNA Level	Protein Level	Mutation Type				Basal	After Fluid Deprivation	After dDAVP	
c.3G>T	p.M1I	Missense	NR	Complete	<6 mo	25	32	31	160
c.85G>A[a]	p.G29S	Missense							
c.64C>G	p.L22V	Missense	Reduced water permeability ER retention	Partial	From infancy	68	442	358	105
c.543C>G	p.C181W	Missense							
c.56C>T	p.A19V	Missense	NR	NR	NR	NR	NR	No response	160,161
c.85G>A[a]	p.G29S	Missense							
c.71T>C	p.V24A	Missense	Intracellular retention	NR	NR	106	NR	NR	162
c.559C>T[a]	p.R187C	Missense	Inadequate PKA-dependent activation						163
c.83T>C	p.L28P	Missense	ER retention	Complete	1 mo	89	NR	No response	164
c.127–128delCA[a]	p.Q43Rfs*63	Frameshift deletion	NR	Complete	1 mo	116	NR	78	165
c.323C>T	p.T108M	Missense							
c.127–128delCA[a]	p.Q43Rfs*63	Frameshift deletion	NR	Complete	<12 mo	100	125	<50	166
c.501–502insC	p.V168Rfs*30	Frameshift insertion							
c.127–128delCA[a]	p.Q43Rfs*63	Frameshift deletion	NR	Complete	2 mo	92	NR	No response	167
c.607-1G>A	NR	Splice site							
c.140C>T	p.A47V	Missense	ER retention	Complete	Early infancy	230	No response	189	164,168

(continued on next page)

Table 4
(continued)

| Mutation | | | | | | Urine Osmolality (mOsm/L) | | | |
cDNA Level	Protein Level	Mutation Type	Pathogenic Mechanism	Phenotype	Age at Onset	Basal	After Fluid Deprivation	After dDAVP	Reference
c.170A>C	p.Q57P	Missense	Intracellular retention	Complete	1 mo	50	NR	No response	169
c.190G>A	p.G64R	Missense	ER retention	Complete	10 wk	56	NR	No response	162,170
c.203A>G	p.N68S	Missense	ER retention	Partial	<6 wk	82	236	450	171
c.209C>A	p.A70D	Missense	NR	Complete	<1 mo	92	87	149	172
c.560G>A	p.R187H	Missense							
c.211G>A	p.V71M	Missense	ER retention	Complete	NR	96	NR	91	164,168
c.253C>T	p.R85*	Nonsense	NR	Complete	2 mo	103	NR	106	173,174
c.257C>T	p.A86V	Missense	NR	NR	NR	51	NR	NR	175
c.287G>A	p.G96E	Missense	NR	Complete	<6 mo	61	66	61	176
c.298G>A	p.G100R	Missense	NR	NR	NR	NR	NR	NR	177
c.298G>T	p.G100*	Nonsense	NR	Complete	Infancy	52	NR	81	178
c.299G>T	p.G100V	Missense	Intracellular retention	Complete	2 mo	50	NR	No response	169
c.320T>A	p.I107N	Missense	NR	Complete	<7 wk	79	NR	No response	179
c.360+3G>A	NR	Splice site	NR	Complete	12 d	337	NR	No response	180
c.369delC	p.N123Lfs*131	Frameshift deletion	NR	Complete	6 wk	NR	150	No response	162
c.374C>T	p.T125M	Missense	Impaired AQP2 water permeability	Complete	4 d	121	No response	No response	181
c.523G>A	p.G175R	Missense							
c.377C>T	p.T126M	Missense	ER retention	Complete	<5 mo	173	NR	No response	171
c.389C>T	p.A130V	Missense	NR	NR	NR	NR	NR	NR	182
c.410T>G	p.L137P	Missense	NR	Complete	NR	89	NR	NR	183
c.439G>A	p.A147T	Missense	ER retention	Complete	<3 mo	50	No response	No response	171

c.450T>A[a]	p.D150E	Missense	Reduced water permeability	Partial	Infancy	160	NR	614	107
c.450T>A[a]	p.D150E	Missense	Reduced water permeability	Complete	NR	77	NR	No response	107
c.587G>A	p.G196D	Missense	Intracellular retention						
c.450T>A[a] c.643G>T	p.D150E p.G215C	Missense Missense	ER retention	Partial	<9 mo	80	202	252	184
c.502G>A[a]	p.V168M	Missense	ER retention	Partial	Birth	76	185	216	106
c.502G>A[a] c.646T>C[a]	p.V168M p.S216P	Missense Missense	ER retention	Complete	3 mo	60	NR	153	106,173
c.526-1G>A	NR	Splice site		NR	NR	NR	NR	NR	185
c.538G>A	p.G180S	Missense		NR	NR	NR	NR	NR	177
c.550A>C	p.N184H	Missense		NR	NR	NR	NR	NR	182
c.553C>G	p.P185A	Missense	ER retention	Complete	5 d	150	NR	150	164
c.559C>T[a]	p.R187C	Missense	ER retention	Complete	<2 wk	NR	No response	No response	162,170
c.559C>T[a] c.646T>C[a]	p.R187C p.S216P	Missense Missense	ER retention	NR	NR	NR	NR	NR	18 186
c.559C>T[a]	p.R187C	Missense	Intracellular retention	NR	<4 mo	NR	283	NR	163
c.682A>G	p.K228E	Missense	Inadequate PKA-dependent activation						
c.559C>T[a] c.785C>T[a]	p.R187C p.P262L	Missense Missense	ER retention Intracellular retention (rescued by coexpression with wild type)	Complete	Birth	<150	NR	NR	162 108

(continued on next page)

Table 4
(continued)

| Mutation | | Mutation Type | Pathogenic Mechanism | Phenotype | Age at Onset | Urine Osmolality (mOsm/L) | | | Reference |
cDNA Level	Protein Level					Basal	After Fluid Deprivation	After dDAVP	
c.568G>A	p.A190T	Missense	ER retention	Complete	Birth	NR	NR	NR	108
c.785C>T[a]	p.P262L	Missense	Intracellular retention (rescued by coexpression with wild type)						
c.601C>T	p.H201Y	Missense	NR	Complete	2 mo	NR	263	300	187
c.631G>C	p.G211R	Missense							
c.606G>T	p.W202C	Missense Possible splice site	NR	Complete	4 wk	NR	NR	<180	188
c.580G>A, c.652delC	p.V194I, p.L218Sfs*236	Missense and frameshift deletion	NR	Complete	1 wk	80	NR	80	164
c.606+1G>A	NR	Splice site							
c.643G>A	p.G215S	Missense	NR	NR	4 mo	157	NR	NR	166
c.647C>T[a]	p.S216F	Missense	NR	Complete	Infancy	58	66	76	189

Patients are homozygous for 1 mutation where only 1 mutation is mentioned; they are compound heterozygous where 2 mutations are stated.
Reference sequence NM_000486.
Abbreviation: NR, not reported.
[a] Same mutation reported in different allelic constellations (homozygous/compound heterozygous).

Table 5
AQP2 mutations, pathogenic mechanisms, and corresponding phenotypes in autosomal dominant nephrogenic diabetes insipidus

| Mutation | | | Pathogenic Mechanism | Phenotype | Age at Onset | Urine Osmolality (mOsm/L) | | | Reference |
| | | | | | | | After Fluid | | |
cDNA Level	Protein Level	Mutation Type				Basal	Deprivation	After dDAVP	
c.721delG	p.E241Sfs*333	Frameshift deletion	Impaired trafficking	Partial	12 mo	91	333	NR	190
c.727delG	p.D243Tfs*333	Frameshift deletion	Misrouting to late endosomes/lysosomes	Complete	NR	116	NR	104	111
c.750delG	p.V251Cfs*334	Frameshift deletion	NR	Complete	NR	NR	NR	No response	161
c.760C>T	p.R254W	Missense	Impaired PKA phosphorylation	Partial	9 mo	32	268	NR	117
c.761G>A	p.R254Q	Missense	Impaired PKA phosphorylation	Partial	18 mo	58	220	258	116
c.761G>T	p.R254L	Missense	Impaired PKA phosphorylation	Partial	<12 mo	NR	452[a]	NR	115
c.763–772del	p.Q255Sfs*330	Frameshift deletion	Impaired trafficking	NR	3 y	NR	120	NR	190
c.772G>A	p.E258K	Missense	Golgi retention	Partial	Birth	100	NR	350	110
c.775delC	p.L259Cfs*334	Frameshift deletion	NR	NR	NR	NR	NR	NR	161
c.779–780insA	p.H260Qfs*285	Frameshift insertion	Misrouting to basolateral membrane	Complete	Birth	<200	NR	NR	112
c.812–818del	p.A270Gfs*331	Frameshift deletion	Impaired trafficking	Partial	16 mo	177	468	551	190

Reference sequence NM_000486.
Abbreviation: NR, not reported.
[a] After 2.5% NaCl infusion.

Mutant AQP2 is initially correctly folded and not retained in the ER; instead, in most mutations causing autosomal dominant nephrogenic diabetes insipidus, mutant AQP2 is intracellularly misrouted and not expressed on the apical surface. AQP2 normally forms homotetramers during trafficking (see **Fig. 2**); in cases of autosomal dominant AQP2 mutations, mutant AQP2 acts in a dominant-negative fashion and heterotetramerizes with wild-type AQP2, which is followed by misrouting of the heterotetramers, thereby preventing the correct trafficking of both wild-type and mutant proteins to the cell surface.[109,110] This aberrant trafficking leads to retention in specific subcellular compartments, including the Golgi complex, late endosomes/lysosomes, or the basolateral membrane in polarized cells.[109–113] Depending on the mutation, however, presumably a small amount of wild-type–only tetramers does form, enabling a small amount of correct AQP2 apical membrane expression; in cases of AQP2 mutations interfering with C-terminal phosphorylation, a minimum of 3 correctly phosphorylated monomers per tetramer were shown to be necessary. Furthermore, the abnormally elevated AVP levels, such as during chronic dehydration, stimulate an increased basal expression of AQP2, which is in agreement with the mild phenotype observed.[36,102,114]

An additional pathogenic mechanism for autosomal dominant nephrogenic diabetes insipidus was identified for the AQP2 p.Arg254Leu, the p.Arg254Gln, and the p.Arg254Trp mutations: Ser256 is normally phosphorylated by the PKA downstream of AVPR2 activation, which stimulates AQP2 cell membrane translocation. In the mutants, this phosphorylation is prevented and the channels are retained in intracellular vesicles.[115–117]

Clinically, autosomal dominant nephrogenic diabetes insipidus often leads to a later disease manifestation than autosomal recessive or X-linked nephrogenic diabetes insipidus, with appearance of polyuria and polydipsia in the second half of the first year or later; patients generally demonstrate a milder phenotype with higher urinary osmolality during fluid deprivation and some response to dDAVP (see **Table 5**).

SUMMARY

This report reviews the genetic causes of central diabetes insipidus and nephrogenic diabetes insipidus in the context of their diagnosis and treatment. After the identification of the first pathogenic mutations in congenital diabetes insipidus in the early 1990s, the research into the contributions of AVP, AVPR2, and AQP2 mutations in the pathophysiology of diabetes insipidus have immensely contributed to the understanding of this disease as well as to the normal physiology of the posterior pituitary-distal tubule axis. Diagnostic challenges can be optimized by an understanding of the distinct phenotypes conferred by different diabetes insipidus–causing mutations. Furthermore, these recent developments have enabled the development of novel rational therapeutic strategies for nephrogenic diabetes insipidus, for which there is currently only partial symptomatic treatment available.

Future challenges in familial forms of diabetes insipidus include the identification of the yet unknown gene causing X-linked familial neurohypophyseal diabetes insipidus, the preclinical and clinical development of novel rational therapies for X-linked nephrogenic diabetes insipidus, and the investigation of strategies preventing or delaying neuronal degeneration in early stages of familial neurohypophyseal diabetes insipidus.

REFERENCES

1. Bockenhauer D, Bichet DG. Pathophysiology, diagnosis and management of nephrogenic diabetes insipidus. Nat Rev Nephrol 2015;11(10):576–88.

2. Land H, Schutz G, Schmale H, et al. Nucleotide sequence of cloned cDNA encoding bovine arginine vasopressin-neurophysin II precursor. Nature 1982; 295(5847):299–303.
3. Land H, Grez M, Ruppert S, et al. Deduced amino acid sequence from the bovine oxytocin-neurophysin I precursor cDNA. Nature 1983;302(5906):342–4.
4. Burbach JP, Luckman SM, Murphy D, et al. Gene regulation in the magnocellular hypothalamo-neurohypophysial system. Physiol Rev 2001;81(3):1197–267.
5. Brownstein MJ, Russell JT, Gainer H. Synthesis, transport, and release of posterior pituitary hormones. Science 1980;207(4429):373–8.
6. Acher R, Chauvet J, Rouille Y. Dynamic processing of neuropeptides: sequential conformation shaping of neurohypophysial preprohormones during intraneuronal secretory transport. J Mol Neurosci 2002;18(3):223–8.
7. Brownstein MJ. Biosynthesis of vasopressin and oxytocin. Annu Rev Physiol 1983;45:129–35.
8. de Bree FM, Burbach JP. Structure-function relationships of the vasopressin prohormone domains. Cell Mol Neurobiol 1998;18(2):173–91.
9. Robertson GL. Physiology of ADH secretion. Kidney Int Suppl 1987;21:S20–6.
10. Bourque CW, Oliet SH. Osmoreceptors in the central nervous system. Annu Rev Physiol 1997;59:601–19.
11. Gutkowska J, Antunes-Rodrigues J, McCann SM. Atrial natriuretic peptide in brain and pituitary gland. Physiol Rev 1997;77(2):465–515.
12. Schrier RW, Berl T, Anderson RJ. Osmotic and nonosmotic control of vasopressin release. Am J Physiol 1979;236(4):F321–32.
13. Birnbaumer M, Seibold A, Gilbert S, et al. Molecular cloning of the receptor for human antidiuretic hormone. Nature 1992;357(6376):333–5.
14. Nonoguchi H, Owada A, Kobayashi N, et al. Immunohistochemical localization of V2 vasopressin receptor along the nephron and functional role of luminal V2 receptor in terminal inner medullary collecting ducts. J Clin Invest 1995; 96(4):1768–78.
15. Nielsen S, Frokiaer J, Marples D, et al. Aquaporins in the kidney: from molecules to medicine. Physiol Rev 2002;82(1):205–44.
16. Fushimi K, Sasaki S, Marumo F. Phosphorylation of serine 256 is required for cAMP-dependent regulatory exocytosis of the aquaporin-2 water channel. J Biol Chem 1997;272(23):14800–4.
17. Sasaki S, Fushimi K, Saito H, et al. Cloning, characterization, and chromosomal mapping of human aquaporin of collecting duct. J Clin Invest 1994;93(3): 1250–6.
18. Deen PM, Verdijk MA, Knoers NV, et al. Requirement of human renal water channel aquaporin-2 for vasopressin-dependent concentration of urine. Science 1994;264(5155):92–5.
19. Ward DT, Hammond TG, Harris HW. Modulation of vasopressin-elicited water transport by trafficking of aquaporin2-containing vesicles. Annu Rev Physiol 1999;61:683–97.
20. Moeller HB, Fuglsang CH, Fenton RA. Renal aquaporins and water balance disorders. Best Pract Res Clin Endocrinol Metab 2016;30(2):277–88.
21. Gilbert ML, Yang L, Su T, et al. Expression of a dominant negative PKA mutation in the kidney elicits a diabetes insipidus phenotype. Am J Physiol Renal Physiol 2015;308(6):F627–38.
22. Bankir L, Fernandes S, Bardoux P, et al. Vasopressin-V2 receptor stimulation reduces sodium excretion in healthy humans. J Am Soc Nephrol 2005;16(7): 1920–8.

23. Ecelbarger CA, Kim GH, Terris J, et al. Vasopressin-mediated regulation of epithelial sodium channel abundance in rat kidney. Am J Physiol Renal Physiol 2000;279(1):F46–53.

24. Zhang C, Sands JM, Klein JD. Vasopressin rapidly increases phosphorylation of UT-A1 urea transporter in rat IMCDs through PKA. Am J Physiol Renal Physiol 2002;282(1):F85–90.

25. Sands JM, Nonoguchi H, Knepper MA. Vasopressin effects on urea and H2O transport in inner medullary collecting duct subsegments. Am J Physiol 1987; 253(5 Pt 2):F823–32.

26. Yasui M, Zelenin SM, Celsi G, et al. Adenylate cyclase-coupled vasopressin receptor activates AQP2 promoter via a dual effect on CRE and AP1 elements. Am J Physiol 1997;272(4 Pt 2):F443–50.

27. Baylis PH. Osmoregulation and control of vasopressin secretion in healthy humans. Am J Physiol 1987;253(5 Pt 2):R671–8.

28. Di Iorgi N, Napoli F, Allegri AE, et al. Diabetes insipidus–diagnosis and management. Horm Res Paediatr 2012;77(2):69–84.

29. Robertson GL. Diabetes insipidus: Differential diagnosis and management. Best Pract Res Clin Endocrinol Metab 2016;30(2):205–18.

30. Maghnie M, Villa A, Arico M, et al. Correlation between magnetic resonance imaging of posterior pituitary and neurohypophyseal function in children with diabetes insipidus. J Clin Endocrinol Metab 1992;74(4):795–800.

31. Fujisawa I. Magnetic resonance imaging of the hypothalamic-neurohypophyseal system. J Neuroendocrinol 2004;16(4):297–302.

32. Faerch M, Christensen JH, Corydon TJ, et al. Partial nephrogenic diabetes insipidus caused by a novel mutation in the AVPR2 gene. Clin Endocrinol 2008; 68(3):395–403.

33. Christ-Crain M, Fenske W. Copeptin in the diagnosis of vasopressin-dependent disorders of fluid homeostasis. Nat Rev Endocrinol 2016;12(3):168–76.

34. Saito T, Ishikawa SE, Sasaki S, et al. Urinary excretion of aquaporin-2 in the diagnosis of central diabetes insipidus. J Clin Endocrinol Metab 1997;82(6): 1823–7.

35. Elias PC, Elias LL, Torres N, et al. Progressive decline of vasopressin secretion in familial autosomal dominant neurohypophyseal diabetes insipidus presenting a novel mutation in the vasopressin-neurophysin II gene. Clin Endocrinol 2003; 59(4):511–8.

36. Babey M, Kopp P, Robertson GL. Familial forms of diabetes insipidus: clinical and molecular characteristics. Nat Rev Endocrinol 2011;7(12):701–14.

37. Repaske DR, Medlej R, Gultekin EK, et al. Heterogeneity in clinical manifestation of autosomal dominant neurohypophyseal diabetes insipidus caused by a mutation encoding Ala-1–>Val in the signal peptide of the arginine vasopressin/ neurophysin II/copeptin precursor. J Clin Endocrinol Metab 1997;82(1):51–6.

38. Jendle J, Christensen JH, Kvistgaard H, et al. Late-onset familial neurohypophyseal diabetes insipidus due to a novel mutation in the AVP gene. Clin Endocrinol 2012;77(4):586–92.

39. Bourdet K, Vallette S, Deladoey J, et al. Early-onset central diabetes insipidus due to compound heterozygosity for AVP mutations. Horm Res Paediatr 2016; 85(4):283–7.

40. Heppner C, Kotzka J, Bullmann C, et al. Identification of mutations of the arginine vasopressin-neurophysin II gene in two kindreds with familial central diabetes insipidus. J Clin Endocrinol Metab 1998;83(2):693–6.

41. McLeod JF, Kovacs L, Gaskill MB, et al. Familial neurohypophyseal diabetes insipidus associated with a signal peptide mutation. J Clin Endocrinol Metab 1993;77(3). 599A–599G.
42. Rutishauser J, Spiess M, Kopp P. Genetic forms of neurohypophyseal diabetes insipidus. Best Pract Res Clin Endocrinol Metab 2016;30(2):249–62.
43. Schernthaner-Reiter MH, Adams D, Trivellin G, et al. A novel AVPR2 splice site mutation leads to partial X-linked nephrogenic diabetes insipidus in two brothers. Eur J Pediatr 2016;175(5):727–33.
44. Miyamoto S, Sasaki N, Tanabe Y. Magnetic resonance imaging in familial central diabetes insipidus. Neuroradiology 1991;33(3):272–3.
45. Rutishauser J, Boni-Schnetzler M, Boni J, et al. A novel point mutation in the translation initiation codon of the pre-pro-vasopressin-neurophysin II gene: co-segregation with morphological abnormalities and clinical symptoms in autosomal dominant neurohypophyseal diabetes insipidus. J Clin Endocrinol Metab 1996;81(1):192–8.
46. Robinson AG. DDAVP in the treatment of central diabetes insipidus. N Engl J Med 1976;294(10):507–11.
47. Repaske DR, Phillips JA 3rd, Kirby LT, et al. Molecular analysis of autosomal dominant neurohypophyseal diabetes insipidus. J Clin Endocrinol Metab 1990;70(3):752–7.
48. Sausville E, Carney D, Battey J. The human vasopressin gene is linked to the oxytocin gene and is selectively expressed in a cultured lung cancer cell line. J Biol Chem 1985;260(18):10236–41.
49. Siggaard C, Christensen JH, Corydon TJ, et al. Expression of three different mutations in the arginine vasopressin gene suggests genotype-phenotype correlation in familial neurohypophyseal diabetes insipidus kindreds. Clin Endocrinol 2005;63(2):207–16.
50. Birk J, Friberg MA, Prescianotto-Baschong C, et al. Dominant pro-vasopressin mutants that cause diabetes insipidus form disulfide-linked fibrillar aggregates in the endoplasmic reticulum. J Cell Sci 2009;122(Pt 21):3994–4002.
51. Russell TA, Ito M, Ito M, et al. A murine model of autosomal dominant neurohypophyseal diabetes insipidus reveals progressive loss of vasopressin-producing neurons. J Clin Invest 2003;112(11):1697–706.
52. Ito M, Jameson JL, Ito M. Molecular basis of autosomal dominant neurohypophyseal diabetes insipidus. Cellular toxicity caused by the accumulation of mutant vasopressin precursors within the endoplasmic reticulum. J Clin Invest 1997;99(8):1897–905.
53. Hagiwara D, Arima H, Morishita Y, et al. Arginine vasopressin neuronal loss results from autophagy-associated cell death in a mouse model for familial neurohypophysial diabetes insipidus. Cell Death Dis 2014;5:e1148.
54. Arima H, Oiso Y. Mechanisms underlying progressive polyuria in familial neurohypophysial diabetes insipidus. J Neuroendocrinol 2010;22(7):754–7.
55. Bergeron C, Kovacs K, Ezrin C, et al. Hereditary diabetes insipidus: an immunohistochemical study of the hypothalamus and pituitary gland. Acta Neuropathol 1991;81(3):345–8.
56. Braverman LE, Mancini JP, McGoldrick DM. hereditary idiopathic diabetes insipidus. A case report with autopsy findings. Ann Intern Med 1965;63:503–8.
57. Ito M, Yu RN, Jameson JL. Mutant vasopressin precursors that cause autosomal dominant neurohypophyseal diabetes insipidus retain dimerization and impair the secretion of wild-type proteins. J Biol Chem 1999;274(13):9029–37.

58. Hiroi M, Morishita Y, Hayashi M, et al. Activation of vasopressin neurons leads to phenotype progression in a mouse model for familial neurohypophysial diabetes insipidus. Am J Physiol Regul Integr Comp Physiol 2010;298(2):R486–93.

59. Willcutts MD, Felner E, White PC. Autosomal recessive familial neurohypophyseal diabetes insipidus with continued secretion of mutant weakly active vasopressin. Hum Mol Genet 1999;8(7):1303–7.

60. Abu Libdeh A, Levy-Khademi F, Abdulhadi-Atwan M, et al. Autosomal recessive familial neurohypophyseal diabetes insipidus: onset in early infancy. Eur J Endocrinol 2010;162(2):221–6.

61. Christensen JH, Kvistgaard H, Knudsen J, et al. A novel deletion partly removing the AVP gene causes autosomal recessive inheritance of early-onset neurohypophyseal diabetes insipidus. Clin Genet 2013;83(1):44–52.

62. Barrett TG, Bundey SE, Macleod AF. Neurodegeneration and diabetes: UK nationwide study of Wolfram (DIDMOAD) syndrome. Lancet 1995;346(8988): 1458–63.

63. Strom TM, Hortnagel K, Hofmann S, et al. Diabetes insipidus, diabetes mellitus, optic atrophy and deafness (DIDMOAD) caused by mutations in a novel gene (wolframin) coding for a predicted transmembrane protein. Hum Mol Genet 1998;7(13):2021–8.

64. Osman AA, Saito M, Makepeace C, et al. Wolframln expression induces novel ion channel activity in endoplasmic reticulum membranes and increases intracellular calcium. J Biol Chem 2003;278(52):52755–62.

65. Thompson CJ, Charlton J, Walford S, et al. Vasopressin secretion in the DIDMOAD (Wolfram) syndrome. Q J Med 1989;71(264):333–45.

66. Perrotta S, Di Iorgi N, Ragione FD, et al. Early-onset central diabetes insipidus is associated with de novo arginine vasopressin-neurophysin II or Wolfram syndrome 1 gene mutations. Eur J Endocrinol 2015;172(4):461–72.

67. Elli FM, Ghirardello S, Giavoli C, et al. A new structural rearrangement associated to Wolfram syndrome in a child with a partial phenotype. Gene 2012; 509(1):168–72.

68. Fonseca SG, Fukuma M, Lipson KL, et al. WFS1 is a novel component of the unfolded protein response and maintains homeostasis of the endoplasmic reticulum in pancreatic beta-cells. J Biol Chem 2005;280(47):39609–15.

69. Gabreels BA, Swaab DF, de Kleijn DP, et al. The vasopressin precursor is not processed in the hypothalamus of Wolfram syndrome patients with diabetes insipidus: evidence for the involvement of PC2 and 7B2. J Clin Endocrinol Metab 1998;83(11):4026–33.

70. Frank GR, Fox J, Candela N, et al. Severe obesity and diabetes insipidus in a patient with PCSK1 deficiency. Mol Genet Metab 2013;110(1–2):191–4.

71. McCabe MJ, Gaston-Massuet C, Tziaferi V, et al. Novel FGF8 mutations associated with recessive holoprosencephaly, craniofacial defects, and hypothalamo-pituitary dysfunction. J Clin Endocrinol Metab 2011;96(10):E1709–18.

72. Habiby RL, Robertson GL, Kaplowitz PB, et al. A novel X-linked form of familial neurohypophyseal diabetes insipidus. Pediatr Res 1997;41:67.

73. Hansen LK, Rittig S, Robertson GL. Genetic basis of familial neurohypophyseal diabetes insipidus. Trends Endocrinol Metab 1997;8(9):363–72.

74. Havard CW. Thiazide-induced antidiuresis in diabetes insipidus. Proc R Soc Med 1965;58(12):1005–7.

75. Libber S, Harrison H, Spector D. Treatment of nephrogenic diabetes insipidus with prostaglandin synthesis inhibitors. J Pediatr 1986;108(2):305–11.

76. Monnens L, Jonkman A, Thomas C. Response to indomethacin and hydrochlorothiazide in nephrogenic diabetes insipidus. Clin Sci (Lond) 1984;66(6): 709–15.

77. Alon U, Chan JC. Hydrochlorothiazide-amiloride in the treatment of congenital nephrogenic diabetes insipidus. Am J Nephrol 1985;5(1):9–13.

78. Moeller HB, Rittig S, Fenton RA. Nephrogenic diabetes insipidus: essential insights into the molecular background and potential therapies for treatment. Endocr Rev 2013;34(2):278–301.

79. Postina R, Ufer E, Pfeiffer R, et al. Misfolded vasopressin V2 receptors caused by extracellular point mutations entail congential nephrogenic diabetes insipidus. Mol Cell Endocrinol 2000;164(1–2):31–9.

80. Rosenthal W, Seibold A, Antaramian A, et al. Molecular identification of the gene responsible for congenital nephrogenic diabetes insipidus. Nature 1992; 359(6392):233–5.

81. Demura M, Takeda Y, Yoneda T, et al. Surgical stress-induced transient nephrogenic diabetes insipidus (NDI) associated with decreased Vasopressin receptor2 (AVPR2) expression linked to nonsense-mediated mRNA decay and incomplete skewed X-inactivation in a female patient with a heterozygous AVPR2 mutation (c. 89-90 delAC). Clin Endocrinol 2004;60(6):773–5.

82. Satoh M, Ogikubo S, Yoshizawa-Ogasawara A. Correlation between clinical phenotypes and X-inactivation patterns in six female carriers with heterozygote vasopressin type 2 receptor gene mutations. Endocr J 2008;55(2):277–84.

83. Nomura Y, Onigata K, Nagashima T, et al. Detection of skewed X-inactivation in two female carriers of vasopressin type 2 receptor gene mutation. J Clin Endocrinol Metab 1997;82(10):3434–7.

84. Spanakis E, Milord E, Gragnoli C. AVPR2 variants and mutations in nephrogenic diabetes insipidus: review and missense mutation significance. J Cell Physiol 2008;217(3):605–17.

85. Robben JH, Knoers NV, Deen PM. Cell biological aspects of the vasopressin type-2 receptor and aquaporin 2 water channel in nephrogenic diabetes insipidus. Am J Physiol Renal Physiol 2006;291(2):F257–70.

86. Robben JH, Knoers NV, Deen PM. Characterization of vasopressin V2 receptor mutants in nephrogenic diabetes insipidus in a polarized cell model. Am J Physiol Renal Physiol 2005;289(2):F265–72.

87. Ala Y, Morin D, Mouillac B, et al. Functional studies of twelve mutant V2 vasopressin receptors related to nephrogenic diabetes insipidus: molecular basis of a mild clinical phenotype. J Am Soc Nephrol 1998;9(10):1861–72.

88. Inaba S, Hatakeyama H, Taniguchi N, et al. The property of a novel v2 receptor mutant in a patient with nephrogenic diabetes insipidus. J Clin Endocrinol Metab 2001;86(1):381–5.

89. Armstrong SP, Seeber RM, Ayoub MA, et al. Characterization of three vasopressin receptor 2 variants: an apparent polymorphism (V266A) and two loss-of-function mutations (R181C and M311V). PLoS One 2013;8(6):e65885.

90. Rochdi MD, Vargas GA, Carpentier E, et al. Functional characterization of vasopressin type 2 receptor substitutions (R137H/C/L) leading to nephrogenic diabetes insipidus and nephrogenic syndrome of inappropriate antidiuresis: implications for treatments. Mol Pharmacol 2010;77(5):836–45.

91. Feldman BJ, Rosenthal SM, Vargas GA, et al. Nephrogenic syndrome of inappropriate antidiuresis. N Engl J Med 2005;352(18):1884–90.

92. van Lieburg AF, Knoers NV, Monnens LA. Clinical presentation and follow-up of 30 patients with congenital nephrogenic diabetes insipidus. J Am Soc Nephrol 1999;10(9):1958–64.

93. Morello JP, Salahpour A, Laperriere A, et al. Pharmacological chaperones rescue cell-surface expression and function of misfolded V2 vasopressin receptor mutants. J Clin Invest 2000;105(7):887–95.

94. Oueslati M, Hermosilla R, Schonenberger E, et al. Rescue of a nephrogenic diabetes insipidus-causing vasopressin V2 receptor mutant by cell-penetrating peptides. J Biol Chem 2007;282(28):20676–85.

95. Cheong HI, Cho HY, Park HW, et al. Molecular genetic study of congenital nephrogenic diabetes insipidus and rescue of mutant vasopressin V2 receptor by chemical chaperones. Nephrology (Carlton) 2007;12(2):113–7.

96. Bernier V, Morello JP, Zarruk A, et al. Pharmacologic chaperones as a potential treatment for X-linked nephrogenic diabetes insipidus. J Am Soc Nephrol 2006; 17(1):232–43.

97. Li JH, Chou CL, Li B, et al. A selective EP4 PGE2 receptor agonist alleviates disease in a new mouse model of X-linked nephrogenic diabetes insipidus. J Clin Invest 2009;119(10):3115–26.

98. Olesen ET, Rutzler MR, Moeller HB, et al. Vasopressin-independent targeting of aquaporin-2 by selective E prostanoid receptor agonists alleviates nephrogenic diabetes insipidus. Proc Natl Acad Sci U S A 2011;108(31):12949–54.

99. Procino G, Milano S, Carmosino M, et al. Combination of secretin and fluvastatin ameliorates the polyuria associated with X-linked nephrogenic diabetes insipidus in mice. Kidney Int 2014;86(1):127–38.

100. Bouley R, Pastor-Soler N, Cohen O, et al. Stimulation of AQP2 membrane insertion in renal epithelial cells in vitro and in vivo by the cGMP phosphodiesterase inhibitor sildenafil citrate (Viagra). Am J Physiol Renal Physiol 2005;288(6): F1103–12.

101. Fushimi K, Uchida S, Hara Y, et al. Cloning and expression of apical membrane water channel of rat kidney collecting tubule. Nature 1993;361(6412):549–52.

102. Kamsteeg EJ, Heijnen I, van Os CH, et al. The subcellular localization of an aquaporin-2 tetramer depends on the stoichiometry of phosphorylated and non-phosphorylated monomers. J Cell Biol 2000;151(4):919–30.

103. Deen PM, Weghuis DO, Sinke RJ, et al. Assignment of the human gene for the water channel of renal collecting duct Aquaporin 2 (AQP2) to chromosome 12 region q12->q13. Cytogenet Cell Genet 1994;66(4):260–2.

104. Saito F, Sasaki S, Chepelinsky AB, et al. Human AQP2 and MIP genes, two members of the MIP family, map within chromosome band 12q13 on the basis of two-color FISH. Cytogenet Cell Genet 1995;68(1–2):45–8.

105. Canfield MC, Tamarappoo BK, Moses AM, et al. Identification and characterization of aquaporin-2 water channel mutations causing nephrogenic diabetes insipidus with partial vasopressin response. Hum Mol Genet 1997;6(11):1865–71.

106. Boccalandro C, De Mattia F, Guo DC, et al. Characterization of an aquaporin-2 water channel gene mutation causing partial nephrogenic diabetes insipidus in a Mexican family: evidence of increased frequency of the mutation in the town of origin. J Am Soc Nephrol 2004;15(5):1223–31.

107. Guyon C, Lussier Y, Bissonnette P, et al. Characterization of D150E and G196D aquaporin-2 mutations responsible for nephrogenic diabetes insipidus: importance of a mild phenotype. Am J Physiol Renal Physiol 2009;297(2):F489–98.

108. de Mattia F, Savelkoul PJ, Bichet DG, et al. A novel mechanism in recessive nephrogenic diabetes insipidus: wild-type aquaporin-2 rescues the apical

membrane expression of intracellularly retained AQP2-P262L. Hum Mol Genet 2004;13(24):3045–56.

109. Kamsteeg EJ, Wormhoudt TA, Rijss JP, et al. An impaired routing of wild-type aquaporin-2 after tetramerization with an aquaporin-2 mutant explains dominant nephrogenic diabetes insipidus. EMBO J 1999;18(9):2394–400.

110. Mulders SM, Bichet DG, Rijss JP, et al. An aquaporin-2 water channel mutant which causes autosomal dominant nephrogenic diabetes insipidus is retained in the Golgi complex. J Clin Invest 1998;102(1):57–66.

111. Marr N, Bichet DG, Lonergan M, et al. Heteroligomerization of an Aquaporin-2 mutant with wild-type Aquaporin-2 and their misrouting to late endosomes/lysosomes explains dominant nephrogenic diabetes insipidus. Hum Mol Genet 2002;11(7):779–89.

112. Kamsteeg EJ, Bichet DG, Konings IB, et al. Reversed polarized delivery of an aquaporin-2 mutant causes dominant nephrogenic diabetes insipidus. J Cell Biol 2003;163(5):1099–109.

113. Hirano K, Zuber C, Roth J, et al. The proteasome is involved in the degradation of different aquaporin-2 mutants causing nephrogenic diabetes insipidus. Am J Pathol 2003;163(1):111–20.

114. Nielsen S, DiGiovanni SR, Christensen EI, et al. Cellular and subcellular immunolocalization of vasopressin-regulated water channel in rat kidney. Proc Natl Acad Sci U S A 1993;90(24):11663–7.

115. de Mattia F, Savelkoul PJ, Kamsteeg EJ, et al. Lack of arginine vasopressin-induced phosphorylation of aquaporin-2 mutant AQP2-R254L explains dominant nephrogenic diabetes insipidus. J Am Soc Nephrol 2005;16(10):2872–80.

116. Savelkoul PJ, De Mattia F, Li Y, et al. p.R254Q mutation in the aquaporin-2 water channel causing dominant nephrogenic diabetes insipidus is due to a lack of arginine vasopressin-induced phosphorylation. Hum Mutat 2009;30(10): E891–903.

117. Dollerup P, Thomsen TM, Nejsum LN, et al. Partial nephrogenic diabetes insipidus caused by a novel AQP2 variation impairing trafficking of the aquaporin-2 water channel. BMC Nephrol 2015;16:217.

118. Ilhan M, Tiryakioglu NO, Karaman O, et al. A novel AVP gene mutation in a Turkish family with neurohypophyseal diabetes insipidus. J Endocrinol Invest 2016; 39(3):285–90.

119. Lindenthal V, Mainberger A, Morris-Rosendahl DJ, et al. Dilatative uropathy as a manifestation of neurohypophyseal diabetes insipidus due to a novel mutation in the arginine vasopressin-neurophysin-II gene. Klin Padiatr 2013;225(7):407–12.

120. Christensen JH, Siggaard C, Corydon TJ, et al. Six novel mutations in the arginine vasopressin gene in 15 kindreds with autosomal dominant familial neurohypophyseal diabetes insipidus give further insight into the pathogenesis. Eur J Hum Genet 2004;12(1):44–51.

121. Rittig S, Robertson GL, Siggaard C, et al. Identification of 13 new mutations in the vasopressin-neurophysin II gene in 17 kindreds with familial autosomal dominant neurohypophyseal diabetes insipidus. Am J Hum Genet 1996;58(1): 107–17.

122. Rittig S, Siggaard C, Ozata M, et al. Autosomal dominant neurohypophyseal diabetes insipidus due to substitution of histidine for tyrosine(2) in the vasopressin moiety of the hormone precursor. J Clin Endocrinol Metab 2002;87(7):3351–5.

123. Kobayashi H, Fujisawa I, Ikeda K, et al. A novel heterozygous missense mutation in the vasopressin moiety is identified in a Japanese person with neurohypophyseal diabetes insipidus. J Endocrinol Invest 2006;29(3):252–6.

124. Wahlstrom JT, Fowler MJ, Nicholson WE, et al. A novel mutation in the preprovasopressin gene identified in a kindred with autosomal dominant neurohypophyseal diabetes insipidus. J Clin Endocrinol Metab 2004;89(4):1963–8.

125. Brachet C, Birk J, Christophe C, et al. Growth retardation in untreated autosomal dominant familial neurohypophyseal diabetes insipidus caused by one recurring and two novel mutations in the vasopressin-neurophysin II gene. Eur J Endocrinol 2011;164(2):179–87.

126. Turkkahraman D, Saglar E, Karaduman T, et al. AVP-NPII gene mutations and clinical characteristics of the patients with autosomal dominant familial central diabetes insipidus. Pituitary 2015;18(6):898–904.

127. Bahnsen U, Oosting P, Swaab DF, et al. A missense mutation in the vasopressin-neurophysin precursor gene cosegregates with human autosomal dominant neurohypophyseal diabetes insipidus. EMBO J 1992;11(1):19–23.

128. Goking NQ, Chertow BS, Robertson GL, et al. Familial neurohypophyseal diabetes insipidus: a novel mutation presenting with enuresis. J Investig Med 1997;45:29a.

129. Calvo B, Bilbao JR, Rodriguez A, et al. Molecular analysis in familial neurohypophyseal diabetes insipidus: early diagnosis of an asymptomatic carrier. J Clin Endocrinol Metab 1999;84(9):3351–4.

130. Stephen MD, Fenwick RG, Brosnan PG. Polyuria and polydipsia in a young child: diagnostic considerations and identification of novel mutation causing familial neurohypophyseal diabetes insipidus. Pituitary 2012;15(Suppl 1):S1–5.

131. Gagliardi PC, Bernasconi S, Repaske DR. Autosomal dominant neurohypophyseal diabetes insipidus associated with a missense mutation encoding Gly23->Val in neurophysin II. J Clin Endocrinol Metab 1997;82(11):3643–6.

132. Repaske DR, Browning JE. A de novo mutation in the coding sequence for neurophysin-II (Pro24->Leu) is associated with onset and transmission of autosomal dominant neurohypophyseal diabetes insipidus. J Clin Endocrinol Metab 1994;79(2):421–7.

133. Wolf MT, Dotsch J, Metzler M, et al. A new missense mutation of the vasopressin-neurophysin II gene in a family with neurohypophyseal diabetes insipidus. Horm Res 2003;60(3):143–7.

134. Skordis N, Patsalis PC, Hettinger JA, et al. A novel arginine vasopressin-neurophysin II mutation causes autosomal dominant neurohypophyseal diabetes insipidus and morphologic pituitary changes. Horm Res 2000;53(5):239–45.

135. Flück CE, Deladoey J, Nayak S, et al. Autosomal dominant neurohypophyseal diabetes insipidus in a Swiss family, caused by a novel mutation (C59Delta/A60W) in the neurophysin moiety of prepro-vasopressin-neurophysin II (AVP-NP II). Eur J Endocrinol 2001;145(4):439–44.

136. Luo Y, Wang B, Qiu Y, et al. Clinical and molecular analysis of a Chinese family with autosomal dominant neurohypophyseal diabetes insipidus associated with a novel missense mutation in the vasopressin-neurophysin II gene. Endocrine 2012;42(1):208–13.

137. Abbes AP, Engel H, Bruggeman EJ, et al. Gene symbol: AVP. Disease: Diabetes insipidus, neurohypophyseal. Accession #Hm0558. Hum Genet 2006;118(6):783.

138. Deniz F, Acar C, Saglar E, et al. Identification of a novel deletion in AVP-NPII gene in a patient with central diabetes insipidus. Ann Clin Lab Sci 2015;45(5):588–92.

139. Pisareva E, Strebkova N, Tiulpakov A. Familial neurohypophyseal diabetes insipidus associated with a novel mutation in the arginine vasopressin (AVP) gene. Horm Res 2012;78(suppl. 1):305.

140. Yuasa H, Ito M, Nagasaki H, et al. Glu-47, which forms a salt bridge between neurophysin-II and arginine vasopressin, is deleted in patients with familial central diabetes insipidus. J Clin Endocrinol Metab 1993;77(3):600–4.

141. Miyakoshi M, Kamoi K, Murase T, et al. Novel mutant vasopressin-neurophysin II gene associated with familial neurohypophyseal diabetes insipidus. Endocr J 2004;51(6):551–6.

142. Grant FD, Ahmadi A, Hosley CM, et al. Two novel mutations of the vasopressin gene associated with familial diabetes insipidus and identification of an asymptomatic carrier infant. J Clin Endocrinol Metab 1998;83(11):3958–64.

143. Ito M, Mori Y, Oiso Y, et al. A single base substitution in the coding region for neurophysin II associated with familial central diabetes insipidus. J Clin Invest 1991;87(2):725–8.

144. Melo ME, Marui S, Brito VN, et al. Autosomal dominant familial neurohypophyseal diabetes insipidus caused by a novel mutation in arginine-vasopressin gene in a Brazilian family. Arq Bras Endocrinol Metabol 2008;52(8):1272–6.

145. Nagasaki H, Ito M, Yuasa H, et al. Two novel mutations in the coding region for neurophysin-II associated with familial central diabetes insipidus. J Clin Endocrinol Metab 1995;80(4):1352–6.

146. Ueta Y, Taniguchi S, Yoshida A, et al. A new type of familial central diabetes insipidus caused by a single base substitution in the neurophysin II coding region of the vasopressin gene. J Clin Endocrinol Metab 1996;81(5):1787–90.

147. Rutishauser J, Kopp P, Gaskill MB, et al. A novel mutation (R97C) in the neurophysin moiety of prepro-vasopressin-neurophysin II associated with autosomal-dominant neurohypophyseal diabetes insipidus. Mol Genet Metab 1999;67(1):89–92.

148. Mundschenk J, Rittig S, Siggaard C, et al. A new mutation of the arginine vasopressin-neurophysin II gene in a family with autosomal dominant neurohypophyseal diabetes insipidus. Exp Clin Endocrinol Diabetes 2001;109(8):406–9.

149. Baglioni S, Corona G, Maggi M, et al. Identification of a novel mutation in the arginine vasopressin-neurophysin II gene affecting the sixth intrachain disulfide bridge of the neurophysin II moiety. Eur J Endocrinol 2004;151(5):605–11.

150. DiMeglio LA, Gagliardi PC, Browning JE, et al. A missense mutation encoding cys(67)–> gly in neurophysin ii is associated with early onset autosomal dominant neurohypophyseal diabetes insipidus. Mol Genet Metab 2001;72(1):39–44.

151. Bruggeman EJ. Gene symbol: AVP. Disease: Diabetes Insipidus, neurohypophyseal. Hum Genet 2008;123(5):545.

152. Santiprabhob J, Browning J, Repaske D. A missense mutation encoding Cys73-Phe in neurophysin II is associated with autosomal dominant neurohypophyseal diabetes insipidus. Mol Genet Metab 2002;77(1–2):112–8.

153. Rutishauser J, Kopp P, Gaskill MB, et al. Clinical and molecular analysis of three families with autosomal dominant neurohypophyseal diabetes insipidus associated with a novel and recurrent mutations in the vasopressin-neurophysin II gene. Eur J Endocrinol 2002;146(5):649–56.

154. Fujii H, Iida S, Moriwaki K. Familial neurohypophyseal diabetes insipidus associated with a novel mutation in the vasopressin-neurophysin II gene. Int J Mol Med 2000;5(3):229–34.

155. de Fost M, van Trotsenburg AS, van Santen HM, et al. Familial neurohypophyseal diabetes insipidus due to a novel mutation in the arginine vasopressin-neurophysin II gene. Eur J Endocrinol 2011;165(1):161–5.

156. Tae HJ, Baek KH, Shim SM, et al. A novel splice site mutation of the arginine vasopressin-neurophysin II gene identified in a kindred with autosomal dominant familial neurohypophyseal diabetes insipidus. Mol Genet Metab 2005; 86(1–2):307–13.

157. Calvo B, Bilbao JR, Urrutia I, et al. Identification of a novel nonsense mutation and a missense substitution in the vasopressin-neurophysin II gene in two Spanish kindreds with familial neurohypophyseal diabetes insipidus. J Clin Endocrinol Metab 1998;83(3):995–7.

158. Bullmann C, Kotzka J, Grimm T, et al. Identification of a novel mutation in the arginine vasopressin-neurophysin II gene in familial central diabetes insipidus. Exp Clin Endocrinol Diabetes 2002;110(3):134–7.

159. Abbes AP, Bruggeman B, van Den Akker EL, et al. Identification of two distinct mutations at the same nucleotide position, concomitantly with a novel polymorphism in the vasopressin-neurophysin II gene (AVP-NP II) in two dutch families with familial neurohypophyseal diabetes insipidus. Clin Chem 2000;46(10): 1699–702.

160. Sahakitrungruang T, Wacharasindhu S, Sinthuwiwat T, et al. Identification of two novel aquaporin-2 mutations in a Thai girl with congenital nephrogenic diabetes insipidus. Endocrine 2008;33(2):210–4.

161. Sasaki S, Chiga M, Kikuchi E, et al. Hereditary nephrogenic diabetes insipidus in Japanese patients: analysis of 78 families and report of 22 new mutations in AVPR2 and AQP2. Clin Exp Nephrol 2013;17(3):338–44.

162. van Lieburg AF, Verdijk MA, Knoers VV, et al. Patients with autosomal nephrogenic diabetes insipidus homozygous for mutations in the aquaporin 2 water-channel gene. Am J Hum Genet 1994;55(4):648–52.

163. Leduc-Nadeau A, Lussier Y, Arthus MF, et al. New autosomal recessive mutations in aquaporin-2 causing nephrogenic diabetes insipidus through deficient targeting display normal expression in Xenopus oocytes. J Physiol 2010; 588(Pt 12):2205–18.

164. Marr N, Bichet DG, Hoefs S, et al. Cell-biologic and functional analyses of five new Aquaporin-2 missense mutations that cause recessive nephrogenic diabetes insipidus. J Am Soc Nephrol 2002;13(9):2267–77.

165. Park YJ, Baik HW, Cheong HI, et al. Congenital nephrogenic diabetes insipidus with a novel mutation in the aquaporin 2 gene. Biomed Rep 2014;2(4):596–8.

166. Cen J, Nie M, Duan L, et al. Novel autosomal recessive gene mutations in aquaporin-2 in two Chinese congenital nephrogenic diabetes insipidus pedigrees. Int J Clin Exp Med 2015;8(3):3629–39.

167. Tajima T, Okuhara K, Satoh K, et al. Two novel aquaporin-2 mutations in a sporadic Japanese patient with autosomal recessive nephrogenic diabetes insipidus. Endocr J 2003;50(4):473–6.

168. Muller D, Marr N, Ankermann T, et al. Desmopressin for nocturnal enuresis in nephrogenic diabetes insipidus. Lancet 2002;359(9305):495–7.

169. Lin SH, Bichet DG, Sasaki S, et al. Two novel aquaporin-2 mutations responsible for congenital nephrogenic diabetes insipidus in Chinese families. J Clin Endocrinol Metab 2002;87(6):2694–700.

170. Deen PM, Croes H, van Aubel RA, et al. Water channels encoded by mutant aquaporin-2 genes in nephrogenic diabetes insipidus are impaired in their cellular routing. J Clin Invest 1995;95(5):2291–6.

171. Mulders SM, Knoers NV, Van Lieburg AF, et al. New mutations in the AQP2 gene in nephrogenic diabetes insipidus resulting in functional but misrouted water channels. J Am Soc Nephrol 1997;8(2):242–8.

172. Cheong HI, Cho SJ, Zheng SH, et al. Two novel mutations in the aquaporin 2 gene in a girl with congenital nephrogenic diabetes insipidus. J Korean Med Sci 2005;20(6):1076–8.

173. Vargas-Poussou R, Forestier L, Dautzenberg MD, et al. Mutations in the vasopressin V2 receptor and aquaporin-2 genes in 12 families with congenital nephrogenic diabetes insipidus. J Am Soc Nephrol 1997;8(12):1855–62.

174. Bircan Z, Karacayir N, Cheong HI. A case of aquaporin 2 R85X mutation in a boy with congenital nephrogenic diabetes insipidus. Pediatr Nephrol 2008;23(4): 663–5.

175. Garcia Castano A, Perez de Nanclares G, Madariaga L, et al. Novel mutations associated with nephrogenic diabetes insipidus. A clinical-genetic study. Eur J Pediatr 2015;174(10):1373–85.

176. Rugpolmuang R, Deeb A, Hassan Y, et al. Novel AQP2 mutation causing congenital nephrogenic diabetes insipidus: challenges in management during infancy. J Pediatr Endocrinol Metab 2014;27(1–2):193–7.

177. Carroll P, Al-Mojalli H, Al-Abbad A, et al. Novel mutations underlying nephrogenic diabetes insipidus in Arab families. Genet Med 2006;8(7):443–7.

178. Hochberg Z, Van Lieburg A, Even L, et al. Autosomal recessive nephrogenic diabetes insipidus caused by an aquaporin-2 mutation. J Clin Endocrinol Metab 1997;82(2):686–9.

179. Zaki M, Schoneberg T, Al Ajrawi T, et al. Nephrogenic diabetes insipidus, thiazide treatment and renal cell carcinoma. Nephrol Dial Transplant 2006;21(4): 1082–6.

180. Bircan Z, Mutlu H, Cheong HI. Differential diagnosis of hereditary nephrogenic diabetes insipidus with desmopressin infusion test. Indian J Pediatr 2010; 77(11):1329–31.

181. Goji K, Kuwahara M, Gu Y, et al. Novel mutations in aquaporin-2 gene in female siblings with nephrogenic diabetes insipidus: evidence of disrupted water channel function. J Clin Endocrinol Metab 1998;83(9):3205–9.

182. Fujimoto M, Okada S, Kawashima Y, et al. Clinical overview of nephrogenic diabetes insipidus based on a nationwide survey in Japan. Yonago Acta Med 2014; 57(2):85–91.

183. Duzenli D, Saglar E, Deniz F, et al. Mutations in the AVPR2, AVP-NPII, and AQP2 genes in Turkish patients with diabetes insipidus. Endocrine 2012;42(3):664–9.

184. Iolascon A, Aglio V, Tamma G, et al. Characterization of two novel missense mutations in the AQP2 gene causing nephrogenic diabetes insipidus. Nephron Physiol 2007;105(3):p33–41.

185. Bichet DG, El Tarazi A, Matar J, et al. Aquaporin-2: new mutations responsible for autosomal-recessive nephrogenic diabetes insipidus-update and epidemiology. Clin Kidney J 2012;5(3):195–202.

186. Yamauchi K, Fushimi K, Yamashita Y, et al. Effects of missense mutations on rat aquaporin-2 in LLC-PK1 porcine kidney cells. Kidney Int 1999;56(1):164–71.

187. Liberatore Junior RD, Carneiro JG, Leidenz FB, et al. Novel compound aquaporin 2 mutations in nephrogenic diabetes insipidus. Clinics (Sao Paulo) 2012;67(1):79–82.

188. Oksche A, Moller A, Dickson J, et al. Two novel mutations in the aquaporin-2 and the vasopressin V2 receptor genes in patients with congenital nephrogenic diabetes insipidus. Hum Genet 1996;98(5):587–9.

189. Moon SS, Kim HJ, Choi YK, et al. Novel mutation of aquaporin-2 gene in a patient with congenital nephrogenic diabetes insipidus. Endocr J 2009;56(7): 905–10.

190. Kuwahara M, Iwai K, Ooeda T, et al. Three families with autosomal dominant nephrogenic diabetes insipidus caused by aquaporin-2 mutations in the C-terminus. Am J Hum Genet 2001;69(4):738–48.

Genetic Aspects of Pituitary Adenomas

Pedro Marques, MD, Márta Korbonits, MD, PhD*

KEYWORDS

- Pituitary tumor • Genetics • FIPA • AIP • XLAG • MEN1 • MEN4 • Carney complex

KEY POINTS

- Most pituitary adenomas are sporadic and histologically benign; nevertheless, they can cause significant burden due to hormonal hypersecretion and tumor mass effects.
- Both gene expression changes and genetic alterations, including germline (for example *MEN1* and *AIP* genes) or somatic (for example in *GNAS* or *USP8* genes) mutational events, can be identified in pituitary adenomas.
- Five percent of the pituitary adenomas arise in a familial setting occurring either isolated or as part of a syndrome.
- Isolated pituitary adenomas can be observed in *AIP* gene mutation-positive cases and in X-linked acrogigantism due to *GPR101* duplications, but in most familial isolated pituitary adenomas, the disease-causing mutations have not been identified.
- Syndromic presentations occur in MEN1, MEN4, Carney complex, McCune-Albright syndrome, and rarely, mutations in *DICER1* and *SDH* genes can also predispose to pituitary adenomas.

INTRODUCTION

Pituitary adenomas (PAs) are common monoclonal tumors arising from adenohypophysis cells.[1] PAs account for 15% of all intracranial tumors, being the third most common type of intracranial neoplasms, after meningiomas and gliomas.[2] The prevalence of PAs is remarkably high in autopsy and radiological studies, ranging from 14.4% to 22.5%,[2–4] although many correspond to lesions with no clinical relevance.[5,6] Clinically relevant PAs are significantly less common, with a prevalence varying from 1:1064 to 1:1470 in the general population.[7–11] PAs are usually benign, but they can cause significant burden to patients, due to excessive or low hormonal secretion and to tumor

Disclosure Statement: Dr P. Marques has nothing to disclose; Dr M. Korbonits had grant support from Pfizer, Ipsen, and Novartis.
Centre for Endocrinology, William Harvey Research Institute, Barts and the London School of Medicine and Dentistry, Queen Mary University of London, Charterhouse Square, London EC1M 6BQ, UK
* Corresponding author.
E-mail address: m.korbonits@qmul.ac.uk

mass effects, including compression and invasion of relevant surrounding structures. The most common PAs are prolactinomas (46.2%–66.2%), followed by nonfunctioning PAs (NFPAs) (14.7%–37%), somatotropinomas (9%–16.5%), corticotropinomas (1.58%–5.9%), and rarely, thyrotropinomas (0%–1.2%).[2,7–11]

Most PAs occur sporadically (95%). They have a lower level of somatic mutation rate compared with other tumors, but have altered expression profile of numerous pathways, including cell cycle proteins and growth factors, often due to epigenetic mechanisms.[12] Genetic alterations in sporadic PAs may include somatic mutations typically in oncogenes, due to point mutations, such as in the guanine nucleotide-activating α-subunit (GNAS) gene, leading to somatotropinomas, or in ubiquitin-specific protease 8 (USP8) gene in corticotropinomas,[1,13–15] or changes in gene copy number, such as in the phosphatidylinositol 3-kinase (PI3K) subunit p110α (PIK3CA).[16,17]

Five percent of PAs occur in a family setting, because of a genetic defect that predisposes to PA development, either isolated or as part of a syndrome (**Fig. 1**). Despite their relative rarity, hereditary PAs are important entities because they often present in younger patients, have a more aggressive course, and are more refractory to therapy.[18] Syndromic presentation occurs in multiple endocrine neoplasia type 1 (MEN1), MEN4, Carney complex (CNC), McCune-Albright syndrome (MAS), and, more rarely, in DICER1 and succinate dehydrogenase (SDH)-related syndromes. Isolated PAs can be observed in aryl hydrocarbon receptor interacting protein (AIP) mutation-positive cases, in X-linked acrogigantism (XLAG) syndrome due to GPR101 duplications and in AIP and GPR101-negative familial isolated PAs (FIPA). Although PRKAR1A,[19] DICER1,[20] and AIP[21] occur as germline mutations, GNAS mutations can occur in a mosaic or pituitary-specific somatic setting.[22,23] GPR101 mutations can be germline and mosaic,[24,25] and MEN1 and SDH mutations are primarily germline but a few somatic mutations have also been described.[26,27]

The aim of this article is to review the current knowledge regarding the genetics of PA, in both sporadic and familial PAs and in associated syndromes, from a genetic, molecular, and clinical point of view.

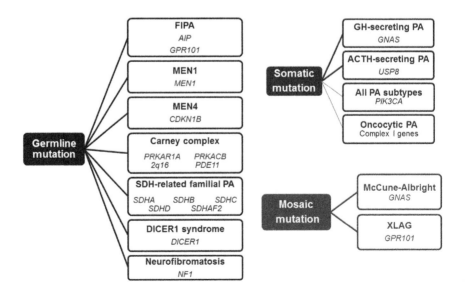

Fig. 1. Pituitary tumors due to genetic origin.

SPORADIC PITUITARY ADENOMAS

PAs are benign and monoclonal in origin, expanding from intrinsic molecular genetic abnormalities in a single somatic pituitary cell.[28] In early tumor clonality studies, namely X-chromosomal inactivation analysis, the monoclonal origin of growth hormone (GH), prolactin, and adrenocorticotropic hormone (ACTH)-secreting PAs and NFPAs was seen in female patients heterozygous for variant alleles of X-linked genes (hypoxanthine phosphoribosyl transferase and phosphoglycerate kinase). PAs have only one X-inactivation type, paternal or maternal, and never both.[28–33] PA monoclonality is also supported by other findings: pituitary tissue surrounding sporadic PAs normally has no features of hyperplasia although this can be seen in some genetic syndromes; complete surgical resection may result in long-term remission; activating or inactivating mutations in hypothalamic hormone receptors have not been reported.[1]

Acquired genetic or epigenetic changes likely confer an advantage to the modified cells, in terms of abnormal cell cycle activation, growth, and proliferation, allowing monoclonal expansion. In contrast, in some PAs with genetic origin, the presence of hyperplasia is well described. Hyperplasia has been commonly described in the context of CNC, MAS, and XLAG, and also in a few AIP cases.[21,25,34,35] Pituitary hyperplasia does not lead to tumor formation in the context of untreated primary hypothyroidism, hypogonadism, or congenital adrenal hyperplasia as well as in cases of ectopic corticotropin-releasing hormone or GH-releasing hormone (GHRH) secretion.[36,37]

Mutational Events

The first somatic mutation identified in sporadic PA is in the *GNAS* gene, which occurs in up to 40% of somatotropinomas. This somatic heterozygous mutation abolishes the GTP-ase activity of the G protein α-subunit, resulting in constitutional activation of adenylyl cyclase, with increased cyclic adenosine monophosphate (cAMP) levels and protein kinase A (PKA) activation. The phosphorylation of cAMP response element-binding protein leads to persistent GH hypersecretion and cell proliferation.[38–41]

A second common somatic mutation was found in the gene encoding USP8 in sporadic corticotropinomas.[14] *USP8* codes for a protein with deubiquitinase activity that inhibits the lysosomal degradation of epidermal growth factor receptor (EGFR). The mutations occur in a single domain of the protein, normally binding protein 14-3-3, which protects USP8 from cleavage to a more active shorter form. The mutations destroy the 14-3-3 binding site leading to increased USP8 cleavage with a more active shorter isoform and therefore gain-of-function. Excessive deubiquitination leads to increased recycling of EGFR to the cell surface, resulting in enhanced EGFR signaling and increased transcription of pro-opiomelanocortin (**Fig. 2**).[42,43] *USP8* mutations are the cause of Cushing disease in about one-third to two-thirds of these patients.[15,42,44,45] Patients with corticotropinomas positive for *USP8* mutations are more frequently women, diagnosed at a younger age, and they also tend to be smaller than *USP8* wild-type corticotropinomas.[14,15,44,45] Moreover, *USP8* mutated corticotropinomas are less associated with parasellar invasion in comparison to wild-type cases (12.7 vs 41.0%, respectively).[15] The degree of hypercortisolism appears to be similar in patients with or without *USP8* mutations.[15,45] In addition, the *USP8* mutational status in ACTH-secreting PAs may predict drug susceptibility, as the frequency of *USP8* mutations was found to be significantly higher in tumors expressing somatostatin receptor type 5 (SSTR5), suggesting more favorable responses to pasireotide.[45]

Single-nucleotide mutations or gene amplifications in the catalytic subunit of PI3K (*PIK3CA*) have been described in a significant percentage (30%) of all types of

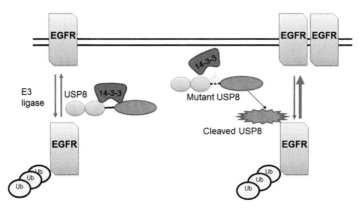

Fig. 2. USP8 and tumorigenesis in corticotropinomas. Normally there is a balance between EGFR ubiquitination—by an E3 ligase enzyme, leading to EGFR degradation, and deubiquitination—by USP8, leading to EGFR recycling. Mutation in the 14-3-3 binding domain of USP8 (represented here by yellow star) leads to inability of 14-3-3 protein binding; therefore, USP8 is cleaved, and the more active shortened protein leads to excessive deubiquitination and increased recycling of EGFR. This results in sustained EGFR activity, leading to ERK1/2 upregulation, enhanced transcription of pro-opiomelanocortin and ACTH, and increased cellular proliferation.

PAs,[16,17] and slightly more commonly in invasive adenomas, according to one of these studies.[16] The PI3K family of enzymes regulates cell proliferation, differentiation, motility, survival, and intracellular trafficking. PI3K is activated by several growth factor signaling pathways, whereas its key downstream effector AKT is known to be upregulated in PAs.[46] Interestingly, however, patients with germline mutation in the PTEN-PI3K-AKT pathway genes, representing Cowden syndrome, do not harbor PA.[47]

Mutations in classical tumor suppressor genes (TSG) such *TP53* and *RB1*, or in oncogenes such *HRAS* and *MYC*, are found rarely and exclusively in aggressive PAs or pituitary carcinomas.[16,18,48,49] In particular, *HRAS* mutations were found mostly in pituitary carcinomas, which has led to the suggestion that this must be important in malignant transformation rather than in initiation of PA.[2,48] On the other hand, less aggressive phenotypes can be found in oncocytic pituitary tumors. Mitochondrial DNA mutations in the components of the respiratory complex I in oncocytic PA lead to the disruption of this protein complex. Respiratory complex mutations have now been suggested to be a somatic modifier for pituitary tumorigenesis, which is associated with low genomic instability, explaining the less aggressive behavior of these adenomas.[50,51] Recently, a patient with Maffucci syndrome due to a commonly occurring mosaic mutation in the isocitrate dehydrogenase 1 (*IDH1*, p.R132C) was identified with a PA; further studies are needed to confirm if this was coincidental or whether the *IDH1* was causative in this case,[52] as a study on 246 PAs did not identify recurring *IDH1* p.R132H mutations.[53]

Gene Expression Changes

The factors that most commonly involved in pituitary tumorigenesis are cell cycle deregulation, altered signaling pathways, epigenetically silenced TSG or overexpressed oncogenes and growth factors, hormonal overstimulation, and an altered intrapituitary microenvironment.[1,29,54,55] The role of environmental factors has also been indicated,[56,57] but further data are needed in this field. Genes with altered expressions in PAs have been summarized in Supplementary Tables 1 and 2.

Cell cycle protein abnormalities have been suggested to be present in 80% of PAs.[58] The main regulators of the cell cycle are cyclin-dependent kinases (CDK) and their inhibitors (CDKI), through the modulation of the G1/S transition. CDKs are activated by cyclins promoting the initiation and progression of cell cycle by phosphorylation and, consequently, inactivation of the retinoblastoma (Rb) protein.[59–61] Rb inactivation results in release of the E2F transcription factor from Rb binding, allowing the transcription of S-phase genes and cycle cell progression.[62] CDKIs such as *CDKN1B* (coding for p27), *CDKN2A* (p16), and *CDKN2C* (p18) suppress cellular proliferation by preventing the inactivation of Rb, therefore acting as a TSG.[63] In sporadic PAs, CDKIs are frequently downregulated as a consequence of epigenetic alterations, such as promoter hypermethylation or histone modification.[12,64–66] Overexpression of cyclins D1, D3, and E has been documented in somatotropinomas, corticotropinomas, and NFPAs.[59,67–69]

Pituitary tumor transforming gene 1 (*PTTG1*) is another important cell cycle regulator, exhibiting oncogenic properties.[70] *PTTG1* encodes a protein with multiple biological effects: stimulation of basic fibroblast growth factor–mediated angiogenesis; enhancement of oncogene *C-MYC* transcription; interaction with *TP53*; and suppression of *p21* expression.[71,72] Overexpression of *PTTG1* was found in many PA subtypes, and it has been proposed as a marker of invasiveness and microvessel density in PAs.[2,73] *ZAC1* and growth arrest and DNA-damage inducible gene-45 gamma (*GADD45*-γ) genes are also important to the cell cycle control, acting as TSGs.[61,74–76] Maternally expressed gene 3 (*MEG3*) encodes a noncoding RNA that act as a TSG through *TP53* and *Rb* pathways. *MEG3* gene has been shown to be downregulated in NFPAs and prolactinomas due to promoter hypermethylation.[77]

Growth factor secretion and/or growth factor receptor expression are commonly altered in PAs (Supplementary Tables 1 and 2). Fibroblast growth factors are complex ligands involved in pituitary development and growth and might have a role in the tumorigenesis.[2] Other growth factors, such as epidermal growth factor and bone morphogenetic protein (BMP4), may be disrupted, predisposing to PAs.[78–80] Signal transduction mediators, such as protein kinase C (*PKC*) and *PIK3CA*,[16,46,81] and transcription factors, like *PTX1*, *PIT1*, and *HMGA2*,[2,82–84] may be overexpressed in some sporadic PAs. The β-catenin pathway has also been implicated in pituitary tumorigenesis.[85,86] Messenger RNA (mRNA) expression studies, where several Wnt pathway inhibitors were shown to be downregulated in PAs in comparison to normal pituitary tissue, together with immunostaining data, suggest that aberrant activation of the canonical Wnt signaling pathway may well be involved in pituitary oncogenesis,[85] and recent data support this for MEN1-related tumorigenesis as well.[87]

The vast majority of pituitary tumors are benign, although they are often locally invasive. It is striking, however, how rarely pituitary carcinomas are encountered.[88] Cellular senescence has been suggested to explain the benign nature of PAs. Cellular senescence is an antiproliferative response, induced by DNA damage, oxidative stress, age-linked telomere shortening, chromosomal instability and aneuploidy, loss of TSG, or, paradoxically, by oncogene activation, which leads to irreversible cell cycle arrest. Senescent pituitary cells are growth constrained by cell cycle inhibitors, and therefore, protected from deleterious consequences of proliferative oncogenes, hormones, or transforming factors, preventing their malignant transformation.[1,18,89] More than 70% of somatotropinomas overexpress *PTTG1* gene, which leads to aneuploidy and induction of senescence markers, including p21 and β-galactosidase.[90–92] Oncogene-induced senescence in corticotropinomas and NFPAs appears to be more related to p27 and p15/p16, respectively.[1,92,93]

MicroRNAs (miRNAs) are small noncoding RNAs that are involved in posttranslational gene expression regulation, mRNA translation, and degradation.[94] miRNAs regulate about 30% of human genes, and they can act as activators or inhibitors of carcinogenesis. Altered expression of miRNAs has been described in PAs, and specific miRNA signatures are related to clinical and therapeutic characteristics of these tumors.[18,94–96] Some miRNAs have antiproliferative properties, such as miR-16-1,[97,98] miR-let-7,[97] or miR-23b and miR-130b.[99] miR-132, miR-15a, and miR-16 inhibit the pituitary tumor cell proliferation, migration, and invasion, acting as TSG in pituitary tumors by directly targeting Sox5.[100] The downregulation of miR-410 has also recently been involved in the pathogenesis of gonadotroph PAs.[101] However, other miRNAs promote pituitary tumorigenesis, such as miR-128a, miR-516-3p, and miR-155.[102] Interestingly, miR-107 has shown both oncogenic and tumor suppression properties, depending on the tissue type.[103] Deregulation of miRNAs expression might be relevant for the biological behavior of some PAs. Recently, it has been shown that the downregulation of miR-183 in prolactinomas confers more aggressive behavior and malignant potential to these tumors. miR-183 has been demonstrated to act as antiproliferative by interfering directly with the expression of key genes such as *KIAA0101*, which in turn is involved in cell cycle activation and inhibition of cell cycle arrest mediated by p53-p21.[104] Moreover, there is evidence that miRNAs may be involved in the mechanism of action of some drugs, such as somatostatin analogs (SSA) and dopamine agonists (DA), and specific miRNAs may predict the response to medical therapy.[18,94] In a study involving patients with somatotropinomas, 13 microRNAs were expressed differently between PAs of patients either pretreated with lanreotide or not, and 7 miRNAs were differentially expressed in tumors of patients who did or did not respond to medical treatment.[105] miRNA analysis in response to medical therapy has also been done in prolactinomas. miR-206, miR-516b, and miR-550 were significantly upregulated, whereas miR-671-5p was downregulated, in bromocriptine-treated prolactinomas.[106] It is thought that in the future, tumor suppressor miRNAs will become available to target and treat specific types of PAs.[94]

FAMILIAL PITUITARY ADENOMAS

Familial PAs have been described for many years, but the field has significantly expanded since the identification of *AIP* as a germline mutation in some families with acromegaly and prolactinoma. Familial PAs occur either isolated or as part of endocrine-related tumor syndromes, such MEN1, MEN4, CNC, or XLAG syndrome. Rarely, germline mutations in *NF1*, *DICER1*, and *SDH* may also predispose to PAs.[107]

Familial Isolated Pituitary Adenomas

FIPA is characterized by the occurrence of 2 or more cases of PA in a family in the absence of other associated tumors.[108] However, germline mutations can also be identified in seemingly sporadic cases due to either de novo mutations, as is common in XLAG, or due to low penetrance and therefore lack of known family history, as often seen in *AIP* mutation-positive cases. FIPA is a heterogeneous condition with significant differences in phenotype among the various subtypes.

FIPA kindreds may have the same PA subtype among affected subjects (homogeneous FIPA), or a mixture of different types of PAs may occur in the same kindred (heterogeneous FIPA).[107] In the authors' cohort, most homogeneous FIPA cases (around half of the families) consist of acromegaly (54% of the homogenous families), prolactinoma (27%), and NFPA (17%).[109] In heterogeneous FIPA families, a combination of different PA subtypes can occur (prolactinomas, somatotropinomas, NFPAs, and corticotropinomas), but the most common phenotype is the combination of acromegaly and prolactinoma (37% of heterogeneous kindreds).[109] Of note, the frequency of prolactinomas is much lower in FIPA than in sporadic adenomas from the general population (22%–38% vs 46.2%–66.2%), which is partially explained by the higher prevalence of somatotropinomas in FIPA patients than in the general population (35%–57.8% vs 9%–16.5%).[107,109]

AIP Mutation-Positive Patients

In 2006, linkage analysis in 2 Finnish FIPA families identified a truncating germline mutation in the *AIP* gene (p.Q14* mutation) as a predisposition for PA.[110] Since then, a flurry of further studies have identified numerous other *AIP* mutations. *AIP* mutations are present in 15% to 30% of FIPA families.[111] A recent large series reported pathogenic or likely pathogenic *AIP* gene mutations in 17.1% of 216 FIPA families and in 8.4% of young (<30 year old) apparently sporadic patients,[109] and similar data were found in previous studies as well.[108] In patients with sporadic pituitary macroadenomas younger than 30 years, germline *AIP* mutations can be found in 11.7%; *AIP* gene is mutated in 20% of apparently sporadic pediatric PAs.[112]

Genetic and Molecular Aspects

AIP was first described in 1996 as an inhibitor of hepatitis B virus X protein–mediated transactivation. The *AIP* gene is located at chromosomal region 11q13.2, has 6 exons, and encodes a protein with 330 amino acids. AIP is a cochaperone protein that contains 3 tetratricopeptide repeats and an α-helix in the C-terminal region, and these 7 α-helices mediate interactions with other proteins.[113,114]

It is postulated that in *AIP*-mutated FIPA, AIP loses its ability to bind its partners, and therefore, loses its activity as a tumor suppressor.[107,108,113] The role of *AIP* as TSG is supported by the association of several loss-of-function mutations with the development of PAs and the presence of loss of heterozygosity (LOH) in 11q13 in *AIP*-mutated PAs. Furthermore, *AIP* overexpression decreases cell proliferation in vitro, whereas *AIP* knockdown increases proliferation.[21,115–117] *AIP*-mutated PAs have low AIP expression at both mRNA and protein levels.[21,117] According to data from a recent study, enhanced proteasomal degradation is the main mechanism for most pathogenic missense mutations.[118] The last exon nonsense mutation p.R304* also undergoes rapid protein degradation, whereas exon 1 to 5 nonsense mutation RNAs are likely to undergo nonsense-mediated decay.[118]

AIP is ubiquitously expressed with some variation among different tissues. In normal pituitary tissue, *AIP* is expressed predominantly in somatotrophs and lactotrophs, normally within cytoplasmic secretory vesicles, but it is absent in normal corticotrophs and gonadotrophs. In sporadic PAs, *AIP* is expressed in all tumor types: in sporadic somatotropinomas, AIP colocalizes with GH in secretory vesicles, but in sporadic prolactinomas, corticotropinomas, or NFPAs, AIP resides in the cytoplasm.[21]

Several binding partners of the AIP protein have been described: aryl hydrocarbon receptor (AHR), heat shock protein 90 (HSP90), phosphodiesterase subtype 4A5 (PDE4A5), PDE2A, heat shock cognate 70, survivin, peroxisome proliferator-activated receptor-α, thyroid hormone receptor β1, estrogen receptor-α, Epstein-Barr virus–encoded nuclear protein-3, hepatitis B virus X protein, rearranged during transfection tyrosine-kinase receptor (RET), along with many other proteins.[108,113] Thus, *AIP* inactivation has the potential to interfere with a wide spectrum of cellular and environmental signals.

The best known AIP binding partner is AHR, which is a ligand-activated transcription factor. It has been originally described as the mediator of the toxic effects of the environmental toxin 2,3,7,8-tetrachloro-*p*-dioxin (TCDD), but endogenous ligands have also been described since. Upon TCDD binding, the cytoplasmic AHR + AIP + HSP90 complex is translocated to the nucleus, where AHR is released from the complex and creates a dimer with the AHR nuclear translator (ARNT) to bind to xenobiotic response element regions of DNA. The role of AHR may include regulation of the activity of other nuclear receptors, transcription factors, and protein kinases, leading to changes in the cell cycle, cell adhesion, migration, and intracellular signaling.

AHR involvement in the pituitary tumorigenesis is still unclear. AHR knockout mice do not develop PAs.[119–122] AHR promotes the cell cycle in the absence of ligand binding,[123] and it interacts with cyclin D1 and CDK4 in breast cancer cells.[124] *AIP* mutation-positive PAs have decreased AHR and ARNT levels, whereas the AHR repressor AHRR has increased expression in sporadic somatotropinomas.[115,117] A recent study suggests that genetic variants in the AHR pathway might be associated with larger somatotroph adenomas and SSA resistance in patients living in highly polluted areas,[56] but further data are needed to confirm these findings.

Disruption of the cAMP-PKA molecular pathway is important for somatotroph tumorigenesis as seen in CNC, MAS, and possibly XLAG. AIP interacts with PDE4A5 (enzyme involved in the inactivation of cAMP), and *AIP* mutations lead to the loss of the AIP-PDE4A5 interaction.[21,125] Recently, it has been shown that AIP deficiency causes a dysfunction in cAMP signaling, leading to elevated concentrations of cAMP through defective $G\alpha$i-2 and $G\alpha$i-3 proteins, which normally inhibit cAMP synthesis. In addition, immunostaining of $G\alpha$i-2 showed that AIP deficiency is associated with decreased $G\alpha$i-2 protein expression in human and mouse GH-secreting PAs, highlighting a defective $G\alpha$i signaling in these tumors. Thus, the failure to inhibit cAMP synthesis through dysfunctional $G\alpha$i signaling may explain the development of GH-secreting PAs in *AIP* mutation carriers.[126] However, there are other potential pathogenic mechanisms, particularly those related to *survivin* and *RET*.[111] Survivin is an inhibitor of apoptosis, through the inactivation of proapoptotic caspases. AIP and HSP90 can stabilize via preventing survivin ubiquitination.[127,128] *RET* is also a possible candidate partner, although mutations in RET or AIP did not seem to change the observed interaction.[129]

More than 100 *AIP* gene variants have now been described, including insertions/deletions, single-nucleotide polymorphisms, nonsense and missense mutations, duplications, promoter and splice-site mutations, and large genomic deletions.[108,109] The most common mutation site in the *AIP* gene is the p.R304 locus (R304* and R304Q), a CpG-type mutation hotspot identified in several independent populations.[108,109] One of these represents a founder mutation in Ireland, as the same haplotype including the R304* mutation was found in 18 families with Irish origin, including a patient with gigantism from the eighteenth century, where DNA collected from the skeleton also harbored the same mutation and haplotype.[130,131] The authors' calculations suggest that their common ancestor lived around 2500 years ago, and this fact explains the rich Irish folklore surrounding giants in the area. The other hotspot mutations in the *AIP* gene affect codons 81 (Refs.[21,109,125,132,133] and M. Korbonits, unpublished data, 2016) and 271 (Refs.[112,125,134–136] and M. Korbonits, unpublished data, 2016), and founder mutations have also been described in Finland, Italy, and France.[110,137,138]

Truncating mutations account for most *AIP* mutations (almost 80% in the familial cohort and 60% in sporadic cohorts), and around 70% of all known *AIP* mutations, cause a disruption in the C-terminus. A genotype-phenotype correlation was found, because truncating mutations are associated with earlier disease onset. No significant differences were found, however, between patients with *AIP* truncating and nontruncating mutations regarding proportion of GH excess cases, number of patients per kindred, tumoral diameter, macroadenoma frequency, extrasellar invasion, or number of treatments received.[109]

Clinical Aspects

The penetrance of PAs among *AIP* mutation-positive carriers is around 12% to 30%. Data from well-studied families found an overall penetrance rate of 22.7%.[109] When patients that were prospectively diagnosed were excluded from that calculation, the total PA penetrance was 12.5%, highlighting the relevance of clinical screening of apparently unaffected carriers.[109] The relatively low penetrance of PAs among *AIP* mutation carriers, together with their variable clinical characteristics, suggests the involvement of other disease-modifying genes.[139,140]

There might be a slight male predominance for AIP cases,[21,125,141] although in a recent large series this was not significant.[109] Male predominance might be influenced by ascertainment bias for gigantism cases, a condition more prevalent in men partially due to the physiologically later puberty and therefore later growth cessation. *AIP* mutation-positive patients typically manifest the disease in the second decade with mean age at diagnosis between 18 and 24 years; almost all *AIP* mutation-positive cases are diagnosed before the age of 40.[108,141,142]

Clinical manifestations are related to hormonal excess or mass effects. Gigantism is particularly frequent, representing over a third of *AIP* mutation-positive patients.[108,109] Among pituitary gigantism, approximately 30% are attributed to *AIP* mutations, whereas other genetic causes are less common: XLAG, MAS, CNC, and MEN1 are responsible for pituitary gigantism in 10%, 5%, 1%, and 1% of the cases, respectively.[143] In another large series of patients with gigantism, *AIP* mutations were identified as the cause of 41.2% of the pituitary gigantism cases, whereas XLAG was responsible for 7.8% of the cases.[35] Still, a genetic cause for pituitary gigantism remains to be found in more than half of the cases of pituitary gigantism.[35,143] *AIP* mutation-positive patients also have an increased risk for pituitary apoplexy,[21,34,109,144] especially childhood pituitary apoplexy.[109]

Most *AIP* mutation-positive PAs are macroadenomas (nearly 90%), commonly invasive and/or with extrasellar extension (in more than 50%). Most of these are GH- and/or prolactin-secreting PAs (around 80%); NFPAs can be also found but often with positive GH or prolactin immunostaining, whereas corticotropinomas and thyrotropinomas are very rare.[107] *AIP*-mutated PAs have more aggressive features in comparison to sporadic PAs[108]: they are more frequently sparsely granulated[21] and have lower AIP protein levels, which are seen as a marker of invasiveness and as a predictor of SSA response even in sporadic PAs.[145,146]

AIP mutation-positive PAs require a multimodal therapeutic approach often including more than one surgery. Prolactinomas often need to be operated possibly due to reduced DA responsiveness,[141] and somatotropinomas are commonly resistant to SSA.[21,112,141] PAs harboring germline *AIP* mutations have less GH and insulin-like growth factor type 1 (IGF-1) reductions to SSA in comparison to acromegaly negative for *AIP* mutation (−40 vs −75% for GH, and −47.4% vs −56% for IGF-1, respectively). Moreover, SSA were associated with a significantly lower tumor shrinkage in *AIP* mutation-positive PAs (0% vs −41.4%, respectively).[141] Interestingly, *AIP* is upregulated in sporadic somatotropinomas treated with SSA before surgery, and the *AIP* expression is a predictor of SSA responsiveness.[116,147] *AIP* is suggested to mediate SSA response in somatotropinomas through *ZAC1*. Upregulation of *AIP* increases *ZAC1* expression, an antiproliferative target of somatostatin, whereas silencing *AIP* results in a reduction of *ZAC1* mRNA.[116,148] Thus, this AIP-ZAC1 pathway together with the AIP-Gαi interaction may explain why *AIP* mutation-positive somatotropinomas have poor responses to SSA.

Sporadic PAs with low AIP were resistant to first-generation SSA (100 vs 60%; $P = .02$), whereas they had similar responsiveness to pasireotide in comparison to tumors with conserved AIP expression (50 vs 40%; $P = .74$). Tumors with low AIP had reduced SSTR2 expression compared with normal AIP expressing sporadic PAs, but no difference regarding the SSTR5.[149]

Genetic screening is now available for selected patients with PA (**Fig. 3**). If a patient with PA has a relative with PA without associated syndromic features, the diagnosis of FIPA is made, and genetic testing for *AIP* mutations could be offered.[150] *AIP* screening is suggested in FIPA cases as well as childhood-onset PAs and young-onset (<30 years) macroadenomas even with no family history of PA. If an *AIP* mutation is identified in a certain kindred, genetic screening should then be offered to the family members at risk. As the youngest known case with large PA presented with symptoms from the age of 3 and diagnosed at the time of pituitary apoplexy at the age of 4,[136] genetic screening is suggested early.[18,109,150,151]

Unaffected carriers should undergo baseline assessments as approximately a quarter of subjects initially thought to be unaffected *AIP* mutation-positive carriers may have pituitary abnormalities. Clinical evaluation, including careful monitoring of growth in children, prolactin and IGF-1 measurements, and a baseline pituitary MRI, is suggested.[109] In children, to avoid the need for anesthesia, baseline pituitary MRI should be performed around the age of 10 years if clinical and biochemical assessment is normal earlier. Annual pituitary function tests are recommended. If a case is prospectively diagnosed, treatment and follow-up should be similar as for sporadic PAs, although it is acknowledged that *AIP* mutation-positive PAs are more refractory to treatment.[109] Ending the follow-up can be considered in older patients, given the low probability of detecting new PA patients after the fifth decade of life.[109,150,151] Earlier interruption of the follow-up is controversial, but the frequency of monitoring may be reduced above the age of 30 years.[18]

AIP Mutation-Negative FIPA Patients

AIP mutation-negative families have age of onset similar to sporadic PA, whereas tumor behavior has been found to be more aggressive. The penetrance is incomplete and even lower than in *AIP* mutation-positive kindreds. The distribution of their adenoma types is depicted in **Fig. 4**. Genetic and clinical screening of FIPA families with no *AIP* mutations is uncertain and more controversial. In these cases, education on symptoms should be provided, and eventually, a baseline screening and follow-up can be considered in some kindreds.[18,109,152] The authors have encountered several prospective diagnoses of PA in *AIP* mutation-negative FIPA families.[109] As PA are relatively common, there is a possibility that at least some of the *AIP* mutation-negative apparent families might be coincidental, or due to more complex pituitary-related mutant gene sets and not to a single gene mutation.

X-linked Acrogigantism Syndrome

The XLAG syndrome was recently identified in patients with very young-onset gigantism and PA or hyperplasia.[25] XLAG syndrome is responsible for approximately 10% of pituitary gigantism cases.[35,143] As no other disease has been identified in XLAG patients to date, this disease also belongs to the FIPA group.

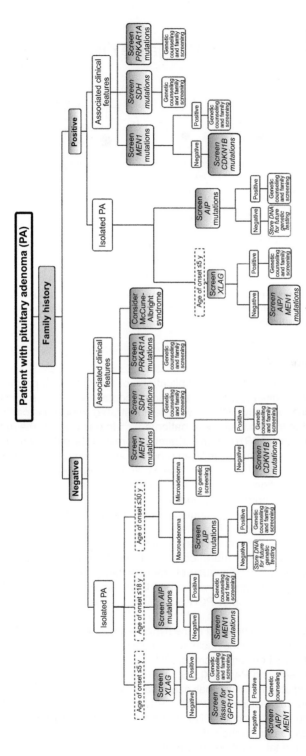

Fig. 3. Suggested approach for genetic testing in a patient with a PA. This flowchart does not consider PitB due to *DICER1* mutation, because strictly speaking these are not "adenomas."

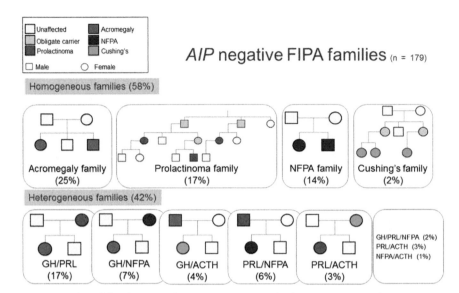

Fig. 4. Examples of family trees of AIP mutation negative homogeneous or heterogeneous FIPA families. Percentages represent proportion in the cohort of 179 AIP mutation-negative FIPA kindreds. PRL, prolactin.

Genetic and Molecular Aspects

XLAG syndrome is caused by microduplications of the orphan G-protein coupled receptor GPR101. Originally, a duplicated region containing 4 genes was identified at the Xq26.3 locus, but only GPR101 was demonstrated to be significantly overexpressed in the pituitary tissue of these patients.[25,35] In one patient, the mutated region involved only the GPR101 gene, therefore proving its pathogenicity.[35] Most patients with XLAG syndrome have been reported as having sporadic de novo mutations with a few having familial germline Xq26.3 microduplications.[143,153,154] In addition, mosaic mutations have also been described in men.[24,35,154] The clinical features are similar in both sexes, and in de novo germline, mosaic, or familial forms. Somatic mosaicism is challenging for the diagnosis of XLAG syndrome, as blood-derived DNA may show false-negative results. Thus, some sporadic men with suspected XLAG syndrome may require sampling from the pituitary or from various tissues and/or more complex laboratory techniques in order to establish the diagnosis.[24,154] Because of the possible small size of the duplicated region, a standard CGH array may show false-negative results, and a high-resolution CGH study or droplet PCR may be necessary to identify the GPR101 microduplication.[35,154]

GPR101 is significantly expressed in the hypothalamus and other parts of the brain with the highest expression in the nucleus accumbens. It may play a role in energy homeostasis and pituitary hormone secretion.[25,155] GPR101 has been found to be highly expressed in GH-secreting PAs in XLAG syndrome patients, in comparison to non-GPR101 duplicated somatotropinomas or normal pituitary tissue, where its expression is low.[25] The exact mechanism by which GPR101 overexpression leads to pituitary hormone secretion and tumorigenesis is not fully understood. GPR101 can activate the cAMP pathway for which the mitogenic effects in pituitary somatotrophs and its involvement in hormonal secretion are well established.[25,156]

Several findings support the involvement of central GHRH in the pathogenesis and progression of XLAG syndrome, at least in some patients.[157] Somatotroph hyperplasia accompanies adenoma formation in XLAG syndrome patients, whereas some patients only have pituitary hyperplasia without adenoma.[24,35,158] Some features seen in these patients resemble pituitary abnormality features seen in ectopic GHRH-excess conditions.[25,153] GHRH staining was demonstrated to be absent in GH-secreting tumors from XLAG syndrome patients, but abundant GHRH-receptor was seen in some hyperplastic and adenomatous tissue.[25,153] Elevated circulating GHRH levels were detected in some, but not in all, XLAG syndrome cases in the absence of peripheral sources.[158] Dynamic pulsatility studies conducted in XLAG syndrome patients showed GHRH, GH, and prolactin elevations.[157] Throughout these studies, GHRH levels were elevated at all study time points, although fluctuations did occur; in turn, prolactin levels varied by <7% from the baseline, but changes in GH levels were more prominent during these dynamic studies (−23.6% to +61.5%).[157] Moreover, GHRH secretion is tightly regulated by integrated central and peripheral signals, and *GPR101* is expressed in the hypothalamus and other brain regions, where the integration of such signals occurs.[154] In vitro studies using tissue from patients with XLAG give further support for a role of GHRH hypersecretion in XLAG syndrome: GH and prolactin secretion were stimulated by GHRH coincubation,[158] whereas a GHRH antagonist was able to reduce basal and stimulated GH and prolactin secretion in a dose-dependent manner.[157]

Despite the original suggestion regarding *GPR101* variant p.E308D, data from large sporadic PA cohorts showed that germline or somatic *GPR101* single nucleotide mutations are very rare, occurring in up to 1.6%[25,35,140] and do not play a role in pituitary tumorigenesis. No digenism with *AIP* was identified.[35,140] Mutations or overexpression of the *GPR101* gene has not been reported in pediatric corticotropinomas; only a rare germline *GPR101* variant was found in one case, but in vitro studies excluded pathogenic effect.[155] Of note, loss-of-function *GPR101* mutations or deletions were not identified as a cause of congenital isolated GH deficiency.[159]

Clinical Aspects

The clinical features of XLAG syndrome are striking.[24,35,143,153] The key manifestation is increased growth (gigantism) starting at a very early age with height remarkably elevated at the time of diagnosis (average +3.9 standard deviation score). Following normal birth weight, rapid growth begins between 1 and 24 months, and overgrowth is always detected before the age of 5 years.[35,143,153] Other features may also be present: acral enlargement, coarsened facial features, and unexpectedly increased appetite (in about one-third of the patients), and less frequently, acanthosis nigricans, sleep apnea/snoring, excessive perspiration, or abdominal distension (**Fig. 5**).[143,153,160]

Most patients are females. Explanation for this could be that (i) they have two X chromosomes, so twice the chance to harbor a mutation; (ii) there could be a higher chance for mutations in the sperm,[161] and ones affecting *GPR101* will obviously manifest in a female baby; and (iii) the predominance of female cases might be due to a potential negative effect of Xq26.3 microduplication on the viability of hemizygous male embryos.[143,153]

Patients with XLAG syndrome may develop pituitary macroadenomas, although some have isolated hyperplasia or hyperplasia in conjunction with PA, together with marked GH/IGF-1 elevations. Hyperprolactinemia accompanies GH elevations in 85% of the cases.[35] From the histopathological point of view, XLAG-related PAs are mostly mixed somatotroph/lactotroph adenomas that show a characteristic sinusoidal and lobular architecture and contain both densely and sparsely granulated

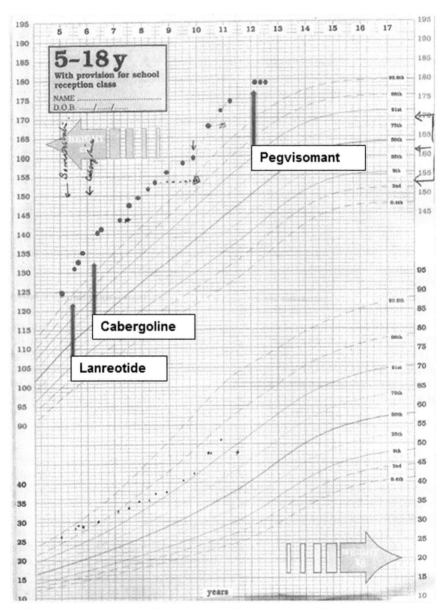

Fig. 5. A typical growth chart of a patient with XLAG syndrome. Of note, the early onset of the disease and also the difficulties in its control despite the multimodal therapy approach. (*Courtesy of* Dr Christine Burren, Bristol, UK.)

somatotrophs; microcalcifications and follicle-like structures are also commonly observed. Moreover, Ki67 index is normally low (less than 3%) and mitotic count often negligible.[35]

Treatment of XLAG syndrome is complex, in most cases multimodal.[35,153] Neurosurgery is normally the first therapeutic approach in cases with PA, but it is often insufficient (sometimes 2 or 3 surgeries are needed), requiring additional medical therapy or radiotherapy. SSA efficacy is poor in XLAG syndrome, with a lack of GH/IGF-1 control in all patients, even using adult doses and despite the presence of moderate- to high-staining levels of SSTR type 2.[153] In a recent study, octreotide showed no inhibitory effect on GH or prolactin in XLAG pituitary cell culture, but pasireotide was found to have a small inhibitory effect on GH secretion, which suggests that some benefit might be obtained with this drug.[157] In 1990, a remarkable case of pituitary gigantism was reported due to somatomammotroph hyperplasia,[158] recently confirmed as an XLAG syndrome patient.[35] In vitro, this patient's pituitary cells were markedly inhibited by octreotide and bromocriptine despite the absence of a satisfactory response in vivo.[158] DAs alone are insufficient to control hormonal hypersecretion, whereas pegvisomant, either alone or combined with SSA/DA, may allow hormonal control in most cases. Although in the past hyperplasia cases had to be treated with complete hypophysectomy, today with the availability of pegvisomant, DAs and SSA, medical therapy is a viable option.[24,35,158] Radiotherapy response is also poor; with a relatively slow onset of effect, it may not be sufficient alone, especially in a rapidly growing child.[143,153]

MULTIPLE ENDOCRINE NEOPLASIA TYPE 1 SYNDROME

MEN1 is an autosomal dominant disorder, characterized by the occurrence of endocrine and nonendocrine tumors. The 3 main components of MEN1 are parathyroid neoplasms causing primary hyperparathyroidism, pancreatic neuroendocrine tumors (pNETs), and PAs. Other neoplasms, such adrenocortical tumors, thymic NETs, gastric carcinoids, facial angiofibromas, lipomas, collagenomas, ependymomas, meningiomas, breast cancer, and rarely, pheochromocytomas (Pheo), may also occur (Table 1).[27,162] The diagnosis of MEN1 is established in one of these scenarios: a patient with 2 or more MEN1-associated tumors; a patient with one MEN1-associated tumor and a first-degree relative with MEN1; a mutant gene carrier, that is, an individual with a MEN1 mutation but no clinical, biochemical, or structural evidence of MEN1.[163]

Genetic and Molecular Aspects

MEN1 gene encodes a 610-amino-acid protein called menin and is regarded as TSG because heterozygous inactivating mutations predispose to neoplasia, and most MEN1-related tumors (around 90%) show LOH at 11q13.[164,165] In MEN-1 tumors with no LOH, it is hypothesized that other mechanisms of gene inactivation may occur, such as hypermethylation, mutations of the promoter, or, in noncoding regions, mRNA regulation.[27,166,167] Menin is ubiquitously expressed and is predominantly located in the nucleus, where it can associate with chromatin, double-stranded DNA, lysine-specific histone methyltransferases, and also components of transcriptional repressor complexes.[162] Menin has several functions, such as transcription regulation, genome stability, cell division and cell cycle control, apoptosis, and epigenetic regulation,[27,167,168] resultant from its interaction with numerous partners.

Menin is a key transcription regulator due to its interaction with many partners, like JunD, NF-kB, pem, SIN3A, HDAC, Smad1, Smad3, Smad5, Runx2, MLL, estrogen receptor-α, host cell factor 2, and RBBP5.[27,87] Menin also interacts with activin in normal pituitary, negatively regulating cell proliferation, and secretion of prolactin, GH, and ACTH. Furthermore, important proliferative factors in endocrine neoplasms are negatively modulated by menin, such as insulin-like growth factor binding protein 2, IGF-2, and parathyroid hormone-related protein.[169,170] In addition, menin acts as a repressor of telomerase activity through the human telomerase reverse transcriptase.[171]

Table 1
Characteristic tumors in multiple endocrine neoplasia type 1 syndrome with suggested biochemical and radiological assessments

Tumors	Estimated Prevalence in MEN1 (%)	Age to Begin the Screening (y)	Biochemical Annual Test	Imaging Test (Time Interval)
Parathyroid adenomas	90	8	Calcium, parathyroid hormone	None
Gastrinomas	40	20	Gastrin (gastric pH)	MRI or computed tomographic (CT) scan or endoscopic ultrasonography (annually)
Insulinomas	10	5	Insulin, fast ng glucose	
Nonfunctioning	20–55	<10	Chromogranin A, glucagon, vasoactive intestinal polypeptide, pancreatic polypeptide	
Other PNETs	<1			
Prolactinomas	20	5	Prolactin	Pituitary MRI (every 3 y)
Somatotropinomas	10	5	IGF-1	
Corticotropinomas	<5	5		
NFPAs	<5	5		
Adrenocortical tumors	40	<10	None, unless symptoms and/or adrenal tumors >1 cm identified on imaging	MRI or CT scan (annually with pancreatic imaging)
Pheo	<1	—	—	—
Bronchopulmonary carcinoid	2	15	None	CT or MRI scan (every 1–2 y)
Thymic carcinoid	2	15	None	CT or MRI scan (every 1–2 y)
Gastric carcinoid	10	—	—	—
Lipomas	30	—	—	—
Angiofibromas	85	—	—	—
Collagenomas	70	—	—	—
Meningiomas	8	—	—	—
Invasive breast cancer	6	—	—	—

Menin may increase or decrease gene expression by epigenetic regulation via histone methylation or acetylation.[27,172] Menin activates the transcription of CDKN1B and CDKN1C by recruiting the histone methyltransferase MLL protein to the promoters and coding regions of those genes. CDKN1B and CDKN1C are predominantly expressed in endocrine organs, which can explain, at least in part, the selectivity of MEN1 tumorigenesis.[173] Recent data suggest that loss of menin activates cell cycle protein CDK4, and this may lead to tumorigenesis in pituitary and pancreatic tissue.[174]

Recently, a model has been proposed, which explains, at least partially, how MEN1 loss may trigger epigenetic modifications and perturb signaling pathways leading to tumorigenesis.[87] It has been demonstrated that loss of MEN1 leads to DNA (cytosine-5)-methyltransferase 1 (DNMT1) activation, which in turn is implicated in DNA hypermethylation, driving the MEN1-related tumorigenesis in endocrine tissues (but not in exocrine tissues). The tissue-specific effects might be due to different cofactors or histone methylation patterns in endocrine and exocrine tissues.[87] The increased activity of DNMT1 mediates global DNA hypermethylation, including the SOX regulatory genes, which in turn results in aberrant activation of the Wnt/β-catenin signaling pathway. Hyperactivation of the Wnt/β-catenin signaling pathway results in increased cell proliferation and expression of oncogenic Wnt-target genes, leading then to MEN1 tumorigenesis.[87]

Thus, these complex interactions and the functional versatility of menin provide numerous mechanisms for tumorigenesis and tissue selectivity of MEN1-associated tumors.[162,168]

More than 1500 MEN1 mutations are known, and they are distributed throughout the whole gene, involving coding regions and splice sites.[167,175] Most MEN1 mutations are deletions or insertions resulting in frameshift or nonsense mutations, leading to truncation or absence of menin.[167,176] Most MEN1 mutations are familial, but 10% of the cases occur sporadically due to de novo MEN1 mutations. It is important to note that between 3% and 25% of patients with clinical MEN1 may not harbor germline mutations in MEN1 gene, which are detectable with Sanger sequencing of the coding region. These cases may have partial or whole gene deletions, which could be detected only by multiplex ligation-dependent probe amplification (MLPA) or long-range PCR amplification[27,177] or could be due to other gene mutations (see later discussion).

The clinical phenotype of MEN1 patients, family members, even identical twins, or unrelated families with same MEN1 mutation may have different MEN1 features.[162,167,178] Epigenetic mechanisms or modifying genes may influence the phenotype of patients harboring the same MEN1 mutation.[162] Although there is no direct genotype-phenotype correlation, a few studies highlighted a trend for a genotype-phenotype correlation[179,180]: it has been shown that patients carrying MEN1 mutations affecting the JunD interacting domain have a 2-fold increased risk of death from MEN1-related cancers.[180] A recent large series, involving 797 patients with MEN1 syndrome from 265 kindreds, found significant intrafamilial correlations for pituitary tumors, adrenal tumors, and thymic NETs, estimating their heritability (proportion of the phenotypic expression that is attributable to gene effects) at 64%, 65%, and 97%.[179] In addition, a recent study found a significant association between a rare MEN1 mutation (p.A541T, rs2959656) and clinically active PAs (odds ratio = 17.8; $P = .0002$).[181]

Clinical Aspects

The prevalence of MEN1 is approximately 1:30,000. MEN1 has been estimated to occur in 1% to 18% of patients with primary hyperparathyroidism, 16% to 38% of patients with gastrinomas, and less than 3% of patients with PAs.[27] The overall penetrance of MEN1 is generally high, with biochemical manifestations present by the fifth decade of life in 95% of cases. However, penetrance depends on patient's age and gender, and it is organ-specific (see **Table 1**). PA penetrance is 30% to 40%.[163,182] MEN1 patients have reduced life expectancy, and the mortality is mostly due to pNETs and thymic carcinoids. A multicenter study reported that near 70% of patients with MEN1 die from a cause directly related to MEN1.[183]

On average, 30% of MEN1 patients develop PAs,[27] although the incidence of PA in individuals with MEN1 varies from 15% to 50%.[182,184–186] Conversely, less than 3% of PA patients have MEN1. The mean age at presentation is 38 years, but these can occur as early as 5 years of age or as late as the ninth decade of life.[163,185,187] In this setting, PAs are more common in women (around 70% of MEN1-related PA patients are women), which is yet unexplained, although estrogen has been suggested as a possible reason due to their stimulatory properties in pituitary cell proliferation.[185,188] PA is the first manifestation of MEN1 in approximately 15% to 20% of cases, and its distribution by subtype is similar to sporadic PA cohorts: prolactinomas occur more commonly (60%), then NFPAs (15%), somatotropinomas (10%), corticotropinomas (5%), and rarely, thyrotropinomas (<1%).[162,163,185] In MEN1 patients, PAs are more frequently multiple, more aggressive, and often macroadenomas (85% of cases, compared with 40% in sporadic PAs).[27,138,184,185] However, Ki67 and mitotic count are not significantly different between MEN1-associated PAs and sporadic PAs.[184]

The diagnosis and management of PAs in patients with MEN1 are similar to those used in sporadic PAs (including neurosurgery, radiotherapy, and medical therapy), but they might be less responsive to treatment. Treatment of hormonally active PAs in MEN1 may be less efficient as shown by a study in which the restoration of PA hormonal secretion was achieved in 42% versus 90% in MEN1 versus non-MEN1 patients, respectively.[185] A separate analysis of 85 MEN1-associated prolactinomas found that 44% were resistant to DA.[162] However, a recent series from the Dutch MEN1 Study Group reported good responses of MEN1-associated prolactinomas to medical therapy (response rate >90%).[182] Moreover, in the same series, MEN1-associated PAs, particularly microadenomas, have shown a relatively indolent behavior (at least equivalent to sporadic PAs), therefore not requiring different follow-up or therapeutic approaches.[182]

MEN1 genetic testing is helpful, allowing clinicians to confirm the diagnosis and identify family members who carry MEN1 mutations and benefit from appropriate screening and monitoring (see **Table 1**).[189] MEN1 mutational analysis should be undertaken in: (i) an index case with 2 or more MEN1-associated endocrine tumors; (ii) asymptomatic first-degree relatives of a known mutation carrier; (iii) a first-degree relative of a mutation carrier expressing familial MEN1; (iv) individuals with suspicious or atypical MEN1: parathyroid tumors before the age of 30 years, multigland parathyroid disease, gastrinoma, or multiple pNETs at any age, existence of 2 or more nonclassical MEN1-associated tumors.[163] Patients with childhood-onset macroprolactinomas, especially with other prolactinomas in the family, could also be considered for screening.[138,190] MEN1 analysis in asymptomatic individuals should be performed in the first decade of life, because there have been endocrine tumors reported by the age of 5 years.[27,163,187]

MULTIPLE ENDOCRINE NEOPLASIA TYPE 4 SYNDROME

The absence of MEN1 mutations in 5% to 10% of patients with MEN1 clinical features led to the investigation of additional loci implicated in this phenotype. A rat model displaying MEN1-like phenotype was discovered to harbor a mutation in *CDKN1B* gene, which resulted in an absence of p27 protein in the observed endocrine tumors.[191] These findings prompted studies in patients with MEN1 who had no *MEN1* mutations.[192,193] Around 3% of patients with MEN1-associated tumors fulfilling the diagnostic criteria for MEN1, but with no *MEN1* mutations, indeed carried *CDKN1B* mutations; this autosomal dominant condition was termed MEN4.[27,168] Mutations in other CDKI (p15 [*CDKN2B*, 1%], p18 [*CDKN2C*, 0.5%], p21 [*CDKN1A*, 0.5%]) have also been identified in rare MEN1-like cases.[194]

Genetic and Molecular Aspects

CDKN1B is a TSG located on chromosome 12q13 in humans and encodes for the CDKI p27.[195] *CDKN1B* transcription is regulated by menin, which enhances the activity of *CDKN1B* promoter through its interaction with histone methyltransferases. p27 levels are also regulated via mitogen-activated protein kinase (MAPK) and *PIK3CA*. Loss-of-function mutations in *CDKN1B* lead to decreased cellular levels of p27 and/or to p27 functional defects, which reduce its binding with interacting partners.[196,197] To date, 8 different heterozygous loss-of-function *CDKN1B* mutations associated with MEN4 have been described.[168]

Clinical Aspects

A comprehensive phenotype of MEN4 patients is not yet established due to the small number of patients identified so far. For the same reasons, the penetrance of MEN4, the frequency of familial and sporadic cases, and phenotype-genotype correlation cannot be determined yet.

Primary hyperparathyroidism is present in all reported MEN4 patients. Other MEN-1-like tumors identified are PAs (corticotropinomas, somatotropinomas, and NFPAs), pNETs, adrenocortical tumors, and meningiomas as well as uterine neoplasms.[194,198–201] To establish whether *CDKN1B* mutations can cause isolated PAs, 124 affected individuals from 88 *AIP* mutation-negative FIPA families were studied: none had a *CDKN1B* germline defect[202]; thus, systematic screening of *CDKN1B* mutations in FIPA patients is currently unjustified.[201,202]

CARNEY COMPLEX

CNC, initially described in 1985 by Carney and colleagues,[203] is a rare multiple neoplasia syndrome associated with cardiocutaneous manifestations.[204,205] CNC is inherited in an autosomal dominant fashion with almost complete penetrance. Approximately 70% of CNC patients have affected family members, whereas others have de novo genetic defects.[206]

Genetic and Molecular Aspects

The genetic basis of CNC is heterogeneous.[207,208] Most CNC cases (73%) are caused by an inactivating germline mutation in the type 1α regulatory subunit of PKA (*PRKAR1A*).[209] *PRKAR1A* is located in the CNC1 loci at 17q24.2, encodes the most widely expressed PKA regulatory subunit, and acts as TSG. CNC-associated tumors often present LOH at 17q22-24 supporting the role of *PRKAR1A* as TSG.[210] PKA is a tetramer composed of 2 regulatory and 2 catalytic subunits, which acts as a main mediator of cAMP signaling. The stimulation of G protein leads to activation of adenylyl cyclase that produces cAMP, which in turn activates PKA by the dissociation of the regulatory subunits from the active sites of catalytic subunits. Active catalytic subunits are then released and phosphorylate downstream targets both in the cytoplasm and in the nucleus, promoting cell proliferation among other functions. Therefore, a reduction of the regulatory subunit type 1α due to *PRKAR1A* mutations leads to an increase of cAMP-stimulated PKA activity, which in turn stimulates MAPK-mediated proliferation, upregulates the signaling of Wnt, and decreases TFG-β-mediated apoptosis (**Fig. 6**).[162,211–214]

More than 125 different *PRKAR1A* mutations have been described to date.[208] Almost all generate a premature stop codon leading to nonsense-mediated mRNA decay and absence of the encoded protein; however, some *PRKAR1A* mutations in CNC patients were demonstrated to express the regulatory subunit but with loss of an inhibitory effect on the PKA pathway.[207,210,215] Large deletions can be detected by comparative genomic hybridization or MLPA in up to 20% of CNC patients previously thought to be *PRKAR1A* mutation-negative on sequencing analysis.[216,217]

A second genetic locus referred to as CNC2 locus, located at 2p16, is also associated with CNC. To date, the gene residing in this region responsible for CNC-associated tumors remains unknown.[218] Recently, duplication of the catalytic subunit gene *PRKACB* was associated with CNC.[219]

There are data suggesting a genotype-phenotype correlation in CNC. *PRKAR1A* mutation carriers have myxomas, thyroid tumors, schwannomas, and large-cell calcifying Sertoli cell tumors (LCCSCT) more frequently and earlier than *PRKAR1A* mutation-negative CNC patients.[209] Patients with large *PRKAR1A* deletions manifest CNC features at an earlier age.[206,216] A small intronic germline deletion in *PRKAR1A* (c.709-7del6) is present in most cases with isolated primary pigmented nodular adrenocortical disease (PPNAD).[220] Of note, in a series of CNC patients caused by *PRKAR1A* mutations, variants of phosphodiesterase type 11A (*PDE11A*) gene were associated with higher incidence of PPNAD and LCCSCT, suggesting that *PDE11A* can modify the CNC phenotype.[221]

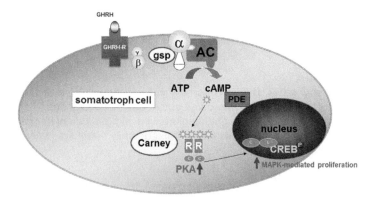

Fig. 6. The cAMP-PKA pathway in somatotroph cells. In normal somatotroph cells, ligand binding to the GHRH receptor activates the stimulatory G protein leading to adenylyl cyclase (AC) activation, which converts adenosine triphosphate (ATP) into cAMP. cAMP binding to PKA regulatory subunits (R) causes dissociation from the catalytic PKA subunit (C), which in turn is released and acts as kinase. The catalytic subunit activates CREB by phosphorylation, which mediates transcription of genes with CRE-containing promoters. In somatic or mosaic alpha G protein subunit mutations, the AC has prolonged activation. In CNC, the reduction of the regulatory subunit type 1α due to *PRKAR1A* mutations leads to an increase of cAMP-stimulated PKA activity, which in turn stimulates MAPK-mediated proliferation. gsp, Gs protein.

Clinical Aspects

The exact prevalence of CNC is unknown. In one of the largest series, 63% of the CNC patients were females.[208,209] The mean age at CNC diagnosis is 20 years, although there are cases diagnosed as early as the second year of life or as late as the fifth decade.[206,222]

Clinical manifestations of CNC are quite variable and include skin lesions, myxomatous tumors, and nonendocrine and endocrine neoplasms, including PAs.[208,209] Diagnostic criteria of CNC are listed in **Table 2**.[208] Genetic testing should be offered to patients with 2 or more CNC diagnostic criteria or relatives of CNC patients. If genetic testing is negative for *PRKAR1A* gene, other candidates are *PRKACA*, *PRKACB*, and PDE genes.[208]

Upregulation of the cAMP pathway affects somatotrophs and lactotrophs in the pituitary.[223] Up to 75% of CNC patients have abnormal GH, IGF-1, or prolactin levels, as well as an abnormal response of GH to the oral glucose tolerance test, but PAs can be detected in only 10%.[224,225] The incidence of acromegaly in CNC is estimated at 10% to 12%, and it is usually apparent by the third decade of life.[208,209] There is a prolonged period of somatomammotroph hyperplasia before PA formation. CNC-associated PAs are mostly GH- or GH/prolactin-secreting ones, frequently multiple and small-sized, essentially microadenomas surrounded by hyperplasia (regarded as putative precursor of the GH-producing PAs), although invasive macroadenomas were also described. Somatotropinomas and/or somatomammotroph hyperplasia might be treated surgically or with SSA.[226] Pure prolactinomas are rare.[227,228] Cushing disease due to ACTH-secreting PAs has not been reported in CNC. Mutations in *PRKAR1A*, *PRKACA*, and *PRKACB* have not been found in sporadic PAs.[19,229]

PHEOCHROMOCYTOMAS/PARAGANGLIOMAS AND PITUITARY ADENOMAS

The first description of coexisting PAs and pheochromocytomas/paragangliomas (Pheo/PGL) dates from 1952.[230] In 2006, a patient with PA and SDHB mutation,[231] and in 2008 a patient with PA and PGL with SDHC mutation, have been described.[232] The coexistence of the 2 diseases could be due to coincidence or a common pathogenic mechanism.

Recently, using tumor DNA analysis to look for LOH and immunohistochemistry for their related gene products, it has been possible to identify causal links between genes predisposing to Pheo/PGL and PAs,[233–235] a clinical scenario named 3PAs (pituitary, Pheo, and PGL).[236] A total of 74 patients having both Pheo/PGL and PA are currently reported: 22 (20%) with identified mutations in predisposing Pheo/PGL or PA genes, 23 (31%) with a personal or family history suggestive of hereditary endocrine syndrome, and 29 (39%) as isolated cases (**Fig. 7**).[237–239]

Genetic, Molecular, and Clinical Aspects

The SDH mitochondrial complex incorporates 4 subunits (A, B, C, and D), which forms the catalytic enzymatic core (A and B) and anchor the complex to the inner mitochondrial (subunits C and D), plus its associated assembly factor (*SDHAF2*). SDH is a part of the tricarboxylic acid and electron transport chain, catalyzing the succinate to fumarate step. Disruption of *SDH* leads to the inhibition of prolyl hydroxylases due to succinate accumulation, which in turn are unable to hydroxylate the transcription factor hypoxia-inducible factor 1-α (HIF1α), generating a pseudohypoxia state with transcription of HIF-responsive genes. Mutations in genes encoding the SDH components can result in hereditary Pheo/PGL and in the Carney-Stratakis syndrome.[240,241]

There is increasing evidence that germline *SDHx* mutations may play a role in pituitary tumorigenesis. Single reports and cohort studies of 3 PAs cases confirmed the

Table 2 Diagnostic criteria for Carney complex	
	Prevalence (%)
Major diagnostic criteria	
1. Spotty skin pigmentation with typical distribution (lips, conjunctiva and inner/outer canthi, genital mucosa)	70–80
2. Cutaneous and mucosal myxoma or heart myxomas	30–50/20–40
3. Breast myxomatosis	20
4. PPNAD or paradoxic positive response of glucocorticoid secretion to dexamethasone given during Liddle's test	Up to 60
5. Acromegaly as resultant of GH-producing adenoma	10–12
6. LCCSCT or characteristic calcifications on testicular ultrasound	Up to 75
7. Thyroid cancer (at any age) or multiple hypoechoic nodules on thyroid ultrasound in prepubertal children	Nodules in up to 75
8. Psammomatous melanocytic schwannomas	10
9. Blue nevus	40
10. Breast ductal adenoma (multiple)	20
11. Osteochondromyxoma	Rare
Supplemental criteria	
1. Affected first-degree relatives 2. Activating pathogenic variants of *PRKAR1A* (single base substitutions and copy number variation) and *PRKACB* 3. Inactivating mutations of the *PRKAR1A* gene	
Minor criteria—findings suggestive of (or possibly associated with) CNC, but no diagnostic for the disease	
1. Intense freckling (without darkly pigment spots or typical distribution) 2. Blue nevus, common type (if multiple) 3. Café-au-lait spots or other "birthmarks" 4. Elevated IGF-1 levels, abnormal glucose tolerance test, or paradoxic GH response to thyrotropin-releasing hormone in the absence of clinical acromegaly 5. Cardiomyopathy 6. History of Cushing syndrome, acromegaly, or sudden death in extended family 7. Pilonidal sinus 8. Colonic polyps (usually associated with acromegaly) 9. Multiple skin tags or other skin lesions; lipomas 10. Hyperprolactinemia 11. Single, benign thyroid nodule in a subject younger than 18 y; multiple thyroid nodules in an individual older than 18 y (on thyroid ultrasound) 12. Family history of carcinoma, particularly of thyroid, colon, pancreas, ovary; other multiple or malignant tumors	

To make the diagnosis of CNC, a patient must either (1) exhibit 2 of the major criteria confirmed by imaging, biochemistry, or histology; or (2) meet one major criteria and one supplemental criteria.

association between PGLs and PAs in patients with germline *SDH* mutations,[232–236,242] in some cases with well-documented LOH at the *SDH* locus along with a reduction of the respective SDH protein expression in PA tissue.[233,235] Heterozygous *Sdhb* knockout mice have abnormal pituitary hyperplasia, providing evidence

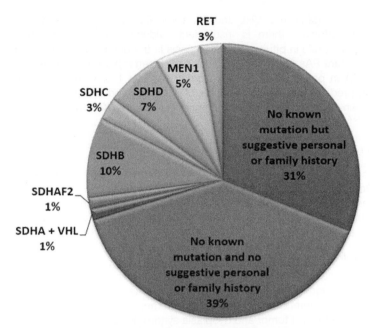

Fig. 7. Summary of the reported cases of coexisting PA and Pheo/PGL. Of the total of 74 patients with coexisting PA and Pheo/PGL published until now, 22 patients have either a confirmed genetic mutation in a recognized PA or a Pheo/PGL-predisposing gene or a variant, which is thought to be pathogenic; 23 patients do not have a confirmed pathogenic genetic mutation in a PA or Pheo/PGL-predisposing gene but have features suggestive of a genetic link; 29 patients have coexistent PA and Pheo/PGL but no known mutation or suggestive personal/family history.

that *SDHx*-deficient cells may be the initial abnormality leading to PA formation. In addition, adenohypophyseal cells in these mice show mitochondrial and nuclear abnormalities and increased *HIF1α* expression, suggesting that hypoxia may be implicated in the tumor transformation process.[236] Moreover, when PA and Pheo/PGL index cases were found in the setting of Pheo/PGL family history, *SDHx* mutations were identified in 75% of cases. Nevertheless, *SDHx* mutations are very rare in unselected sporadic PAs, and therefore, genetic screening is not justified routinely in patients with PA, unless there is coexistence of Pheo/PGL and/or family history of Pheo/PGL.[233,236,243]

SHDx mutation-associated PAs are more common among familial cases, can lead to multiple pituitary tumor phenotypes (somatotropinoma, prolactinoma, and NFPA), and present more frequently as macroadenomas displaying aggressive behavior, more often requiring surgery, and being more resistant to SSA.[233,234,236] Interestingly, the PAs of patients harboring *SHDx* alterations have a unique histologic feature with extensive vacuolization of the cytoplasm.[233]

Coexistence of Pheo/PGL and PAs has been described in only 4 patients with *MEN1* mutations (3 had Pheo and 1 had abdominal PGL). The demonstration LOH at the *MEN1* locus together with absent menin staining in the Pheo samples suggests a pathogenic role rather than just a coincidence.[233]

There are 2 cases of PA in Von Hippel–Lindau (VHL) syndrome,[233] but LOH was described in these PA cases at the *VHL* locus. Together with the low number of reported PAs in patients with VHL syndrome who undergo regular surveillance brain imaging, this suggests that VHL and PA association is rare and can be a coincidence.[237] In addition, there is insufficient evidence to conclude whether *RET* mutations play a role in pituitary tumorigenesis in the described patients with MEN2 and concomitant PAs.[237,244,245] No cases have been reported of a coexisting Pheo/PGL and PA in patients with neurofibromatosis type 1 or with other mutations in Pheo/PGL predisposing genes, such as MYC-associated factor (*MAX*), transmembrane protein 127 (*TMEM127*), kinesin family member 1B (*KIF1B*), or fumarate hydratase (*FH*).[237]

PITUITARY BLASTOMA AND *DICER1* MUTATIONS

The first case of pituitary blastoma (PitB) was described in 2008 in a 13-month-old female child who presented with Cushing disease and diabetes insipidus. The "blastoma" designation was given to reflect the embryonic-primordial appearance and neonatal presentation,[246] and other similar clinical presentations and histopathologic features were also reported.[247]

Genetic and Molecular Aspects

The genetic basis for PitB was uncovered in 2011, when an infant with PitB who had a family history suggestive of DICER1 syndrome was recognized as harboring an inherited *DICER1* mutation.[20,248] DICER1 syndrome, also known as pleuropulmonary blastoma (PPB)-familial tumor and dysplasia syndrome, is caused by a heterozygous germline mutation in the *DICER1* gene. *DICER1* encodes a small RNA processing endoribonuclease that cleaves precursor miRNAs into mature miRNAs, which in turn regulate the mRNA expression.[20,249]

PitB pathogenesis encompasses the existence of a loss-of-function germline *DICER1* mutation plus the occurrence of a second somatic "hit" (most often affecting an RNase IIIb metal ion-binding residue of DICER1), which are crucial to initiate the tumor development in the embryonic pituitary.[20,249]

Clinical Aspects

The main manifestations are PPB, cystic nephroma, Sertoli-Leydig cell tumors, goiter, and more rarely, sarcomas, dysplasias, and PitB.[250–252] The elements of this syndrome are characterized by age-specific manifestation. PitB, currently seen as a pathognomonic feature of DICER1 syndrome, is very rare with low penetrance (<1%), but potentially lethal in early childhood.[20] The median age at the appearance of the first PitB symptoms is 8 months (range 7 and 24 months). Cushing's disease (an exceedingly rare endocrinopathy in infancy) and ophthalmoplegia are the most common presenting symptoms of PitB. Even in the absence of a formal genetic diagnosis, this clinical presentation should lead the clinician to consider PitB as a strong diagnostic hypothesis and trigger the evaluation of other DICER1 syndrome-related disorders in either the patient or the family. Many PitBs have aggressive biological behavior and may well metastasize or be fatal in approximately 40% of the cases.[20,249]

MCCUNE-ALBRIGHT SYNDROME

MAS is a rare disorder, with estimated prevalence ranging between 1/100,000 and 1/1,000,000, reported for the first time in 1937 by McCune and shortly thereafter by Albright.[253] It is classically defined by the triad polyostotic fibrous dysplasia, café-au-lait skin pigmentation, and precocious puberty. Later, it was recognized that other endocrinopathies can be associated with MAS, such as GH excess, hyperthyroidism, Cushing's syndrome, and hyperparathyroidism, as well as nonendocrine organ disorders.[254,255] Those disorders can occur alone or in combination and encompass a wide range of severity due to the variable level of mosaicism.[256]

Genetic and Molecular Aspects

Activating *GNAS* mutations that stimulate adenylate cyclase have been confirmed as the molecular cause of MAS,[22] in most cases involving a substitution of arginine at position 201 by histidine or cysteine. The variable involvement of endocrine glands, the sporadic occurrence of MAS, and the characteristic pattern of bone and skin lesions, which follows lines of embryologic development, are all in accordance with the mosaic distribution of abnormal cells due to the postzygotic occurrence of *GNAS* mutation (ie, somatic mutation).[253,255] Detection of *GNAS* mutations in the affected tissues is high (90%), whereas peripheral lymphocytes show 21% to 27% positivity in patients with MAS.[256] Germline *GNAS* mutations have not been described, as they are probably lethal to the embryo.[257,258]

The *GNAS* locus displays a complex genomic imprinting, generating multiple alternative products from the paternal and maternal alleles. In humans, tissue-specific imprinting has been demonstrated in the pituitary, where Gsα is exclusively expressed from the maternal allele. In *GNAS* mutation-positive somatotropinomas in MAS, mutations are almost always located in the maternal allele; therefore, acromegaly only occurs in MAS patients with an affected maternal allele.[18,259]

Clinical Aspects

Pituitary disease in MAS is characterized by elevated GH levels, which can be seen in 21% of the cases, and it is often accompanied by hyperprolactinemia; however, only 33% to 65% of MAS with GH excess harbor PAs detectable by imaging studies.[260–262] Pituitary involvement in MAS includes somatotroph hyperplasia (most common) as well as somatotroph, lactotroph, or somatomammotroph adenomas.[260,261] Surgical treatment in MAS-related acromegaly can be difficult due to the presence of craniofacial bone, sphenoidal sinus, and sella turcica lesions (complicating surgical approaches) or absence of PA in the imaging studies. Medical therapies with SSA and DA may lead to disease control, although often only partially, and additional benefit can be obtained with pegvisomant, whereas the role of radiotherapy is controversial.[262,263]

SUMMARY

PAs are relatively common tumors, mostly benign. Pituitary tumorigenesis is determined by inherited and acquired genetic defects as well as epigenetic changes. Most PAs occur sporadically, but around 5% occur in a family setting due to a genetic defect that predispose to adenomas either in isolation or as part of a tumor syndrome. Remarkable advances have been achieved in the past few years in the field of pituitary tumor genetics, with a deeper understanding of their pathophysiology, discovery of new conditions, such as XLAG syndrome, new disease causing mutations (*USP8*), and the recognition of PAs as part of previously known tumor syndromes, such as SDH- or DICER1-related disease. Genetic screening and clinical follow-up of carriers may lead to better long-term outcomes, whereas better understanding of pituitary tumorigenesis can lead to further improvements in terms of diagnosis, treatment, and follow-up for both familiar and sporadic cases of PAs.

SUPPLEMENTARY DATA

Supplementary data related to this article can be found at http://dx.doi.org/10.1016/j.ecl.2017.01.004.

REFERENCES

1. Melmed S. Pituitary tumors. Endocrinol Metab Clin North Am 2015;44(1):1–9.
2. Aflorei ED, Korbonits M. Epidemiology and etiopathogenesis of pituitary adenomas. J Neurooncol 2014;117(3):379–94.
3. Scheithauer BW, Gaffey TA, Lloyd RV, et al. Pathobiology of pituitary adenomas and carcinomas. Neurosurgery 2006;59(2):341–53.
4. Ezzat S, Asa SL, Couldwell WT, et al. The prevalence of pituitary adenomas: a systematic review. Cancer 2004;101(3):613–9.
5. Freda PU, Beckers AM, Katznelson L, et al. Pituitary incidentaloma: an Endocrine Society clinical practice guideline. J Clin Endocrinol Metab 2011;96(4): 894–904.
6. Vasilev V, Rostomyan L, Daly AF, et al. MANAGEMENT OF ENDOCRINE DISEASE: pituitary "incidentaloma": neuroradiological assessment and differential diagnosis. Eur J Endocrinol 2016;175(4):R171–84.
7. Daly AF, Rixhon M, Adam C, et al. High prevalence of pituitary adenomas: a cross-sectional study in the province of Liege, Belgium. J Clin Endocrinol Metab 2006;91(12):4769–75.
8. Fernandez A, Karavitaki N, Wass JA. Prevalence of pituitary adenomas: a community-based, cross-sectional study in Banbury (Oxfordshire, UK). Clin Endocrinol (Oxf) 2010;72(3):377–82.
9. Fontana E, Gaillard R. Epidemiology of pituitary adenoma: results of the first Swiss study. Rev Med Suisse 2009;5(223):2172–4 [in French].
10. Gruppetta M, Mercieca C, Vassallo J. Prevalence and incidence of pituitary adenomas: a population based study in Malta. Pituitary 2013;16(4):545–53.
11. Raappana A, Koivukangas J, Ebeling T, et al. Incidence of pituitary adenomas in Northern Finland in 1992-2007. J Clin Endocrinol Metab 2010;95(9):4268–75.
12. Pease M, Ling C, Mack WJ, et al. The role of epigenetic modification in tumorigenesis and progression of pituitary adenomas: a systematic review of the literature. PLoS One 2013;8(12):e82619.
13. Melmed S. Pathogenesis of pituitary tumors. Nat Rev Endocrinol 2011;7(5): 257–66.
14. Reincke M, Sbiera S, Hayakawa A, et al. Mutations in the deubiquitinase gene USP8 cause Cushing's disease. Nat Genet 2015;47(1):31–8.
15. Ma ZY, Song ZJ, Chen JH, et al. Recurrent gain-of-function USP8 mutations in Cushing's disease. Cell Res 2015;25(3):306–17.
16. Lin Y, Jiang X, Shen Y, et al. Frequent mutations and amplifications of the PIK3CA gene in pituitary tumors. Endocr Relat Cancer 2009;16(1):301–10.
17. Murat CB, Braga PB, Fortes MA, et al. Mutation and genomic amplification of the PIK3CA proto-oncogene in pituitary adenomas. Braz J Med Biol Res 2012;45(9): 851–5.
18. Gadelha MR, Trivellin G, Hernandez Ramirez LC, et al. Genetics of pituitary adenomas. Front Horm Res 2013;41:111–40.
19. Kaltsas GA, Kola B, Borboli N, et al. Sequence analysis of the PRKAR1A gene in sporadic somatotroph and other pituitary tumours. Clin Endocrinol (Oxf) 2002; 57(4):443–8.

20. de Kock L, Sabbaghian N, Plourde F, et al. Pituitary blastoma: a pathognomonic feature of germ-line DICER1 mutations. Acta Neuropathol 2014;128(1):111–22.

21. Leontiou CA, Gueorguiev M, van der Spuy J, et al. The role of the aryl hydrocarbon receptor-interacting protein gene in familial and sporadic pituitary adenomas. J Clin Endocrinol Metab 2008;93(6):2390–401.

22. Weinstein LS, Shenker A, Gejman PV, et al. Activating mutations of the stimulatory G protein in the McCune-Albright syndrome. N Engl J Med 1991;325(24): 1688–95.

23. Landis CA, Masters SB, Spada A, et al. GTPase inhibiting mutations activate the alpha chain of Gs and stimulate adenylyl cyclase in human pituitary tumours. Nature 1989;340(6236):692–6.

24. Rodd C, Millette M, Iacovazzo D, et al. Somatic GPR101 duplication causing X-linked acrogigantism (XLAG)-diagnosis and management. J Clin Endocrinol Metab 2016;101(5):1927–30.

25. Trivellin G, Daly AF, Faucz FR, et al. Gigantism and acromegaly due to Xq26 microduplications and GPR101 mutation. N Engl J Med 2014;371(25):2363–74.

26. Gill AJ, Hes O, Papathomas T, et al. Succinate dehydrogenase (SDH)-deficient renal carcinoma: a morphologically distinct entity: a clinicopathologic series of 36 tumors from 27 patients. Am J Surg Pathol 2014;38(12):1588–602.

27. Thakker RV. Multiple endocrine neoplasia type 1 (MEN1) and type 4 (MEN4). Mol Cell Endocrinol 2014;386(1–2):2–15.

28. Herman V, Fagin J, Gonsky R, et al. Clonal origin of pituitary adenomas. J Clin Endocrinol Metab 1990;71(6):1427–33.

29. Zhou Y, Zhang X, Klibanski A. Genetic and epigenetic mutations of tumor suppressive genes in sporadic pituitary adenoma. Mol Cell Endocrinol 2014; 386(1–2):16–33.

30. Alexander JM, Biller BM, Bikkal H, et al. Clinically nonfunctioning pituitary tumors are monoclonal in origin. J Clin Invest 1990;86(1):336–40.

31. Biller BM, Alexander JM, Zervas NT, et al. Clonal origins of adrenocorticotropin-secreting pituitary tissue in Cushing's disease. J Clin Endocrinol Metab 1992; 75(5):1303–9.

32. Gicquel C, Le Bouc Y, Luton JP, et al. Monoclonality of corticotroph macroadenomas in Cushing's disease. J Clin Endocrinol Metab 1992;75(2):472–5.

33. Jacoby LB, Hedley-Whyte ET, Pulaski K, et al. Clonal origin of pituitary adenomas. J Neurosurg 1990;73(5):731–5.

34. Villa C, Lagonigro MS, Magri F, et al. Hyperplasia-adenoma sequence in pituitary tumorigenesis related to aryl hydrocarbon receptor interacting protein gene mutation. Endocr Relat Cancer 2011;18(3):347–56.

35. Iacovazzo D, Caswell R, Bunce B, et al. Germline or somatic GPR101 duplication leads to X-linked acrogigantism: a clinico-pathological and genetic study. Acta Neuropathol Commun 2016;4(1):56.

36. Joshi AS, Woolf PD. Pituitary hyperplasia secondary to primary hypothyroidism: a case report and review of the literature. Pituitary 2005;8(2):99–103.

37. Lois K, Santhakumar A, Vaikkakara S, et al. Phaeochromocytoma and ACTH-dependent Cushing's syndrome: tumor CRF-secretion can mimic pituitary Cushing's disease. Clin Endocrinol (Oxf) 2016;84(2):177–84.

38. Tada M, Kobayashi H, Moriuchi T. Molecular basis of pituitary oncogenesis. J Neurooncol 1999;45(1):83–96.

39. Spada A, Vallar L. G-protein oncogenes in acromegaly. Horm Res 1992;38(1–2): 90–3.

40. Lania A, Mantovani G, Spada A. Genetics of pituitary tumors: focus on G-protein mutations. Exp Biol Med (Maywood) 2003;228(9):1004–17.

41. Ronchi CL, Peverelli E, Herterich S, et al. Landscape of somatic mutations in sporadic GH-secreting pituitary adenomas. Eur J Endocrinol 2016;174(3): 363–72.

42. Theodoropoulou M, Reincke M, Fassnacht M, et al. Decoding the genetic basis of Cushing's disease: USP8 in the spotlight. Eur J Endocrinol 2015;173(4): M73–83.

43. Mizuno E, Iura T, Mukai A, et al. Regulation of epidermal growth factor receptor down-regulation by UBPY-mediated deubiquitination at endosomes. Mol Biol Cell 2005;16(11):5163–74.

44. Perez-Rivas LG, Theodoropoulou M, Ferrau F, et al. The gene of the ubiquitin-specific protease 8 is frequently mutated in adenomas causing Cushing's disease. J Clin Endocrinol Metab 2015;100(7):997–1004.

45. Hayashi K, Inoshita N, Kawaguchi K, et al. The USP8 mutational status may predict drug susceptibility in corticotroph adenomas of Cushing's disease. Eur J Endocrinol 2016;174(2):213–26.

46. Dworakowska D, Wlodek E, Leontiou CA, et al. Activation of RAF/MEK/ERK and PI3K/AKT/mTOR pathways in pituitary adenomas and their effects on downstream effectors. Endocr Relat Cancer 2009;16(4):1329–38.

47. Orloff MS, He X, Peterson C, et al. Germline PIK3CA and AKT1 mutations in Cowden and Cowden-like syndromes. Am J Hum Genet 2013;92(1):76–80.

48. Cai WY, Alexander JM, Hedley-Whyte ET, et al. ras mutations in human prolactinomas and pituitary carcinomas. J Clin Endocrinol Metab 1994;78(1):89–93.

49. Karga HJ, Alexander JM, Hedley-Whyte ET, et al. Ras mutations in human pituitary tumors. J Clin Endocrinol Metab 1992;74(4):914–9.

50. Kurelac I, MacKay A, Lambros MB, et al. Somatic complex I disruptive mitochondrial DNA mutations are modifiers of tumorigenesis that correlate with low genomic instability in pituitary adenomas. Hum Mol Genet 2013;22(2): 226–38.

51. Niveiro M, Aranda FI, Paya A, et al. Oncocytic transformation in pituitary adenomas: immunohistochemical analyses of 65 cases. Arch Pathol Lab Med 2004;128(7):776–80.

52. Hao S, Hong CS, Feng J, et al. Somatic IDH1 mutation in a pituitary adenoma of a patient with Maffucci syndrome. J Neurosurg 2016;124(6):1562–7.

53. Casar-Borota O, Oystese KA, Sundstrom M, et al. A high-throughput analysis of the IDH1(R132H) protein expression in pituitary adenomas. Pituitary 2016;19(4): 407–14.

54. Asa SL, Ezzat S. The pathogenesis of pituitary tumors. Annu Rev Pathol 2009;4: 97–126.

55. Yoshida S, Kato T, Kato Y. EMT involved in migration of stem/progenitor cells for pituitary development and regeneration. J Clin Med 2016;5(4):43–59.

56. Cannavo S, Ragonese M, Puglisi S, et al. Acromegaly is more severe in patients with AHR or AIP gene variants living in highly polluted areas. J Clin Endocrinol Metab 2016;101(4):1872–9.

57. Cannavo S, Ferrau F, Ragonese M, et al. Increased prevalence of acromegaly in a highly polluted area. Eur J Endocrinol 2010;163(4):509–13.

58. Sapochnik M, Nieto LE, Fuertes M, et al. Molecular mechanisms underlying pituitary pathogenesis. Biochem Genet 2016;54(2):107–19.

59. Jordan S, Lidhar K, Korbonits M, et al. Cyclin D and cyclin E expression in normal and adenomatous pituitary. Eur J Endocrinol 2000;143(1):R1–6.

60. Moreno CS, Evans CO, Zhan X, et al. Novel molecular signaling and classification of human clinically nonfunctional pituitary adenomas identified by gene expression profiling and proteomic analyses. Cancer Res 2005;65(22): 10214–22.
61. Vandeva S, Jaffrain-Rea ML, Daly AF, et al. The genetics of pituitary adenomas. Best Pract Res Clin Endocrinol Metab 2010;24(3):461–76.
62. Quereda V, Malumbres M. Cell cycle control of pituitary development and disease. J Mol Endocrinol 2009;42(2):75–86.
63. Franklin DS, Godfrey VL, Lee H, et al. CDK inhibitors p18(INK4c) and p27(Kip1) mediate two separate pathways to collaboratively suppress pituitary tumorigenesis. Genes Dev 1998;12(18):2899–911.
64. Bamberger CM, Fehn M, Bamberger AM, et al. Reduced expression levels of the cell-cycle inhibitor p27Kip1 in human pituitary adenomas. Eur J Endocrinol 1999;140(3):250–5.
65. Ogino A, Yoshino A, Katayama Y, et al. The p15(INK4b)/p16(INK4a)/RB1 pathway is frequently deregulated in human pituitary adenomas. J Neuropathol Exp Neurol 2005;64(5):398–403.
66. Simpson DJ, Hibberts NA, McNicol AM, et al. Loss of pRb expression in pituitary adenomas is associated with methylation of the RB1 CpG island. Cancer Res 2000;60(5):1211–6.
67. Simpson DJ, Frost SJ, Bicknell JE, et al. Aberrant expression of G(1)/S regulators is a frequent event in sporadic pituitary adenomas. Carcinogenesis 2001; 22(8):1149–54.
68. Hibberts NA, Simpson DJ, Bicknell JE, et al. Analysis of cyclin D1 (CCND1) allelic imbalance and overexpression in sporadic human pituitary tumors. Clin Cancer Res 1999;5(8):2133–9.
69. Saeger W, Schreiber S, Ludecke DK. Cyclins D1 and D3 and topoisomerase II alpha in inactive pituitary adenomas. Endocr Pathol 2001;12(1):39–47.
70. Pei L, Melmed S. Isolation and characterization of a pituitary tumor-transforming gene (PTTG). Mol Endocrinol 1997;11(4):433–41.
71. Salehi F, Kovacs K, Scheithauer BW, et al. Pituitary tumor-transforming gene in endocrine and other neoplasms: a review and update. Endocr Relat Cancer 2008;15(3):721–43.
72. Vlotides G, Eigler T, Melmed S. Pituitary tumor-transforming gene: physiology and implications for tumorigenesis. Endocr Rev 2007;28(2):165–86.
73. Xiao JQ, Liu XH, Hou B, et al. Correlations of pituitary tumor transforming gene expression with human pituitary adenomas: a meta-analysis. PLoS One 2014; 9(3):e90396.
74. Pagotto U, Arzberger T, Theodoropoulou M, et al. The expression of the antiproliferative gene ZAC is lost or highly reduced in nonfunctioning pituitary adenomas. Cancer Res 2000;60(24):6794–9.
75. Zhang X, Sun H, Danila D, et al. Loss of expression of GADD45 gamma, a growth inhibitory gene, in human pituitary adenomas: implications for tumorigenesis. J Clin Endocrinol Metab 2002;87(3):1262–7.
76. Neto L, Wildemberg LE, Colli LM, et al. ZAC1 and SSTR2 are downregulated in non-functioning pituitary adenomas but not in somatotropinomas. PLoS One 2013;8(10):e77406.
77. Gejman R, Batista DL, Zhong Y, et al. Selective loss of MEG3 expression and intergenic differentially methylated region hypermethylation in the MEG3/DLK1 locus in human clinically nonfunctioning pituitary adenomas. J Clin Endocrinol Metab 2008;93(10):4119–25.

78. Missale C, Boroni F, Losa M, et al. Nerve growth factor suppresses the transforming phenotype of human prolactinomas. Proc Natl Acad Sci U S A 1993; 90(17):7961–5.

79. Shorts-Cary L, Xu M, Ertel J, et al. Bone morphogenetic protein and retinoic acid-inducible neural specific protein-3 is expressed in gonadotrope cell pituitary adenomas and induces proliferation, migration, and invasion. Endocrinology 2007;148(3):967–75.

80. Theodoropoulou M, Arzberger T, Gruebler Y, et al. Expression of epidermal growth factor receptor in neoplastic pituitary cells: evidence for a role in corticotropinoma cells. J Endocrinol 2004;183(2):385–94.

81. Schiemann U, Assert R, Moskopp D, et al. Analysis of a protein kinase C-alpha mutation in human pituitary tumours. J Endocrinol 1997;153(1):131–7.

82. Palmieri D, Valentino T, De Martino I, et al. PIT1 upregulation by HMGA proteins has a role in pituitary tumorigenesis. Endocr Relat Cancer 2012;19(2):123–35.

83. Pellegrini I, Barlier A, Gunz G, et al. Pit-1 gene expression in the human pituitary and pituitary adenomas. J Clin Endocrinol Metab 1994;79(1):189–96.

84. Fedele M, Visone R, De Martino I, et al. HMGA2 induces pituitary tumorigenesis by enhancing E2F1 activity. Cancer Cell 2006;9(6):459–71.

85. Elston MS, Gill AJ, Conaglen JV, et al. Wnt pathway inhibitors are strongly downregulated in pituitary tumors. Endocrinology 2008;149(3):1235–42.

86. Gueorguiev M, Grossman AB. Pituitary gland and beta-catenin signaling: from ontogeny to oncogenesis. Pituitary 2009;12(3):245–55.

87. Yuan Z, Sanchez Claros C, Suzuki M, et al. Loss of MEN1 activates DNMT1 implicating DNA hypermethylation as a driver of MEN1 tumorigenesis. Oncotarget 2016;7(11):12633–50.

88. Heaney AP. Clinical review: pituitary carcinoma: difficult diagnosis and treatment. J Clin Endocrinol Metab 2011;96(12):3649–60.

89. Chesnokova V, Zonis S, Ben-Shlomo A, et al. Molecular mechanisms of pituitary adenoma senescence. Front Horm Res 2010;38:7–14.

90. Chesnokova V, Melmed S. Pituitary senescence: the evolving role of Pttg. Mol Cell Endocrinol 2010;326(1–2):55–9.

91. Manojlovic-Gacic E, Skender-Gazibara M, Popovic V, et al. Oncogene-induced senescence in pituitary adenomas-an immunohistochemical Study. Endocr Pathol 2016;27(1):1–11.

92. Alexandraki KI, Khan MM, Chahal HS, et al. Oncogene-induced senescence in pituitary adenomas and carcinomas. Hormones (Athens) 2012;11(3):297–307.

93. Chesnokova V, Zonis S, Zhou C, et al. Lineage-specific restraint of pituitary gonadotroph cell adenoma growth. PLoS One 2011;6(3):e17924.

94. Gadelha MR, Kasuki L, Denes J, et al. MicroRNAs: suggested role in pituitary adenoma pathogenesis. J Endocrinol Invest 2013;36(10):889–95.

95. Di Ieva A, Butz H, Niamah M, et al. MicroRNAs as biomarkers in pituitary tumors. Neurosurgery 2014;75(2):181–9 [discussion: 8–9].

96. Li XH, Wang EL, Zhou HM, et al. MicroRNAs in human pituitary adenomas. Int J Endocrinol 2014;2014:435171.

97. Sivapragasam M, Rotondo F, Lloyd RV, et al. MicroRNAs in the human pituitary. Endocr Pathol 2011;22(3):134–43.

98. Bottoni A, Piccin D, Tagliati F, et al. miR-15a and miR-16-1 down-regulation in pituitary adenomas. J Cell Physiol 2005;204(1):280–5.

99. Leone V, Langella C, D'Angelo D, et al. Mir-23b and miR-130b expression is downregulated in pituitary adenomas. Mol Cell Endocrinol 2014;390(1–2):1–7.

100. Renjie W, Haiqian L. MiR-132, miR-15a and miR-16 synergistically inhibit pituitary tumor cell proliferation, invasion and migration by targeting Sox5. Cancer Lett 2015;356(2 Pt B):568–78.

101. Mussnich P, Raverot G, Jaffrain-Rea ML, et al. Downregulation of miR-410 targeting the cyclin B1 gene plays a role in pituitary gonadotroph tumors. Cell Cycle 2015;14(16):2590–7.

102. Butz H, Liko I, Czirjak S, et al. Down-regulation of Wee1 kinase by a specific subset of microRNA in human sporadic pituitary adenomas. J Clin Endocrinol Metab 2010;95(10):E181–91.

103. Trivellin G, Butz H, Delhove J, et al. MicroRNA miR-107 is overexpressed in pituitary adenomas and inhibits the expression of aryl hydrocarbon receptor-interacting protein in vitro. Am J Physiol Endocrinol Metab 2012;303(6): E708–19.

104. Roche M, Wierinckx A, Croze S, et al. Deregulation of miR-183 and KIAA0101 in aggressive and malignant pituitary tumors. Front Med (lausanne) 2015;2:54.

105. Mao ZG, He DS, Zhou J, et al. Differential expression of microRNAs in GH-secreting pituitary adenomas. Diagn Pathol 2010;5:79.

106. Wang C, Su Z, Sanai N, et al. microRNA expression profile and differentially-expressed genes in prolactinomas following bromocriptine treatment. Oncol Rep 2012;27(5):1312–20.

107. Daly AF, Beckers A. Familial isolated pituitary adenomas (FIPA) and mutations in the aryl hydrocarbon receptor interacting protein (AIP) gene. Endocrinol Metab Clin North Am 2015;44(1):19–25.

108. Beckers A, Aaltonen LA, Daly AF, et al. Familial isolated pituitary adenomas (FIPA) and the pituitary adenoma predisposition due to mutations in the aryl hydrocarbon receptor interacting protein (AIP) gene. Endocr Rev 2013;34(2): 239–77.

109. Hernandez-Ramirez LC, Gabrovska P, Denes J, et al. Landscape of familial isolated and young-onset pituitary adenomas: prospective diagnosis in AIP mutation carriers. J Clin Endocrinol Metab 2015;100(9):E1242–54.

110. Vierimaa O, Georgitsi M, Lehtonen R, et al. Pituitary adenoma predisposition caused by germline mutations in the AIP gene. Science 2006;312(5777): 1228–30.

111. Lloyd C, Grossman A. The AIP (aryl hydrocarbon receptor-interacting protein) gene and its relation to the pathogenesis of pituitary adenomas. Endocrine 2014;46(3):387–96.

112. Tichomirowa MA, Barlier A, Daly AF, et al. High prevalence of AIP gene mutations following focused screening in young patients with sporadic pituitary macroadenomas. Eur J Endocrinol 2011;165(4):509–15.

113. Trivellin G, Korbonits M. AIP and its interacting partners. J Endocrinol 2011; 210(2):137–55.

114. Stockinger B, Di Meglio P, Gialitakis M, et al. The aryl hydrocarbon receptor: multitasking in the immune system. Annu Rev Immunol 2014;32:403–32.

115. Heliovaara E, Raitila A, Launonen V, et al. The expression of AIP-related molecules in elucidation of cellular pathways in pituitary adenomas. Am J Pathol 2009;175(6):2501–7.

116. Chahal HS, Trivellin G, Leontiou CA, et al. Somatostatin analogs modulate AIP in somatotroph adenomas: the role of the ZAC1 pathway. J Clin Endocrinol Metab 2012;97(8):E1411–20.

117. Jaffrain-Rea ML, Angelini M, Gargano D, et al. Expression of aryl hydrocarbon receptor (AHR) and AHR-interacting protein in pituitary adenomas: pathological and clinical implications. Endocr Relat Cancer 2009;16(3):1029–43.

118. Hernandez-Ramirez LC, Martucci F, Morgan RM, et al. Rapid proteasomal degradation of mutant proteins is the primary mechanism leading to tumorigenesis in patients with missense AIP mutations. J Clin Endocrinol Metab 2016; 101(8):3144–54.

119. Lahvis GP, Pyzalski RW, Glover E, et al. The aryl hydrocarbon receptor is required for developmental closure of the ductus venosus in the neonatal mouse. Mol Pharmacol 2005;67(3):714–20.

120. Lin BC, Nguyen LP, Walisser JA, et al. A hypomorphic allele of aryl hydrocarbon receptor-associated protein-9 produces a phenocopy of the AHR-null mouse. Mol Pharmacol 2008;74(5):1367–71.

121. Fernandez-Salguero PM, Hilbert DM, Rudikoff S, et al. Aryl-hydrocarbon receptor-deficient mice are resistant to 2,3,7,8-tetrachlorodibenzo-p-dioxin-induced toxicity. Toxicol Appl Pharmacol 1996;140(1):173–9.

122. Gonzalez FJ, Fernandez-Salguero P. The aryl hydrocarbon receptor: studies using the AHR-null mice. Drug Metab Dispos 1998;26(12):1194–8.

123. Peng L, Mayhew CN, Schnekenburger M, et al. Repression of Ah receptor and induction of transforming growth factor-beta genes in DEN-induced mouse liver tumors. Toxicology 2008;246(2–3):242–7.

124. Barhoover MA, Hall JM, Greenlee WF, et al. Aryl hydrocarbon receptor regulates cell cycle progression in human breast cancer cells via a functional interaction with cyclin-dependent kinase 4. Mol Pharmacol 2010;77(2):195–201.

125. Igreja S, Chahal HS, King P, et al. Characterization of aryl hydrocarbon receptor interacting protein (AIP) mutations in familial isolated pituitary adenoma families. Hum Mutat 2010;31(8):950–60.

126. Tuominen I, Heliovaara E, Raitila A, et al. AIP inactivation leads to pituitary tumorigenesis through defective $G\alpha i$-cAMP signaling. Oncogene 2015;34(9): 1174–84.

127. Fortugno P, Beltrami E, Plescia J, et al. Regulation of survivin function by Hsp90. Proc Natl Acad Sci U S A 2003;100(24):13791–6.

128. Kang BH, Altieri DC. Regulation of survivin stability by the aryl hydrocarbon receptor-interacting protein. J Biol Chem 2006;281(34):24721–7.

129. Canibano C, Rodriguez NL, Saez C, et al. The dependence receptor Ret induces apoptosis in somatotrophs through a Pit-1/p53 pathway, preventing tumor growth. EMBO J 2007;26(8):2015–28.

130. Chahal HS, Stals K, Unterlander M, et al. AIP mutation in pituitary adenomas in the 18th century and today. N Engl J Med 2011;364(1):43–50.

131. Radian S, Diekmann Y, Gabrovska P, et al. Increased population risk of AIP-related acromegaly and gigantism in Ireland. Human Mutation 2017;38:78–85.

132. Guaraldi F, Corazzini V, Gallia GL, et al. Genetic analysis in a patient presenting with meningioma and familial isolated pituitary adenoma (FIPA) reveals selective involvement of the R81X mutation of the AIP gene in the pathogenesis of the pituitary tumor. Pituitary 2012;15(Suppl):61–7.

133. Toledo RA, Mendonca BB, Fragoso MC, et al. Isolated familial somatotropinoma: 11q13-loh and gene/protein expression analysis suggests a possible involvement of AIP also in non-pituitary tumorigenesis. Clinics (Sao Paulo) 2010; 65(4):407–15.

134. Daly AF, Vanbellinghen JF, Khoo SK, et al. Aryl hydrocarbon receptor-interacting protein gene mutations in familial isolated pituitary adenomas: analysis in 73 families. J Clin Endocrinol Metab 2007;92(5):1891–6.

135. Jennings JE, Georgitsi M, Holdaway I, et al. Aggressive pituitary adenomas occurring in young patients in a large Polynesian kindred with a germline R271W mutation in the AIP gene. Eur J Endocrinol 2009;161(5):799–804.

136. Korbonits M, Dutta P, Reddy KS, et al. Exome sequencing reveals double hit by *AIP* gene mutation and copy loss of chromosome 11 but negative X-LAG in a pituitary adenoma of a 4 years child with gigantism treated with multimodal therapy. Paper presented at the Endocrine Society. Boston, April 2, 2016. Available at: https://endo.confex.com/endo/2016endo/webprogram/Paper28082.html.

137. Occhi G, Jaffrain-Rea ML, Trivellin G, et al. The R304X mutation of the aryl hydrocarbon receptor interacting protein gene in familial isolated pituitary adenomas: mutational hot-spot or founder effect? J Endocrinol Invest 2010; 33(11):800–5.

138. Cuny T, Pertuit M, Sahnoun-Fathallah M, et al. Genetic analysis in young patients with sporadic pituitary macroadenomas: besides AIP don't forget MEN1 genetic analysis. Eur J Endocrinol 2013;168(4):533–41.

139. Khoo SK, Pendek R, Nickolov R, et al. Genome-wide scan identifies novel modifier loci of acromegalic phenotypes for isolated familial somatotropinoma. Endocr Relat Cancer 2009;16(3):1057–63.

140. Lecoq AL, Bouligand J, Hage M, et al. Very low frequency of germline GPR101 genetic variation and no biallelic defects with AIP in a large cohort of patients with sporadic pituitary adenomas. Eur J Endocrinol 2016;174(4):523–30.

141. Daly AF, Tichomirowa MA, Petrossians P, et al. Clinical characteristics and therapeutic responses in patients with germ-line AIP mutations and pituitary adenomas: an international collaborative study. J Clin Endocrinol Metab 2010; 95(11):E373–83.

142. Beckers A, Daly AF. The clinical, pathological, and genetic features of familial isolated pituitary adenomas. Eur J Endocrinol 2007;157(4):371–82.

143. Rostomyan L, Daly AF, Petrossians P, et al. Clinical and genetic characterization of pituitary gigantism: an international collaborative study in 208 patients. Endocr Relat Cancer 2015;22(5):745–57.

144. Xekouki P, Mastroyiannis SA, Avgeropoulos D, et al. Familial pituitary apoplexy as the only presentation of a novel AIP mutation. Endocr Relat Cancer 2013; 20(5):L11–4.

145. Kasuki L, Vieira Neto L, Armondi Wildemberg LE, et al. Low aryl hydrocarbon receptor-interacting protein expression is a better marker of invasiveness in somatotropinomas than Ki-67 and p53. Neuroendocrinology 2011;94(1):39–48.

146. Kasuki L, Vieira Neto L, Wildemberg LE, et al. AIP expression in sporadic somatotropinomas is a predictor of the response to octreotide LAR therapy independent of SSTR2 expression. Endocr Relat Cancer 2012;19(3):L25–9.

147. Jaffrain-Rea ML, Rotondi S, Turchi A, et al. Somatostatin analogues increase AIP expression in somatotropinomas, irrespective of Gsp mutations. Endocr Relat Cancer 2013;20(5):753–66.

148. Gadelha MR, Kasuki L, Korbonits M. Novel pathway for somatostatin analogs in patients with acromegaly. Trends Endocrinol Metab 2013;24(5):238–46.

149. Iacovazzo D, Carlsen E, Lugli F, et al. Factors predicting pasireotide responsiveness in somatotroph pituitary adenomas resistant to first-generation somatostatin analogues: an immunohistochemical study. Eur J Endocrinol 2016; 174(2):241–50.

150. Korbonits M, Storr H, Kumar AV. Familial pituitary adenomas—who should be tested for AIP mutations? Clin Endocrinol (Oxf) 2012;77(3):351–6.

151. Williams F, Hunter S, Bradley L, et al. Clinical experience in the screening and management of a large kindred with familial isolated pituitary adenoma due to an aryl hydrocarbon receptor interacting protein (AIP) mutation. J Clin Endocrinol Metab 2014;99(4):1122–31.

152. Schofl C, Honegger J, Droste M, et al. Frequency of AIP gene mutations in young patients with acromegaly: a registry-based study. J Clin Endocrinol Metab 2014;99(12):E2789–93.

153. Beckers A, Lodish MB, Trivellin G, et al. X-linked acrogigantism syndrome: clinical profile and therapeutic responses. Endocr Relat Cancer 2015;22(3):353–67.

154. Daly AF, Yuan B, Fina F, et al. Somatic mosaicism underlies X-linked acrogigantism syndrome in sporadic male subjects. Endocr Relat Cancer 2016;23(4):221–33.

155. Trivellin G, Correa RR, Batsis M, et al. Screening for GPR101 defects in pediatric pituitary corticotropinomas. Endocr Relat Cancer 2016;23(5):357–65.

156. Peverelli E, Mantovani G, Lania AG, et al. cAMP in the pituitary: an old messenger for multiple signals. J Mol Endocrinol 2014;52(1):R67–77.

157. Daly AF, Lysy PA, Desfilles C, et al. GHRH excess and blockade in X-LAG syndrome. Endocr Relat Cancer 2016;23(3):161–70.

158. Moran A, Asa SL, Kovacs K, et al. Gigantism due to pituitary mammosomatotroph hyperplasia. N Engl J Med 1990;323(5):322–7.

159. Castinetti F, Daly AF, Stratakis CA, et al. GPR101 mutations are not a frequent cause of congenital isolated growth hormone deficiency. Horm Metab Res 2016;48(6):389–93.

160. Naves LA, Daly AF, Dias LA, et al. Aggressive tumor growth and clinical evolution in a patient with X-linked acro-gigantism syndrome. Endocrine 2016;51(2):236–44.

161. Kong A, Frigge ML, Masson G, et al. Rate of de novo mutations and the importance of father's age to disease risk. Nature 2012;488(7412):471–5.

162. Schernthaner-Reiter MH, Trivellin G, Stratakis CA. MEN1, MEN4, and Carney complex: pathology and molecular genetics. Neuroendocrinology 2016;103(1):18–31.

163. Thakker RV, Newey PJ, Walls GV, et al. Clinical practice guidelines for multiple endocrine neoplasia type 1 (MEN1). J Clin Endocrinol Metab 2012;97(9):2990–3011.

164. Chandrasekharappa SC, Guru SC, Manickam P, et al. Positional cloning of the gene for multiple endocrine neoplasia-type 1. Science 1997;276(5311):404–7.

165. Lemmens I, Van de Ven WJ, Kas K, et al. Identification of the multiple endocrine neoplasia type 1 (MEN1) gene. The European Consortium on MEN1. Hum Mol Genet 1997;6(7):1177–83.

166. Luzi E, Marini F, Giusti F, et al. The negative feedback-loop between the oncomir Mir-24-1 and menin modulates the Men1 tumorigenesis by mimicking the "Knudson's second hit". PLoS One 2012;7(6):e39767.

167. Lemos MC, Thakker RV. Multiple endocrine neoplasia type 1 (MEN1): analysis of 1336 mutations reported in the first decade following identification of the gene. Hum Mutat 2008;29(1):22–32.

168. Thakker RV. Genetics of parathyroid tumours. J Intern Med 2016;280(6):574–83.

169. Fontaniere S, Tost J, Wierinckx A, et al. Gene expression profiling in insulinomas of Men1 beta-cell mutant mice reveals early genetic and epigenetic events

involved in pancreatic beta-cell tumorigenesis. Endocr Relat Cancer 2006; 13(4):1223–36.

170. La P, Schnepp RW, D Petersen C, et al. Tumor suppressor menin regulates expression of insulin-like growth factor binding protein 2. Endocrinology 2004; 145(7):3443–50.

171. Hashimoto M, Kyo S, Hua X, et al. Role of menin in the regulation of telomerase activity in normal and cancer cells. Int J Oncol 2008;33(2):333–40.

172. Hughes CM, Rozenblatt-Rosen O, Milne TA, et al. Menin associates with a tri-thorax family histone methyltransferase complex and with the hoxc8 locus. Mol Cell 2004;13(4):587–97.

173. Wu T, Hua X. Menin represses tumorigenesis via repressing cell proliferation. Am J Cancer Res 2011;1(6):726–39.

174. Gillam MP, Nimbalkar D, Sun L, et al. MEN1 tumorigenesis in the pituitary and pancreatic islet requires Cdk4 but not Cdk2. Oncogene 2015;34(7):932–8.

175. Concolino P, Costella A, Capoluongo E. Multiple endocrine neoplasia type 1 (MEN1): an update of 208 new germline variants reported in the last nine years. Cancer Genet 2016;209(1–2):36–41.

176. Machens A, Schaaf L, Karges W, et al. Age-related penetrance of endocrine tu-mours in multiple endocrine neoplasia type 1 (MEN1): a multicentre study of 258 gene carriers. Clin Endocrinol (Oxf) 2007;67(4):613–22.

177. Cavaco BM, Domingues R, Bacelar MC, et al. Mutational analysis of Portuguese families with multiple endocrine neoplasia type 1 reveals large germline dele-tions. Clin Endocrinol (Oxf) 2002;56(4):465–73.

178. Bassett JH, Forbes SA, Pannett AA, et al. Characterization of mutations in pa-tients with multiple endocrine neoplasia type 1. Am J Hum Genet 1998;62(2): 232–44.

179. Thevenon J, Bourredjem A, Faivre L, et al. Unraveling the intrafamilial correla-tions and heritability of tumor types in MEN1: a Groupe d'etude des Tumeurs En-docrines study. Eur J Endocrinol 2015;173(6):819–26.

180. Thevenon J, Bourredjem A, Faivre L, et al. Higher risk of death among MEN1 patients with mutations in the JunD interacting domain: a Groupe d'etude des Tumeurs Endocrines (GTE) cohort study. Hum Mol Genet 2013;22(10):1940–8.

181. Peculis R, Balcere I, Rovite V, et al. Polymorphisms in MEN1 and DRD2 genes are associated with the occurrence and characteristics of pituitary adenomas. Eur J Endocrinol 2016;175(2):145–53.

182. de Laat JM, Dekkers OM, Pieterman CR, et al. Long-term natural course of pi-tuitary tumors in patients with MEN1: results from the DutchMEN1 Study Group (DMSG). J Clin Endocrinol Metab 2015;100(9):3288–96.

183. Goudet P, Murat A, Binquet C, et al. Risk factors and causes of death in MEN1 disease. A GTE (Groupe d'Etude des Tumeurs Endocrines) cohort study among 758 patients. World J Surg 2010;34(2):249–55.

184. Trouillas J, Labat-Moleur F, Sturm N, et al. Pituitary tumors and hyperplasia in multiple endocrine neoplasia type 1 syndrome (MEN1): a case-control study in a series of 77 patients versus 2509 non-MEN1 patients. Am J Surg Pathol 2008;32(4):534–43.

185. Verges B, Boureille F, Goudet P, et al. Pituitary disease in MEN type 1 (MEN1): data from the France-Belgium MEN1 multicenter study. J Clin Endocrinol Metab 2002;87(2):457–65.

186. Sakurai A, Suzuki S, Kosugi S, et al. Multiple endocrine neoplasia type 1 in Japan: establishment and analysis of a multicentre database. Clin Endocrinol (Oxf) 2012;76(4):533–9.

187. Stratakis CA, Schussheim DH, Freedman SM, et al. Pituitary macroadenoma in a 5-year-old: an early expression of multiple endocrine neoplasia type 1. J Clin Endocrinol Metab 2000;85(12):4776–80.

188. Shull JD, Birt DF, McComb RD, et al. Estrogen induction of prolactin-producing pituitary tumors in the Fischer 344 rat: modulation by dietary-energy but not protein consumption. Mol Carcinog 1998;23(2):96–105.

189. Newey PJ, Thakker RV. Role of multiple endocrine neoplasia type 1 mutational analysis in clinical practice. Endocr Pract 2011;17(Suppl 3):8–17.

190. Gan HW, Bulwer C, Jeelani O, et al. Treatment-resistant pediatric giant prolactinoma and multiple endocrine neoplasia type 1. Int J Pediatr Endocrinol 2015; 2015(1):15.

191. Pellegata NS, Quintanilla-Martinez L, Siggelkow H, et al. Germ-line mutations in p27Kip1 cause a multiple endocrine neoplasia syndrome in rats and humans. Proc Natl Acad Sci U S A 2006;103(42):15558–63.

192. Igreja S, Chahal H, Akker S, et al. Assessment of p27 (cyclin-dependent kinase inhibitor 1B) and aryl hydrocarbon receptor-interacting protein (AIP) genes in multiple endocrine neoplasia (MEN1) syndrome patients without any detectable MEN1 gene mutations. Clin Endocrinol (Oxf) 2009;70(2):259–64.

193. Occhi G, Regazzo D, Trivellin G, et al. A novel mutation in the upstream open reading frame of the CDKN1B gene causes a MEN4 phenotype. PLoS Genet 2013;9(3):e1003350.

194. Agarwal SK, Mateo C, Marx SJ. Rare germline mutations in cyclin-dependent kinase inhibitor genes in multiple endocrine neoplasia type 1 and related states. J Clin Endocrinol Metab 2009;94(5):1826–34.

195. James MK, Ray A, Leznova D, et al. Differential modification of p27Kip1 controls its cyclin D-cdk4 inhibitory activity. Mol Cell Biol. 2008;28(1):498–510.

196. Andreu EJ, Lledo E, Poch E, et al. BCR-ABL induces the expression of Skp2 through the PI3K pathway to promote p27Kip1 degradation and proliferation of chronic myelogenous leukemia cells. Cancer Res 2005;65(8):3264–72.

197. Donovan JC, Milic A, Slingerland JM. Constitutive MEK/MAPK activation leads to p27(Kip1) deregulation and antiestrogen resistance in human breast cancer cells. J Biol Chem 2001;276(44):40888–95.

198. Bugalho MJ, Domingues R. Uncommon association of cerebral meningioma, parathyroid adenoma and papillary thyroid carcinoma in a patient harbouring a rare germline variant in the CDKN1B gene. BMJ Case Rep 2016.

199. Malanga D, De Gisi S, Riccardi M, et al. Functional characterization of a rare germline mutation in the gene encoding the cyclin-dependent kinase inhibitor p27Kip1 (CDKN1B) in a Spanish patient with multiple endocrine neoplasia-like phenotype. Eur J Endocrinol 2012;166(3):551–60.

200. Molatore S, Marinoni I, Lee M, et al. A novel germline CDKN1B mutation causing multiple endocrine tumors: clinical, genetic and functional characterization. Hum Mutat 2010;31(11):E1825–35.

201. Georgitsi M, Raitila A, Karhu A, et al. Germline CDKN1B/p27Kip1 mutation in multiple endocrine neoplasia. J Clin Endocrinol Metab 2007;92(8):3321–5.

202. Tichomirowa MA, Lee M, Barlier A, et al. Cyclin-dependent kinase inhibitor 1B (CDKN1B) gene variants in AIP mutation-negative familial isolated pituitary adenoma kindreds. Endocr Relat Cancer 2012;19(3):233–41.

203. Carney JA, Gordon H, Carpenter PC, et al. The complex of myxomas, spotty pigmentation, and endocrine overactivity. Medicine (Baltimore) 1985;64(4): 270–83.

204. Bertherat J. Carney complex (CNC). Orphanet J Rare Dis 2006;1:21.

205. Stratakis CA. Clinical genetics of multiple endocrine neoplasias, Carney complex and related syndromes. J Endocrinol Invest 2001;24(5):370–83.
206. Stratakis CA, Kirschner LS, Carney JA. Clinical and molecular features of the Carney complex: diagnostic criteria and recommendations for patient evaluation. J Clin Endocrinol Metab 2001;86(9):4041–6.
207. Kirschner LS, Sandrini F, Monbo J, et al. Genetic heterogeneity and spectrum of mutations of the PRKAR1A gene in patients with the Carney complex. Hum Mol Genet 2000;9(20):3037–46.
208. Correa R, Salpea P, Stratakis CA. Carney complex: an update. Eur J Endocrinol 2015;173(4):85–97.
209. Bertherat J, Horvath A, Groussin L, et al. Mutations in regulatory subunit type 1A of cyclic adenosine 5'-monophosphate-dependent protein kinase (PRKAR1A): phenotype analysis in 353 patients and 80 different genotypes. J Clin Endocrinol Metab 2009;94(6):2085–91.
210. Kirschner LS, Carney JA, Pack SD, et al. Mutations of the gene encoding the protein kinase A type I-alpha regulatory subunit in patients with the Carney complex. Nat Genet 2000;26(1):89–92.
211. Horvath A, Bossis I, Giatzakis C, et al. Large deletions of the PRKAR1A gene in Carney complex. Clin Cancer Res 2008;14(2):388–95.
212. Ragazzon B, Cazabat L, Rizk-Rabin M, et al. Inactivation of the Carney complex gene 1 (protein kinase A regulatory subunit 1A) inhibits SMAD3 expression and TGF beta-stimulated apoptosis in adrenocortical cells. Cancer Res 2009;69(18): 7278–84.
213. Robinson-White A, Hundley TR, Shiferaw M, et al. Protein kinase-A activity in PRKAR1A-mutant cells, and regulation of mitogen-activated protein kinases ERK1/2. Hum Mol Genet 2003;12(13):1475–84.
214. Robinson-White AJ, Leitner WW, Aleem E, et al. PRKAR1A inactivation leads to increased proliferation and decreased apoptosis in human B lymphocytes. Cancer Res 2006;66(21):10603–12.
215. Horvath A, Bertherat J, Groussin L, et al. Mutations and polymorphisms in the gene encoding regulatory subunit type 1-alpha of protein kinase A (PRKAR1A): an update. Hum Mutat 2010;31(4):369–79.
216. Salpea P, Horvath A, London E, et al. Deletions of the PRKAR1A locus at 17q24.2-q24.3 in Carney complex: genotype-phenotype correlations and implications for genetic testing. J Clin Endocrinol Metab 2014;99(1):E183–8.
217. Salpea P, Stratakis CA. Carney complex and McCune Albright syndrome: an overview of clinical manifestations and human molecular genetics. Mol Cell Endocrinol 2014;386(1–2):85–91.
218. Matyakhina L, Pack S, Kirschner LS, et al. Chromosome 2 (2p16) abnormalities in Carney complex tumours. J Med Genet 2003;40(4):268–77.
219. Forlino A, Vetro A, Garavelli L, et al. PRKACB and Carney complex. N Engl J Med 2014;370(11):1065–7.
220. Groussin L, Horvath A, Jullian E, et al. A PRKAR1A mutation associated with primary pigmented nodular adrenocortical disease in 12 kindreds. J Clin Endocrinol Metab 2006;91(5):1943–9.
221. Libe R, Horvath A, Vezzosi D, et al. Frequent phosphodiesterase 11A gene (PDE11A) defects in patients with Carney complex (CNC) caused by PRKAR1A mutations: PDE11A may contribute to adrenal and testicular tumors in CNC as a modifier of the phenotype. J Clin Endocrinol Metab 2011;96(1):208–14.
222. Boikos SA, Stratakis CA. Carney complex: the first 20 years. Curr Opin Oncol 2007;19(1):24–9.

223. Kirschner LS. PRKAR1A and the evolution of pituitary tumors. Mol Cell Endocrinol 2010;326(1–2):3–7.
224. Boikos SA, Stratakis CA. Pituitary pathology in patients with Carney Complex: growth-hormone producing hyperplasia or tumors and their association with other abnormalities. Pituitary 2006;9(3):203–9.
225. Courcoutsakis NA, Tatsi C, Patronas NJ, et al. The complex of myxomas, spotty skin pigmentation and endocrine overactivity (Carney complex): imaging findings with clinical and pathological correlation. Insights Imaging 2013;4(1):119–33.
226. Watson JC, Stratakis CA, Bryant-Greenwood PK, et al. Neurosurgical implications of Carney complex. J Neurosurg 2000;92(3):413–8.
227. Pack SD, Kirschner LS, Pak E, et al. Genetic and histologic studies of somatomammotropic pituitary tumors in patients with the "complex of spotty skin pigmentation, myxomas, endocrine overactivity and schwannomas" (Carney complex). J Clin Endocrinol Metab 2000;85(10):3860–5.
228. Stratakis CA, Matyakhina L, Courkoutsakis N, et al. Pathology and molecular genetics of the pituitary gland in patients with the 'complex of spotty skin pigmentation, myxomas, endocrine overactivity and schwannomas' (Carney complex). Front Horm Res 2004;32:253–64.
229. Larkin SJ, Ferrau F, Karavitaki N, et al. Sequence analysis of the catalytic subunit of PKA in somatotroph adenomas. Eur J Endocrinol 2014;171(6):705–10.
230. Iversen K. Acromegaly associated with phaeochromocytoma. Acta Med Scand 1952;142(1):1–5.
231. Benn DE, Gimenez-Roqueplo AP, Reilly JR, et al. Clinical presentation and penetrance of pheochromocytoma/paraganglioma syndromes. J Clin Endocrinol Metab 2006;91(3):827–36.
232. Lopez-Jimenez E, de Campos JM, Kusak EM, et al. SDHC mutation in an elderly patient without familial antecedents. Clin Endocrinol (Oxf) 2008;69(6):906–10.
233. Denes J, Swords F, Rattenberry E, et al. Heterogeneous genetic background of the association of pheochromocytoma/paraganglioma and pituitary adenoma: results from a large patient cohort. J Clin Endocrinol Metab 2015;100(3):E531–41.
234. Papathomas TG, Gaal J, Corssmit EP, et al. Non-pheochromocytoma (PCC)/paraganglioma (PGL) tumors in patients with succinate dehydrogenase-related PCC-PGL syndromes: a clinicopathological and molecular analysis. Eur J Endocrinol 2014;170(1):1–12.
235. Xekouki P, Pacak K, Almeida M, et al. Succinate dehydrogenase (SDH) D subunit (SDHD) inactivation in a growth-hormone-producing pituitary tumor: a new association for SDH? J Clin Endocrinol Metab 2012;97(3):E357–66.
236. Xekouki P, Szarek E, Bullova P, et al. Pituitary adenoma with paraganglioma/pheochromocytoma (3PAs) and succinate dehydrogenase defects in humans and mice. J Clin Endocrinol Metab 2015;100(5):E710–9.
237. O'Toole SM, Denes J, Robledo M, et al. 15 YEARS OF PARAGANGLIOMA: the association of pituitary adenomas and phaeochromocytomas or paragangliomas. Endocr Relat Cancer 2015;22(4):T105–22.
238. Johnston PC, Kennedy L, Recinos PF, et al. Cushing's disease and co-existing phaeochromocytoma. Pituitary 2016;19(6):654–6.
239. Skoura E, Datseris IE, Xekouki P, et al. SPECT and 18F-FDG PET/CT imaging of multiple paragangliomas and a growth hormone-producing pituitary adenoma as phenotypes from a novel succinate dehydrogenase subunit D mutation. Clin Nucl Med 2014;39(1):81–3.

240. Gimenez-Roqueplo AP, Dahia PL, Robledo M. An update on the genetics of paraganglioma, pheochromocytoma, and associated hereditary syndromes. Horm Metab Res 2012;44(5):328–33.
241. Selak MA, Armour SM, MacKenzie ED, et al. Succinate links TCA cycle dysfunction to oncogenesis by inhibiting HIF-alpha prolyl hydroxylase. Cancer Cell 2005;7(1):77–85.
242. Brahma A, Heyburn P, Swords F. Familial prolactinoma occurring in association with SDHB mutation positive paraganglioma. Endocr Abstr Spring 2009;19:P239.
243. Gill AJ, Toon CW, Clarkson A, et al. Succinate dehydrogenase deficiency is rare in pituitary adenomas. Am J Surg Pathol 2014;38(4):560–6.
244. Heinlen JE, Buethe DD, Culkin DJ, et al. Multiple endocrine neoplasia 2a presenting with pheochromocytoma and pituitary macroadenoma. ISRN Oncol 2011;2011:732452.
245. Naziat A, Karavitaki N, Thakker R, et al. Confusing genes: a patient with MEN2A and Cushing's disease. Clin Endocrinol (Oxf) 2013;78(6):966–8.
246. Scheithauer BW, Kovacs K, Horvath E, et al. Pituitary blastoma. Acta Neuropathol 2008;116(6):657–66.
247. Scheithauer BW, Horvath E, Abel TW, et al. Pituitary blastoma: a unique embryonal tumor. Pituitary 2012;15(3):365–73.
248. Wildi-Runge S, Bahubeshi A, Carret S, et al. New phenotype in the familial DICER1 tumor syndrome: pituitary blastoma presenting at age 9 months. Endocr Rev 2011;32(03_MeetingAbstracts):P1–777.
249. Sahakitrungruang T, Srichomthong C, Pornkunwilai S, et al. Germline and somatic DICER1 mutations in a pituitary blastoma causing infantile-onset Cushing's disease. J Clin Endocrinol Metab 2014;99(8):E1487–92.
250. Bahubeshi A, Bal N, Rio Frio T, et al. Germline DICER1 mutations and familial cystic nephroma. J Med Genet 2010;47(12):863–6.
251. Foulkes WD, Bahubeshi A, Hamel N, et al. Extending the phenotypes associated with DICER1 mutations. Hum Mutat 2011;32(12):1381–4.
252. Hill DA, Ivanovich J, Priest JR, et al. DICER1 mutations in familial pleuropulmonary blastoma. Science 2009;325(5943):965.
253. Dumitrescu CE, Collins MT. McCune-Albright syndrome. Orphanet J Rare Dis 2008;3:12.
254. Collins MT, Singer FR, Eugster E. McCune-Albright syndrome and the extraskeletal manifestations of fibrous dysplasia. Orphanet J Rare Dis 2012;7(Suppl 1):S4.
255. Weinstein LS, Yu S, Warner DR, et al. Endocrine manifestations of stimulatory G protein alpha-subunit mutations and the role of genomic imprinting. Endocr Rev 2001;22(5):675–705.
256. Lumbroso S, Paris F, Sultan C, European Collaborative Study. Activating Gsalpha mutations: analysis of 113 patients with signs of McCune-Albright syndrome–a European Collaborative Study. J Clin Endocrinol Metab 2004;89(5):2107–13.
257. Happle R. The McCune-Albright syndrome: a lethal gene surviving by mosaicism. Clin Genet 1986;29(4):321–4.
258. Weinstein LS, Liu J, Sakamoto A, et al. Minireview: GNAS: normal and abnormal functions. Endocrinology 2004;145(12):5459–64.
259. Hayward BE, Barlier A, Korbonits M, et al. Imprinting of the G(s)alpha gene GNAS1 in the pathogenesis of acromegaly. J Clin Invest 2001;107(6):R31–6.

260. Akintoye SO, Chebli C, Booher S, et al. Characterization of gsp-mediated growth hormone excess in the context of McCune-Albright syndrome. J Clin Endocrinol Metab 2002;87(11):5104–12.
261. Vortmeyer AO, Glasker S, Mehta GU, et al. Somatic GNAS mutation causes widespread and diffuse pituitary disease in acromegalic patients with McCune-Albright syndrome. J Clin Endocrinol Metab 2012;97(7):2404–13.
262. Salenave S, Boyce AM, Collins MT, et al. Acromegaly and McCune-Albright syndrome. J Clin Endocrinol Metab 2014;99(6):1955–69.
263. Galland F, Kamenicky P, Affres H, et al. McCune-Albright syndrome and acromegaly: effects of hypothalamopituitary radiotherapy and/or pegvisomant in somatostatin analog-resistant patients. J Clin Endocrinol Metab 2006;91(12):4957–61.

Defects of Thyroid Hormone Synthesis and Action

Zeina C. Hannoush, MD, Roy E. Weiss, MD, PhD*

KEYWORDS

- Thyroid hormone receptors • Deiodinase • Resistance to thyroid hormone
- Congenital hypothyroidism • Goiter • Dyshormonogenesis • Dysgenesis

KEY POINTS

- Diagnosis of thyroid disease has evolved to involve sophisticated genetic testing of candidate genes to confirm the cause of the thyroid disease.
- Congenital hypothyroidism in the absence of a goiter points to thyroid-stimulating hormone receptor (*TSHR*), Paired Box Gene 8 (*PAX8*), *TTF1*, *FOXE1*, *NKX2-5*, and *DUOX2* gene mutations.
- Congenital hypothyroidism in the presence of a goiter and a low radioactive iodine uptake suggest a sodium iodine symporter mutation.
- Congenital hypothyroidism in the presence of a goiter and high uptake suggests a thyroperoxidase (*TPO*), thyroglobulin (*Tg*), *DUOX2* and *DUOXA2* and *DEHALI*, or *PDS* gene defect.
- Knowledge of the physiologic consequences of genetic mutations can help lead to rational recognition plans and treatment.

INTRODUCTION

In the beginning (before the genomic revolution) thyroid disorders were primarily diagnosed by the presence of a goiter and thought to be due to either deficiency or excess of iodine. Many years later, in 1956, an autoimmune cause was proposed.[1] The clinical tools available to the physicians in those years consisted of measurement of protein-bound iodine (PBI) in the serum as a marker of thyroid hormone (TH) concentration, use of a Geiger counter to measure iodine uptake into the gland with radioactive iodine, as well as measurements of radioiodine discharge after treatment with perchlorate and basal metabolic rates as a surrogate for TH action. Remarkably clinician

The authors have nothing to disclose.
Funded by the National Institutes of Health, grant number: DK015070; NIHMS-ID: 842766.
Department of Medicine, University of Miami Miller School of Medicine, 1120 NW 14th Street, Suite 310F, Miami, FL 33136, USA
* Corresponding author.
E-mail address: rweiss@med.miami.edu

Endocrinol Metab Clin N Am 46 (2017) 375–388
http://dx.doi.org/10.1016/j.ecl.2017.01.005

scientists have mapped most pathways involved in TH synthesis and action based on these rudimentary tests. The sentinel observations of astute physicians more than 50 years ago are responsible for our current outlook on diagnosis and treatment of thyroid disease. Such individuals are Vaughan Pendred[2] who reported 2 sisters having goiter and deafness; John Stanbury and A.N. Hedge[3] who described 3 siblings with congenital hypothyroidism (CH) and goiter, likely due to a defect in organification of iodine; and Samuel Refetoff, Leslie DeGroot, and Laurence DeWind[4] who described a family with insensitivity to TH. As biochemical techniques developed and a clearer understanding of TH synthesis ensued, new pathways were discovered relating to TH synthesis and action. However, the notion that a defect was inherited predated any knowledge of molecular biology. Additionally, in so much as understanding the physiology has been informative with regard to identifying candidate genes (defects in TH receptors, defects in peroxidase), gene linkage and analysis has led to a deeper understanding of new mechanisms and pathways of TH synthesis and action (eg, *DUOXA,* Paired Box Gene 8 [*PAX8*], monocarboxylate transporter 8 [*MCT8*]). Furthermore, when discovering the involvement of a particular gene mutation as the cause of a thyroid defect, there needs to be convincing evidence of the structure-function relationship of the gene and proof that it is responsible for the phenotype (**Figs. 1** and **2**).

We are at a crossroad in diagnosing thyroid disease having evolved from PBI and iodine uptake to sophisticated chips that screen patients' DNA samples for a variety of common binding protein abnormalities or receptor mutations whether it be the TH receptor beta (*THRB*), thyroid-stimulating hormone (TSH) receptors (*TSHRs*), or something else. The purpose of this article is to present a succinct review of the genetic causes of abnormalities in TH synthesis and action exclusive of thyroid cancer,

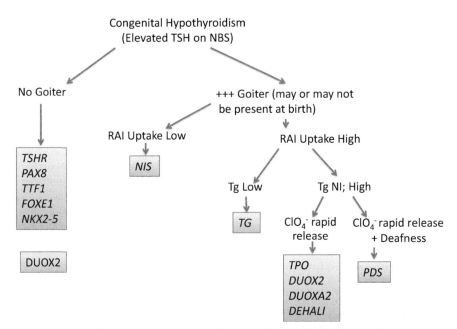

Fig. 1. Algorithm for genetic screening for disorders of TH synthesis. NBS, newborn screening; NI, normal; *NIS*, sodium iodine symporter; *PAX8*, Paired Box Gene 8; RAI, radioactive iodine; *Tg*, serum thyroglobulin; *TPO*, thyroperoxidase; TSH, thyroid-stimulating hormone; *TSHR*, thyroid-stimulating hormone receptor.

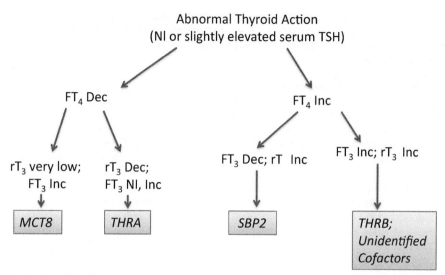

Fig. 2. Algorithm for genetic screening for disorders of TH action. Dec, decrease; FT₃, free T₃; FT₄, free T₄; Inc, increase; *MCT8*, monocarboxylate transporter 8; Nl, normal; rT₃, reverse T₃; *THRB*, TH receptor beta; TSH, thyroid-stimulating hormone.

which is covered in Andrew J. Bauer's article, "Molecular Genetics of Thyroid Cancer in Children and Adolescents," in this issue.

TH is essential for the development and regulation of metabolism and function of virtually all human tissue.[5,6] Inherited disorders of TH synthesis and action are by definition present at birth and can usually be diagnosed then, but the clinical manifestations may not occur until later in life. CH is defined as functional inactivity of TH from birth. It can be in the absence or in the presence of a goiter. Phenotypes based on thyroid function tests can show various permutations from elevated TSH and low 3,5,3',5'-tetra-iodo-L-thyronine (T_4) serum concentrations to other derangements, such as elevated TH levels and nonsuppressed TSH (syndromes of TH unresponsiveness). CH is the most common inborn endocrine disorder with a prevalence of 3000 to 4000 newborns.[7] In absence of adequate treatment, CH is characterized by signs and symptoms of impaired metabolism and by motor and mental developmental delays. Before the introduction of neonatal screening programs, which allowed for early diagnosis and treatment, CH was one of the most common causes of mental retardation.[8] CH can be caused by abnormalities of thyroid gland development and migration (dysgenesis), by inherited defects in one of the steps of TH synthesis (dyshormonogenesis), by problems in intracellular TH transport, metabolism, or at the level of its action as a regulator of gene transcription in the target tissue. The molecular basis of the defects has been elucidated in only a small portion of patients with CH.

Agoitrous Congenital Hypothyroidism: Defects in Thyroid Development

Thyroid dysgenesis accounts for 80% to 85% of the cases of CH. These defects may take the form of complete absence of one or both of the lobes of the thyroid or failure of the gland to descend properly during embryologic development (ectopic). The gold standard for differentiating between the various forms of thyroid dysgenesis is the scintigraphy with ^{99m}sodium (Na^+) pertechnetate or ^{123}iodine (I), as ultrasound examination generally fails to reveal an ectopic thyroid, which is the most common cause of thyroid dysgenesis.[9]

Thyroid dysgenesis is generally a sporadic disease, and in about 5% of the cases a molecular basis has been identified.[8] The most common genes reported to be associated with alteration in thyroid morphogenesis are *TSHR, PAX8, TTF1, FOXE1, NKX2-5*, and *HHEX* (**Table 1**).

Thyroid-stimulating hormone receptor gene
TSHR encodes a transmembrane receptor present on the surface of follicular cells, which mediates the effects of TSH secreted by the anterior pituitary and is critical for the development and function of the thyroid gland.[7] Several cases with homozygous or compound heterozygous loss-of-function *TSHR* mutations have been reported.[8,10] The phenotype of these patients is very variable, ranging from asymptomatic hyperthyrotropinemia to severe CH. The disease is classically inherited in an autosomal recessive trait, although it has become apparent that heterozygotes can have a mild phenotype, which is transmitted in a dominant fashion. Patients are characterized by elevated serum TSH, absence of goiter with a normal hypoplastic gland that does not trap pertechnetate, and surprisingly detectable thyroglobulin (TG) levels with normal to very low levels of TH.[9]

Paired Box Gene 8 gene
PAX8 is a transcriptional factor that plays an important role in the initiation of thyrocyte differentiation and maintenance of follicular cells; furthermore, it regulates the expression of TG, thyroperoxidase (TPO), and the Na^+ I symporter (NIS) (see later discussion) by binding to the respective promoter regions.[11,12]

The involvement of PAX8 has been described in sporadic and familial cases of CH with thyroid dysgenesis. Autosomal dominant transmission with incomplete penetrance and variable expressivity has been described for the familial cases. This extreme variability supports the hypothesis that many factors modulate the phenotypic expression of *PAX8* gene mutations.

Table 1
Causes of nongoitrous congenital hypothyroidism (dysgenesis)

Gene	Chr Location	FT_4	TSH	TG	Mode of Inherit	Comments
TSHR	14q31.1	Dec	Inc	Detectable	AR, sporadic	Normal-hypoplastic thyroid gland that does not trap TCO_4^-
PAX8	2q14.1	Dec	Inc	Dec	AD, sporadic	Variable thyroid phenotype from partial to complete agenesis
TTF1 (NKX2-1)	14q13.3	Dec	Inc	Dec	AD	Brain-thyroid-lung syndrome
FOXE1 (TTF2; FKHL15)	9q22.33	Dec	Inc	Dec	AR	Cleft palate Choanal atresia Spiky hair
NKX2-5	5q35.1	Dec	Inc	Dec	AD, imprinting	Heart disease Ectopic thyroid

Abbreviations: AD, autosomal dominant; AR, autosomal recessive; chr, chromosome; dec; decrease; Inc, increase; TCO_4^-, pertechnetate.

TTF1 gene

TTF1 (also known as NKX2-1 or thyroid-specific enhancer binding protein) is a member of the homeobox domain type of transcription factors. It is expressed in the lungs and vertebral forebrain, in addition to the thyroid gland.[13] It is known to regulate the transcription of TG, TPO, and TSHR genes in the thyroid follicular cells and the surfactant protein B gene in epithelial lung cells.[14–16] The essential role of TTF1 in the development of thyroid, lung, and brain development was first shown in animal models[17]; this was later confirmed by several human case reports of NKX2-1 mutations presenting with primary CH, respiratory distress, and benign hereditary chorea, which are manifestations of the brain-thyroid-lung-syndrome.[18,19] In most cases haploinsufficiency has been considered to be responsible for the phenotype; the clinical features are very variable.[20]

FOXE1 gene

Forkhead box protein E1 (FOXE1) also known, as TTF2 or FKHL15, is a transcription factor member of the forkhead/winged helix domain protein family, many of which are key regulators of embryonic pattern formation and regional specification. It regulates the transcription of TG and TPO.[21] Homozygous mutations in the FOXE1 gene have been reported in patients affected by Bamforth-Lazarus syndrome. This syndrome is characterized by cleft palate, bilateral choanal atresia, spiky hair, and athyreosis.[22]

NKX2-5 gene

In addition to NKX2-1, other genes of the NKX2 family are present in the primitive pharynx and the thyroid anlage, such as NKX2-3, NKX2-5, and NKX2-6. In humans, NKX2-5 is essential for normal heart morphogenesis, myogenesis, and function.[23] Several loss-of-function mutations in NKX2-5 have been described in patients with congenital heart disease,[24] and heterozygous mutations have been associated with human ectopic thyroid.[25] Patients carrying NKX2-5 mutations show a phenotypic variability of both heart and thyroid malformations; this could be a consequence of haploinsufficiency, monoallelic expression, or imprinting factors.[26]

Goitrous Congenital Hypothyroidism: Defects in Thyroid Hormone Synthesis (Dyshormonogenesis)

Approximately 15% to 20% of the cases of CH are caused by thyroid dyshormonogenesis, which can occur at any of the steps involved in TH production. These forms of CH are characterized by an enlargement of the thyroid gland (goiter), and they usually show a classic Mendelian recessive inheritance pattern (**Table 2**).

The synthesis of TH starts with the active transportation of I into the follicular thyroid cells by the NIS present in the basolateral membrane of the cells. Subsequently, I is oxidized by hydrogen peroxidase and bound to tyrosine residues in TG to form iodotyrosine (iodine organification). Some of these hormonally inert iodotyrosines residues, monoiodotyrosine (MIT) and diiodotyrosine (DIT), couple to form the hormonally active iodothyronines T_4 and 3,5,3'-tri-iodo-L-thyronine (T_3). TPO catalyzes the oxidation, organification, and coupling reactions involved in this process.[27] Defects in any of these steps can lead to thyroid dyshormonogenesis. Common known mutations include NIS, SLC26A4, TG, TPO, DUOX2, DUOXA2, and IYD.[28]

Sodium iodine symporter, SLC5A5: defect in iodine uptake

Iodine (I) the oxidized for of Iodide (I^-) is an essential constituent of THs, which are phenolic rings joined by an ether link iodinated at 3 positions (T_3) or 4 positions (T_4).[28] The uptake of I through the basolateral membrane of the follicular thyroid cells is a key point in the biosynthesis of TH. This process is mediated by the NIS (official gene symbol SLC5A5), a 13-transmembrane domain glycoprotein that relies on the

Table 2
Causes of goitrous congenital hypothyroidism (dyshormonogenesis)

Gene	Chr Location	FT$_4$	TSH	Tg	Mode of Inherit	Comments
NIS (SLC5A5)	19p13.11	Dec	Inc	Inc	AR; 13 cases	Saliva: plasma ^{125}I ratio <20
PDS (SLC26A4)	7q22.3	N	N, Inc	Inc	AR; 7.5–10.0 in 100,000	Sensorineuronal hearing loss
TG	8q24.22	Dec	Inc	Dec	AR; 40 cases (1:67,000)	High uptake on scintigraphy
TPO	2p25.3	Dec	N, Inc	N, Inc	AR	Positive CLO$_4^-$ discharge test Iodination and coupling defect
DUOX2 (THOX2)	15q21.1	Dec	Inc	N, Inc	AR	NADPH oxidase Can be transient hypothyroid that corrects
DUOXA2	15q21.1	Dec	Inc	N, Inc	AR	—
IYD (DEHALI)	6q25.1	Dec	Inc	N, Inc	AR	Elevated urinary DIT and MIT levels

Abbreviations: AR autosomal recessive; chr, chromosome; dec, decrease; DIT, diiodotyrosine; Inc, increase; MIT, monoiodotyrosine; N, normal; NADPH, nicotinamide adenine dinucleotide phosphate; *IYD*, iodotyrosine deiodinase.

Na$^+$ electrochemical gradient created by the Na$^+$/potassium (K$^+$) ATPase and allows to actively concentrate I by electrogenic symport of Na$^+$ (2:1 Na$^+$ to I stoichiometry).[28,29] NIS is also expressed in several other differentiated epithelia where it is not regulated by TSH, such as salivary glands, lachrymal glands, gastric mucosa, choroid plexus, and lactating mammary glands.[29]

Since the cloning of *NIS* in 1996,[30] NIS research has become a major field of interest with considerable clinical implications. CH resulting from mutations in *SLCA5A* is specifically referred to as I transport defect (ITD). It follows an autosomal recessive pattern of inheritance. Although it is a rare disorder, to date, 13 such mutations have been reported in the *NIS* coding region (V59E,[31] G93R,[32] R124H,[33] Δ143–323, Q267E,[34] C272X, Δ287–288,[35] T354P,[36] Δ439–443,[37] G395R,[32] G543E,[38] 515X, and Y531X) and 1 in the 5′ untranslated region.[39]

When untreated ITD is clinically characterized by hypothyroidism, goiter, and mental impairment of varying degrees.[28] Diagnostic workup will show a reduced or absent thyroid I uptake. It should be noted that the lack of thyroidal I uptake could lead to the erroneous diagnosis of athyreosis unless TG level is measured. Because the loss of NIS is generalized, it also involves reduced salivary glands and gastric parietal cell uptake of I. A reliable test is the measurement of radioactivity in the equal volumes of saliva and plasma obtained 1 hour after the oral administration of 5 μCi of ^{125}I. A saliva-to-plasma ratio close to unity (normal 20) is diagnostic of an NIS defect. These patients should be managed with levothyroxine replacement therapy; I supplementation could be considered in patients with residual NIS activity as it can improve thyroid function.[29]

Pendred syndrome, SLC26A4: defects in iodine efflux

Pendrin is a highly hydrophobic membrane glycoprotein located at the apical membrane of thyrocytes. It is thought to function as an apical I transporter.[40]

Pendrin is also expressed in the kidney and in the inner ear, where it plays an important role in acid-base metabolism and in the generation of endocochlear potential, respectively.[41,42] It is encoded by the *SLC26A4* gene. Mutations in this gene lead to Pendred syndrome, an autosomal recessive disorder characterized by sensorineural deafness, goiter, and partial defect in I organification.[43,44] The incidence of the disease is estimated to be 7.5 to 10.0 in 100,000; it is thought to account for as many as 10% of cases of hereditary deafness, making it the most common cause of syndromic deafness. About half of these patients do not manifest any thyroid abnormalities; when they do, it is usually not evident until the second decade of life.[45]

Affected patients usually have a positive perchlorate discharge test, with more than 15%, but not complete-release of radiolabeled I following perchlorate administration, indicating a mild thyroid organification defect. A normal discharge test, on the other hand, does not exclude the diagnosis, as this diagnostic tool has a relatively high false-negative rate (5%).[46]

Before performing systematic mutation scanning in suspected cases, targeted screening for the most common, recurrent mutations can be considered. L236P, T416P, and IVS8+1G$\geq$A account for 50% of known *SLC26A4* mutations in Caucasians of Northern Europe descent,[47,48] whereas H723R represents 53% of reported mutant alleles among Japanese.[49]

Thyroglobulin: defects in the follicular matrix protein providing tyrosyl groups for iodine organification

TG is a homodimer of 660 kDa, synthesized exclusively in the thyroid gland. It is secreted into the follicular lumen where it functions as matrix for hormone synthesis providing tyrosyl groups, the non-I component of TH. Iodinated TG constitutes the storage pool for TH and I.[29] At least 40 distinct inactivation *TG* gene mutations have been described[50]; they are associated with moderate to severe CH, usually with low serum TG levels. Affected individuals often have abnormal iodoproteins in their serum, especially iodinated albumin; they excrete iodopeptides of low molecular weight in the urine. The coupling defect results in ineffective formation of T_4 and T_3.[7] Scintigraphy shows high uptake (due to induction of NIS expression by TSH stimulation) in a typically enlarged thyroid gland.

Thyroid peroxidase: defect in the enzyme catalyzing iodide organification

TPO is the enzyme responsible for iodide oxidation, organification, and iodotyrosine coupling. It is a heme containing glycated protein bound to the apical membrane of the follicular thyroid cells. The most prevalent cause of congenital thyroid dyshormonogenesis with permanent hypothyroidism seems to be inactivating biallelic defects in the *TPO* gene.[51,52] Although heterozygous *TPO* mutations do not directly result in abnormal thyroid function, such monoallelic defects may play a role as genetic susceptibility factors in transient hypothyroidism. Neonates with CH found to have a *TPO* mutation require lifelong treatment with TH.[29]

DUOX2: defects in the nicotinamide adenine dinucleotide phosphate–oxidase providing hydrogen peroxidase for thyroid peroxidase

The dual oxidase *DUOX1* and 2 genes (also termed *THOX1* and *THOX2*) encode the nicotinamide adenine dinucleotide phosphate (NADPH) oxidases located at the apical membrane of thyrocytes. They constitute the catalytic core of the calcium ion–dependent hydrogen peroxide generator required for TPO activity and TH synthesis.[53] Since the initial description of *DUOX2* in 2002, 26 different mutations have been reported.[54–62] About half of them are nonsense, frameshift or splice site mutations predicting a dysfunctional enzyme. Although most dyshormonogenesis defects are inherited in an autosomal recessive fashion, a single defective *DUOX2* allele mutation is sufficient to cause CH. With an increasing number of reported cases, phenotype-genotype correlations in patients with these mutations are becoming more complex. The expressivity of *DUOX2* defects is likely influenced by genetic background (eg, *DUOX1*) and may, at least in part, depend on the I intake.[29]

DUOXA2: defect in the DUOX2 cofactor

DUOXA2, a resident endoplasmic reticulum (ER) protein, is required for ER to Golgi transition, maturation, and translocation to the plasma membrane of functional DUOX enzymes. There are 3 reported cases whereby mutations of the *DUOXA2* gene have been identified; in all 3, the loss of a single allele did not lead to abnormal thyroid function.[63–65] Because *DUOXA2* defects lead to secondary deficiency of functional DUOX2 enzymes, one can anticipate that expressivity will be similarly modulated by nutritional I as described for *DUOX2* defects.[29]

Iodotyrosine dehydrogenase: defects in iodine recycling

In addition to the active I transport from the extracellular fluid, intracellular I is also generated by the action of the DEAHLA1 or iodotyrosine deiodinase (IYD) enzymes. MIT and DIT are subjects of NADPH-dependent reductive deiodination by IYD from T_4 and T_3, leading to formation of free iodide and tyrosine, both of which can be reutilized in hormone synthesis.[27] Mutations in homozygosity in the *IYD* gene have been identified in patients with hypothyroidism, goiter, and an elevated DIT level.[66,67]

Loss of IYD activity prevents the normal intrathyroidal I recycling and leads to excessive urinary secretion of DIT and MIT. Because the resulting I deficiency does not manifest at birth, patients with biallelic *IYD* mutations tested normal at neonatal screening for CH. They subsequently came to medical attention at 1.5 to 8.0 years of age. On scintigraphy, a very rapid and high initial uptake of ^{123}I in an enlarged thyroid is observed, followed by a relatively rapid decline of the accumulated I without the administration of perchlorate.[29]

Defects in Thyroid Hormone Action

Impaired sensitivity to thyroid describes a process that interferes with the effectiveness of TH and includes defects in TH action, transport, or metabolism.[68] Clinicians should include these disorders in the differential diagnosis of patients presenting with the appropriate clinical scenario and thyroid function test abnormalities that do not reflect the expected physiologic inverse relationship between TSH and THs (**Table 3**).

Thyroid hormone cell transport defects: monocarboxylate transporter 8

TH is transported across the cell membranes by several molecules. Defective cell-transport proteins may not reach the cell membrane or may not be able to transport the hormone and cause reduced levels of intracellular TH.[69] The importance of these molecules was most convincingly demonstrated with the identification of the first inherited TH cell transport defect caused by mutations in the monocarboxylate transporter 8 (*MCT8*) gene (also known as *SCL16A2*). This molecule plays an important role in the transport of TH into the brain and, therefore, in the effect of TH on brain development.[70] Its mutation is responsible for the Allan-Herndon-Dudley syndrome, an X-linked disease presenting with severe psychomotor deficit and elevated serum concentrations of T_3 and low levels of T_4 and rT_3.[71,72]

Given the existence of other types of TH transporters and their different tissue distribution, it is anticipated that defects in each molecule would result in a distinct

Table 3
Causes of abnormalities in thyroid hormone action (syndromes of impaired sensitivity to thyroid hormone)

Gene	Chr Location	FT_4	TSH	rT_3	FT_3	Goiter	Mode of Inherit	Comments
MCT8	Xq13.2	Dec	Inc	Dec	Inc	No	X-linked	Severe neuropsychiatriac abnormalities
SBP2 (SECISBP2)	9q22.2	Inc	N, Inc	Inc	Dec	No	Unknown	Defect in deiodination of T_4 to T_3
THRB	3p24.2	Inc	N, Inc	Inc	Inc	Yes	AD; >400 cases	Goiter; ADHD; some growth issues
THRA	17q21.1	Dec	N, Inc	Dec	N, Inc	No	AD	Cleft palate Choanal atresia Spiky hair

Abbreviations: AD, autosomal dominant; ADHD, attention-deficit/hyperactivity disorder; chr, chromosome; dec, decrease; Inc, increase; N, normal.

phenotype, some of which can be predicted based on the evidence available from the generation of mice deficient in specific transporters.[73] Current treatment options for patients with *MCT8* mutations are limited; the use of TH analogues that may bypass the molecular defect by using alternative transporters has been studied with promising outcomes that need further investigation.[74,75]

Thyroid hormone metabolism abnormalities: selenocysteine-binding protein 2
T_4, the major product secreted by the thyroid gland, is a prohormone that must be activated by conversion to T_3 in the cell cytoplasm. Defects in any of the factors involved in this enzymatic deiodination reaction can cause a diminished production of T_3 and, thus, reduced sensitivity to TH. The only known inherited defect of TH metabolism defect involves the gene for selenocysteine insertion sequence-binding protein 2 (*SECISBP2*, also known as *SBP2*), 1 of the 12 known genes involved in deiodinase synthesis and degradation. The mutation interferes with conversion of T_4 to T_3, resulting in a low T_3, and high T_4 and rT_3.[76]

Defect in thyroid hormone action: thyroid hormone receptor beta, and alpha and non– thyroid hormone receptor–resistance to thyroid hormone
The genomic action of TH within the nucleus is mediated through the TH receptor (TR). Mutant TR proteins have reduced ability to bind cognate ligand or protein cofactors or to bind to DNA and can result in resistance to TH (RTH). The disorder is characterized by high serum concentrations of free T_4 and usually free T_3, accompanied by normal or slightly high serum TSH concentrations.[68] The most common known cause of resistance to TH is an inherited defect in the *THRB* gene; this condition is termed RTH-beta. Affected patients have persistent elevations of all 3 serum iodothyronines with nonsuppressed TSH. In contrast, patients with mutations of the gene encoding TR-alpha have low serum T_4 and rT_3, borderline high T_3, and normal or slightly elevated TSH; this disorder is termed RTH-alpha.[77] Some individuals have a phenotype that mimics that of a *TR-beta* gene mutation but have no identifiable *TR* gene mutation. This disorder has been termed non–TR-TRH and is thought to be caused by defects in TR cofactors.[78,79]

ACKNOWLEDGMENTS

The authors thank Rabbi Morris Esformes Thyroid Research Fund for support in this work.

REFERENCES

1. Roitt IM, Doniach D, Campbell PN, et al. Auto-antibodies in Hashimoto's disease (lymphadenoid goitre). Lancet 1956;271(6947):820–1.
2. Pendred V. Deaf-mutism and goitre. Lancet 1896;148(3808):532.
3. Stanbury JB, Hedge AN. A study of a family of goitrous cretins. J Clin Endocrinol Metab 1950;10(11):1471–84.
4. Refetoff S, DeWind LT, DeGroot LJ. Familial syndrome combining deaf-mutism, stuppled epiphyses, goiter and abnormally high PBI: possible target organ refractoriness to thyroid hormone. J Clin Endocrinol Metab 1967;27(2):279–94.
5. Medici M, van der Deure WM, Verbiest M, et al. A large-scale association analysis of 68 thyroid hormone pathway genes with serum TSH and FT4 levels. Eur J Endocrinol 2011;164(5):781–8.
6. Peeters RP, van der Deure WM, Visser TJ. Genetic variation in thyroid hormone pathway genes; polymorphisms in the TSH receptor and the iodothyronine deiodinases. Eur J Endocrinol 2006;155(6):655 62.
7. Park SM, Chatterjee VK. Genetics of congenital hypothyroidism. J Med Genet 2005;42(5):379–89.
8. Nettore IC, Cacace V, De Fusco C, et al. The molecular causes of thyroid dysgenesis: a systematic review. J Endocrinol Invest 2013;36(8):654–64.
9. Pohlenz J, Vliet GV, Deladoëy J. Chapter 8-developmental abnormalities of the thyroid A2. In: Weiss RE, Refetoff S, editors. Genetic diagnosis of endocrine disorders. 2nd edition. San Diego (CA): Academic Press; 2016. p. 127–36.
10. Biebermann H, Schöneberg T, Krude H, et al. Mutations of the human thyrotropin receptor gene causing thyroid hypoplasia and persistent congenital hypothyroidism. J Clin Endocrinol Metab 1997;82(10):3471–80.
11. Plachov D, Chowdhury K, Walther C, et al. Pax8, a murine paired box gene expressed in the developing excretory system and thyroid gland. Development 1990;110(2):643–51.
12. De Felice M, Di Lauro R. Thyroid development and its disorders: genetics and molecular mechanisms. Endocr Rev 2004;25(5):722–46.
13. Lazzaro D, Price M, de Felice M, et al. The transcription factor TTF-1 is expressed at the onset of thyroid and lung morphogenesis and in restricted regions of the foetal brain. Development 1991;113(4):1093–104.
14. Civitareale D, Lonigro R, Sinclair AJ, et al. A thyroid-specific nuclear protein essential for tissue-specific expression of the thyroglobulin promoter. EMBO J 1989;8(9):2537–42.
15. Francis-Lang H, Price M, Polycarpou-Schwarz M, et al. Cell-type-specific expression of the rat thyroperoxidase promoter indicates common mechanisms for thyroid-specific gene expression. Mol Cell Biol 1992;12(2):576–88.
16. Bruno MD, Bohinski RJ, Huelsman KM, et al. Lung cell-specific expression of the murine surfactant protein A (SP-A) gene is mediated by interactions between the SP-A promoter and thyroid transcription factor-1. J Biol Chem 1995;270(12):6531–6.
17. Kimura S, Hara Y, Pineau T, et al. The T/ebp null mouse: thyroid-specific enhancer-binding protein is essential for the organogenesis of the thyroid, lung, ventral forebrain, and pituitary. Genes Dev 1996;10(1):60–9.

18. Willemsen MA, Breedveld GJ, Wouda S, et al. Brain-thyroid-lung syndrome: a patient with a severe multi-system disorder due to a de novo mutation in the thyroid transcription factor 1 gene. Eur J Pediatr 2005;164(1):28–30.
19. Carre A, Szinnai G, Castanet M, et al. Five new TTF1/NKX2.1 mutations in brain-lung-thyroid syndrome: rescue by PAX8 synergism in one case. Hum Mol Genet 2009;18(12):2266–76.
20. Ferrara AM, De Michele G, Salvatore E, et al. A novel NKX2.1 mutation in a family with hypothyroidism and benign hereditary chorea. Thyroid 2008;18(9):1005–9.
21. Zannini M, Avantaggiato V, Biffali E, et al. TTF-2, a new forkhead protein, shows a temporal expression in the developing thyroid which is consistent with a role in controlling the onset of differentiation. EMBO J 1997;16(11):3185–97.
22. Bamforth JS, Hughes IA, Lazarus JH, et al. Congenital hypothyroidism, spiky hair, and cleft palate. J Med Genet 1989;26(1):49–51.
23. Tanaka M, Schinke M, Liao HS, et al. Nkx2.5 and Nkx2.6, homologs of Drosophila tinman, are required for development of the pharynx. Mol Cell Biol 2001;21(13):4391–8.
24. Hirayama-Yamada K, Kamisago M, Akimoto K, et al. Phenotypes with GATA4 or NKX2.5 mutations in familial atrial septal defect. Am J Med Genet A 2005;135(1):47–52.
25. Dentice M, Cordeddu V, Rosica A, et al. Missense mutation in the transcription factor NKX2-5: a novel molecular event in the pathogenesis of thyroid dysgenesis. J Clin Endocrinol Metab 2006;91(4):1428–33.
26. Vassart G, Dumont JE. Thyroid dysgenesis: multigenic or epigenetic... or both? Endocrinology 2005;146(12):5035–7.
27. Salvatore D, Davies TF, Schlumberger M, et al. CHAPTER 11-thyroid physiology and diagnostic evaluation of patients with thyroid disorders A2-Kronenberg. In: Melmed S, Polonsky K, Reed Larsen P, et al, editors. Williams textbook of endocrinology. 12th edition. Philadelphia: Content Repository Only!; 2011. p. 327–61.
28. Portulano C, Paroder-Belenitsky M, Carrasco N. The Na+/I- symporter (NIS): mechanism and medical impact. Endocr Rev 2014;35(1):106–49.
29. Grasberger H, Refetoff S. Chapter 7 – Congenital defects of thyroid hormone synthesis. In: Weiss RE, Refetoff S, editors. Genetic diagnosis of endocrine disorders. Second edition. San Diego (CA): Academic Press; 2016. p. 117–25.
30. Dai G, Levy O, Carrasco N. Cloning and characterization of the thyroid iodide transporter. Nature 1996;379(6564):458–60.
31. Reed-Tsur MD, De la Vieja A, Ginter CS, et al. Molecular characterization of V59E NIS, a Na+/I- symporter mutant that causes congenital I- transport defect. Endocrinology 2008;149(6):3077–84.
32. Dohan O, Gavrielides MV, Ginter C, et al. Na(+)/I(-) symporter activity requires a small and uncharged amino acid residue at position 395. Mol Endocrinol 2002;16(8):1893–902.
33. Paroder V, Nicola JP, Ginter CS, et al. The iodide-transport-defect-causing mutation R124H: a delta-amino group at position 124 is critical for maturation and trafficking of the Na+/I- symporter. J Cell Sci 2013;126(Pt 15):3305–13.
34. De La Vieja A, Ginter CS, Carrasco N. The Q267E mutation in the sodium/iodide symporter (NIS) causes congenital iodide transport defect (ITD) by decreasing the NIS turnover number. J Cell Sci 2004;117(Pt 5):677–87.
35. Montanelli L, Agretti P, Marco GD, et al. Congenital hypothyroidism and late-onset goiter: identification and characterization of a novel mutation in the sodium/iodide symporter of the proband and family members. Thyroid 2009;19(12):1419–25.

36. De la Vieja A, Reed MD, Ginter CS, et al. Amino acid residues in transmembrane segment IX of the Na+/I- symporter play a role in its Na+ dependence and are critical for transport activity. J Biol Chem 2007;282(35):25290–8.

37. Li W, Nicola JP, Amzel LM, et al. Asn441 plays a key role in folding and function of the Na+/I- symporter (NIS). FASEB J 2013;27(8):3229–38.

38. De la Vieja A, Ginter CS, Carrasco N. Molecular analysis of a congenital iodide transport defect: G543E impairs maturation and trafficking of the Na+/I- symporter. Mol Endocrinol 2005;19(11):2847–58.

39. Nicola JP, Nazar M, Serrano-Nascimento C, et al. Iodide transport defect: functional characterization of a novel mutation in the Na+/I- symporter 5'-untranslated region in a patient with congenital hypothyroidism. J Clin Endocrinol Metab 2011; 96(7):E1100–7.

40. Everett LA, Green ED. A family of mammalian anion transporters and their involvement in human genetic diseases. Hum Mol Genet 1999;8(10):1883–91.

41. Everett LA, Morsli H, Wu DK, et al. Expression pattern of the mouse ortholog of the Pendred's syndrome gene (Pds) suggests a key role for pendrin in the inner ear. Proc Natl Acad Sci U S A 1999;96(17):9727–32.

42. Royaux IE, Wall SM, Karniski LP, et al. Pendrin, encoded by the Pendred syndrome gene, resides in the apical region of renal intercalated cells and mediates bicarbonate secretion. Proc Natl Acad Sci U S A 2001;98(7):4221–6.

43. Morgans ME, Trotter WR. Association of congenital deafness with goitre; the nature of the thyroid defect. Lancet 1958;1(7021):607–9.

44. Kopp P, Pesce L, Solis SJ. Pendred syndrome and iodide transport in the thyroid. Trends Endocrinol Metab 2008;19(7):260–8.

45. Reardon W, Trembath RC. Pendred syndrome. J Med Genet 1996;33(12): 1037–40.

46. Ladsous M, Vlaeminck-Guillem V, Dumur V, et al. Analysis of the thyroid phenotype in 42 patients with Pendred syndrome and nonsyndromic enlargement of the vestibular aqueduct. Thyroid 2014;24(4):639–48.

47. Campbell C, Cucci RA, Prasad S, et al. Pendred syndrome, DFNB4, and PDS/SLC26A4 identification of eight novel mutations and possible genotype-phenotype correlations. Hum Mutat 2001;17(5):403–11.

48. Coyle B, Reardon W, Herbrick JA, et al. Molecular analysis of the PDS gene in Pendred syndrome. Hum Mol Genet 1998;7(7):1105–12.

49. Tsukamoto K, Suzuki H, Harada D, et al. Distribution and frequencies of PDS (SLC26A4) mutations in Pendred syndrome and nonsyndromic hearing loss associated with enlarged vestibular aqueduct: a unique spectrum of mutations in Japanese. Eur J Hum Genet 2003;11(12):916–22.

50. Targovnik HM, Citterio CE, Rivolta CM. Thyroglobulin gene mutations in congenital hypothyroidism. Horm Res Paediatr 2011;75(5):311–21.

51. Rodrigues C, Jorge P, Soares JP, et al. Mutation screening of the thyroid peroxidase gene in a cohort of 55 Portuguese patients with congenital hypothyroidism. Eur J Endocrinol 2005;152(2):193–8.

52. Avbelj M, Tahirovic H, Debeljak M, et al. High prevalence of thyroid peroxidase gene mutations in patients with thyroid dyshormonogenesis. Eur J Endocrinol 2007;156(5):511–9.

53. Ris-Stalpers C. Physiology and pathophysiology of the DUOXes. Antioxid Redox Signal 2006;8(9–10):1563–72.

54. Moreno JC, Bikker H, Kempers MJ, et al. Inactivating mutations in the gene for thyroid oxidase 2 (THOX2) and congenital hypothyroidism. N Engl J Med 2002; 347(2):95–102.

55. Vigone MC, Fugazzola L, Zamproni I, et al. Persistent mild hypothyroidism associated with novel sequence variants of the DUOX2 gene in two siblings. Hum Mutat 2005;26(4):395.

56. Varela V, Rivolta CM, Esperante SA, et al. Three mutations (p.Q36H, p.G418fsX482, and g.IVS19-2A>C) in the dual oxidase 2 gene responsible for congenital goiter and iodide organification defect. Clin Chem 2006;52(2):182–91.

57. Pfarr N, Korsch E, Kaspers S, et al. Congenital hypothyroidism caused by new mutations in the thyroid oxidase 2 (THOX2) gene. Clin Endocrinol (Oxf) 2006; 65(6):810–5.

58. Ohye H, Fukata S, Hishinuma A, et al. A novel homozygous missense mutation of the dual oxidase 2 (DUOX2) gene in an adult patient with large goiter. Thyroid 2008;18(5):561–6.

59. Maruo Y, Takahashi H, Soeda I, et al. Transient congenital hypothyroidism caused by biallelic mutations of the dual oxidase 2 gene in Japanese patients detected by a neonatal screening program. J Clin Endocrinol Metab 2008;93(11):4261–7.

60. Hoste C, Rigutto S, Van Vliet G, et al. Compound heterozygosity for a novel hemizygous missense mutation and a partial deletion affecting the catalytic core of the H2O2-generating enzyme DUOX2 associated with transient congenital hypothyroidism. Hum Mutat 2010;31(4):E1304–19.

61. Grasberger H. Defects of thyroidal hydrogen peroxide generation in congenital hypothyroidism. Mol Cell Endocrinol 2010;322(1–2):99–106.

62. Yoshizawa-Ogasawara A, Ogikubo S, Satoh M, et al. Congenital hypothyroidism caused by a novel mutation of the dual oxidase 2 (DUOX2) gene. J Pediatr Endocrinol Metab 2013;26(1–2):45–52.

63. Zamproni I, Grasberger H, Cortinovis F, et al. Biallelic inactivation of the dual oxidase maturation factor 2 (DUOXA2) gene as a novel cause of congenital hypothyroidism. J Clin Endocrinol Metab 2008;93(2):605–10.

64. Yi RH, Zhu WB, Yang LY, et al. A novel dual oxidase maturation factor 2 gene mutation for congenital hypothyroidism. Int J Mol Med 2013;31(2):467–70.

65. Hulur I, Hermanns P, Nestoris C, et al. A single copy of the recently identified dual oxidase maturation factor (DUOXA) 1 gene produces only mild transient hypothyroidism in a patient with a novel biallelic DUOXA2 mutation and monoallelic DUOXA1 deletion. J Clin Endocrinol Metab 2011;96(5):E841–5.

66. Moreno JC, Klootwijk W, van Toor H, et al. Mutations in the iodotyrosine deiodinase gene and hypothyroidism. N Engl J Med 2008;358(17):1811–8.

67. Afink G, Kulik W, Overmars H, et al. Molecular characterization of iodotyrosine dehalogenase deficiency in patients with hypothyroidism. J Clin Endocrinol Metab 2008;93(12):4894–901.

68. Refetoff S, Weiss RE, Usala SJ. The syndromes of resistance to thyroid hormone. Endocr Rev 1993;14(3):348–99.

69. Hennemann G, Docter R, Friesema EC, et al. Plasma membrane transport of thyroid hormones and its role in thyroid hormone metabolism and bioavailability. Endocr Rev 2001;22(4):451–76.

70. Ceballos A, Belinchon MM, Sanchez-Mendoza E, et al. Importance of monocarboxylate transporter 8 for the blood-brain barrier-dependent availability of 3,5,3′-triiodo-L-thyronine. Endocrinology 2009;150(5):2491–6.

71. Dumitrescu AM, Liao XH, Best TB, et al. A novel syndrome combining thyroid and neurological abnormalities is associated with mutations in a monocarboxylate transporter gene. Am J Hum Genet 2004;74(1):168–75.

72. Friesema EC, Grueters A, Biebermann H, et al. Association between mutations in a thyroid hormone transporter and severe X-linked psychomotor retardation. Lancet 2004;364(9443):1435–7.
73. Refetoff S, Dumitrescu AM. Syndromes of reduced sensitivity to thyroid hormone: genetic defects in hormone receptors, cell transporters and deiodination. Best Pract Res Clin Endocrinol Metab 2007;21(2):277–305.
74. Di Cosmo C, Liao XH, Dumitrescu AM, et al. A thyroid hormone analog with reduced dependence on the monocarboxylate transporter 8 for tissue transport. Endocrinology 2009;150(9):4450–8.
75. Verge CF, Konrad D, Cohen M, et al. Diiodothyropropionic acid (DITPA) in the treatment of MCT8 deficiency. J Clin Endocrinol Metab 2012;97(12):4515–23.
76. Dumitrescu AM, Liao XH, Abdullah MS, et al. Mutations in SECISBP2 result in abnormal thyroid hormone metabolism. Nat Genet 2005;37(11):1247–52.
77. Bochukova E, Schoenmakers N, Agostini M, et al. A mutation in the thyroid hormone receptor alpha gene. N Engl J Med 2012;366(3):243–9.
78. Weiss RE, Hayashi Y, Nagaya T, et al. Dominant inheritance of resistance to thyroid hormone not linked to defects in the thyroid hormone receptor alpha or beta genes may be due to a defective cofactor. J Clin Endocrinol Metab 1996;81(12):4196–203.
79. Reutrakul S, Sadow PM, Pannain S, et al. Search for abnormalities of nuclear corepressors, coactivators, and a coregulator in families with resistance to thyroid hormone without mutations in thyroid hormone receptor beta or alpha genes. J Clin Endocrinol Metab 2000;85(10):3609–17.

Molecular Genetics of Thyroid Cancer in Children and Adolescents

Andrew J. Bauer, MD

KEYWORDS

- Thyroid cancer • Molecular markers • Oncogene • Mutation • Gene fusion
- Indeterminate cytology

KEY POINTS

- There are clinical differences for how differentiated thyroid cancer (DTC) behaves when diagnosed in pediatric patients compared with adults even within the same histologic variant.
- Pediatric patients with thyroid nodules have a similar likelihood of indeterminate cytology and a higher likelihood of malignancy.
- Mutations in *BRAF* are common in pediatric papillary thyroid carcinoma (PTC) but may not portend an increased risk of invasive or refractory disease.
- There are several familial forms of thyroid cancer that present with clinical disease within the pediatric population, including medullary thyroid cancer and DTC.
- Exploring the integrated genomic landscape of pediatric PTC holds great promise to increase the preoperative diagnosis as well as optimize stratification of care so that a more aggressive approach is pursued only for patients with an increased risk for persistent, recurrent, or refractory disease.

INTRODUCTION

In the simplest approach, thyroid cancer is divided into 2 major categories: follicular-derived tumors, including follicular thyroid carcinoma (FTC) and papillary thyroid carcinoma (PTC), and the parafollicular-derived tumor, medullary thyroid carcinoma (MTC). FTC and PTC are often classified as forms of differentiated thyroid cancer (DTC) because they typically maintain nonmalignant cellular physiology, including the ability to respond to thyroid stimulatory hormone (TSH), transport iodine via the sodium-iodine symporter, and produce thyroglobulin (Tg). In both pediatric patients

Disclosure: The author has nothing to disclose.
Division of Endocrinology and Diabetes, The Thyroid Center, The Children's Hospital of Philadelphia, The Perelman School of Medicine, The University of Pennsylvania, 3401 Civic Center Boulevard, Philadelphia, PA 19104, USA
E-mail address: bauera@chop.edu

Endocrinol Metab Clin N Am 46 (2017) 389–403
http://dx.doi.org/10.1016/j.ecl.2017.01.014
0889-8529/17/© 2017 Elsevier Inc. All rights reserved.

endo.theclinics.com

and adults, these tumors may present as sporadic lesions or be associated with a familial pattern of inheritance. In pediatrics, with decreasing frequency, DTC is most commonly sporadic, followed by radiation induced, associated with treatment of a nonthyroid malignancy, and lastly associated with a familial tumor predisposition syndrome. In contrast, MTC is most commonly associated with an autosomal dominantly inherited disorder, multiple endocrine neoplasia (MEN) type 2, and rarely presents as a sporadic tumor within the pediatric population. This article covers the genetic alterations associated with these two forms of thyroid cancer and provides recommendations for how to incorporate this information into clinical practice.

DIFFERENTIATED THYROID CARCINOMA

Thyroid tumorigenesis and progression are associated with somatic point mutations of *BRAF* and the *RAS* genes, as well as fusions involving the rearranged during transfection (*RET*) and *NTRK1* tyrosine kinases, with resultant constitutive activation of the mitogen-activated protein kinase (MAPK) and phosphoinositide 3-kinase (PI3K) signaling pathways.[1,2] With uncommon exceptions, these mutations are mutually exclusive events and there is a fairly predictable relationship between oncogenic genotype and histopathologic phenotype, with *RET-PTC* rearrangements[3,4] and B-rapidly accelerated fibrosarcoma (*RAF*) point mutations common in PTC,[5] paired-box gene 8 (*PAX8*)-peroxisome proliferator-activated receptor gamma (*PPARG*) common in FTC,[6,7] and *RAS* mutations found in both FTC and follicular variant of PTC (fvPTC).[8,9] With improved technologies, additional point mutations and fusions have been reported (**Table 1**).

The Cancer Genome Atlas (TCGA) project provided a major step forward in defining the genomic landscape of PTC via comprehensive multiplatform analysis of nearly 500 adult tumors.[10] The combined analysis of genomic variants, gene expression, microRNA (miR) expression, alterations in methylation, and proteomic profiles revealed that mutations in *BRAF* and the *RAS* genes were the most common driver events, with gene fusions involving *RET*, neurotrophic tyrosine kinase receptor (*NTRK*), and anaplastic lymphoma receptor tyrosine kinase (*ALK*) found in only 15% of tumors.[10] A thyroid differentiation score was determined by analyzing the expression of 16 thyroid-specific metabolism and function genes and, combining all the data, the investigators suggested a molecular classification into 2 distinct subgroups: *BRAF*-like PTC (BVL-PTC) and *RAS*-like PTC (RL-PTC). Tumors with *RET* fusions followed a molecular pattern and clinical phenotype within the BVL-PTC subgroup and displayed predominant activation of the MAPK signaling pathway, whereas RL-PTC tumors were associated with concurrent activation of the PI3K/AKT and MAPK signaling pathways. The importance of the TCGA results is expansive and clinically applicable with anticipated improvements in diagnostic accuracy as well as stratification of treatment, including selection of tumor-specific systemic therapy. Similar oncogenic variants are found in pediatric PTC; however, a thorough and comprehensive investigation of the genomic landscape across all molecular platforms needs to be performed to determine where crossover in molecular signaling exists before extending the TCGA data into clinical practice for children and adolescents.

GENETIC MUTATIONS AND REARRANGEMENTS OF ONCOGENES

Mutations in *BRAF* and *RAS*, and *RET-PTC* fusions, represent the most common genetic alterations in PTC and FTC. The spectrum of somatic genetic alterations seems to be different between pediatric and adult patients comparing tumors with similar histology, with gene fusions found in a higher percentage of pediatric tumors compared with point mutations. Gene fusions involving *RET* and *NTRK* and point mutations involving *BRAF*

Table 1
Summary of oncogene analysis in pediatric differentiated thyroid cancer

Author, Year	Number Patients <19 y Old	BRAF % (# Tumors)	RAS % (# Tumors)	RET-PTC % (# Tumors)	NTRK Fusion % (# Tumors)	Other: # Tumors
Kumagai et al,[12] 2004	48: post-Chernobyl	17 (8)	4 (2)	35 (17)	NE	None
	31: sporadic	1	0	NE	NE	
Penko et al,[13] 2005	14	0	0	58 (7)	NE	None
Rosenbaum et al,[22] 2005	20	20	NE	NE	NE	NE
Monaco et al,[17] 2012	66 FNA samples	3 (2)	11 (7)	5 (3)	NE	PAX8-PPARG: 2
Sassolas et al,[23] 2012	28	7 (2)	3 (1)	28 (8)	0	None
Ricarte-Filho et al,[21] 2013	26: radiation exposed	12 (3)	0	58 (15)	12 (3)	AGK-BRAF: 1 AKAP9-BRAF: 1 PAX8-PPARG: 1 CREB3L2-PPARG: 1 TSHR: 1
	27: sporadic	26 (7)	7 (2)	26 (7)	7 (2)	Wild type: 9
Henke et al,[16] 2014	27	61 (17)	NE	NE	NE	NE
Givens et al,[15] 2014	19	37 (7)	NE	NE	NE	NE
Ballester et al,[14] 2016	27	37 (10)	0	22 (6)	0	CDKN2A: 1 CTNNB1: 1 TERT promoter: 0
Picarsic et al,[19] 2016	18	17 (3)	17 (3)	17 (3)	22 (4)	NTRK3-ETV6: 3 NTRK1-TPR: 1 PAX8-PPARG: 1
Prasad et al,[20] 2016	27	48 (13)	0	22 (6)	26 (7)	NTRK3-ETV6: 5 NTRK1-TPR: 1 NTRK1-unknown: 1
Nikita et al,[18] 2016	28	32 (9)	4 (1)	(6)	NE	None

Abbreviations: AGK, acylglycerol kinase; AKAP9, A-kinase anchoring protein; AKAP9, A-kinase anchoring protein 9; CREB, cAMP responsive element binding protein; CTNNB1, catenin (cadherin associated protein) beta 1; ETV6, ETS variant 6; FNA, fine-needle aspiration; NE, not examined; TPR, translocated promoter region nuclear basket protein; TSHR, thyrotropin receptor.

and *RAS* occur with highest frequency for both populations; however, approximately 50% of pediatric PTCs have a gene fusion compared with 15% of PTC in adults and point mutations are found in approximately 30% of pediatric PTC compared with 70% in adult PTC. In contrast with earlier reports of mutations in *BRAF* V600E in less than 5% of pediatric PTC,[11–13] more recent reports using newer detection methods report *BRAF* V600E in approximately 30% of pediatric PTC (range, 17%–61%; **Table 2**).[14–23] The incidence and spectrum of genetic events is also influenced by familial forms of DTC and radiation exposure as well as the undefined impact of the anabolic microenvironment of pediatric patients compared with adults. The molecular differences as well as the differences in the microenvironment likely explain why pediatric patients with DTC are more likely to maintain tumor differentiation and display low disease-specific mortality even when they present with invasive and metastatic disease. The development of unique guidelines for the evaluation and management of children and adolescents with thyroid nodules and DTC was an important step forward in caring for the pediatric population[24]; however, studies defining the differences in the genomic landscape between pediatric and adult PTC are critical to improve care as well as in garnering a greater understanding of the events that influence DTC differentiation.

BRAF

BRAF mutations are the most common genetic alterations in PTC from adults and are found in approximately 60% of PTC (range, 29%–87%).[10,25,26] Although more than 40 mutations have been identified to date, 95% of mutations involve nucleotide 1799 with a substitution of valine to glutamate at residue 600 (V600E).[26] Importantly, *BRAF* mutations have not been found in benign thyroid neoplasms, but have been found in up to one-third of anaplastic thyroid cancers.[27,28]

Most mutations lead to constitutive activation of the BRAF kinase and subsequent dysregulated signaling of the MAPK pathway.[29–31] Mutations of *BRAF* are thought to be both an early event of thyroid tumorigenesis, through induction of chromosomal instability, and an important event in proliferation and progression.[32,33] In adults, detection of a *BRAF* mutation in PTC is an independent risk factor for disease progression and recurrence as well as decreased response to radioiodine therapy secondary to *BRAF*-induced decreased expression of the sodium-iodide symporter.[34–37] A similar correlation has not been found in pediatric PTC harboring a somatic mutation in *BRAF* (see **Table 2**),[14–23] although additional studies with a larger number of patients across the spectrum of American Joint Committee on Cancer (AJCC) TNM (tumor, lymph node, metastasis) tumor classifications[38] are needed to more accurately assess whether these observations represent differences in tumor biology or selection bias. Although the presence of a *BRAF* mutation decreases the utility of using Radioactive iodine (RIA) for surveillance and therapy, mutations in *BRAF* are associated with increased expression of the glucose type-1 transporter gene improving the sensitivity of using (18)F-fluorodeoxyglucose positron emission tomography (PET) for surveillance in this difficult group of patients.[39]

Rearranged During Transfection-Papillary Thyroid Carcinoma

RET (rearranged during transfection) is a tyrosine kinase cell membrane receptor that is not expressed in normal thyroid follicular cells. There are approximately 20 *RET* gene fusions and *RET-PTC* is typically associated with both sporadic and radiation-induced PTCs that have classic PTC (cPTC), solid PTC, or diffuse sclerosing variant PTC morphology with frequent psammoma bodies (microcalcifications on ultrasonography [US] imaging).[11,40] They are found in young patients and patients after radiation exposure, and are associated with an increased risk of extrathyroidal extension,

Table 2
The incidence of *BRAF* mutations in pediatric papillary thyroid carcinoma

Author, Year	Number Patients <19 y Old	Detection Method (*BRAF*)	*BRAF* (%)	Clinical Correlation
Kumagai et al,[12] 2004	48: post-Chernobyl	PCR, sequencing	0	Not applicable
	31: sporadic		0	
Penko et al,[13] 2005	14	PCR, sequencing	0	Not applicable
Rosenbaum et al,[22] 2005	20	PCR, shifted termination assay	20	Not reported
Monaco et al,[17] 2012	66 FNA samples	PCR-RFLP	3	Not reported
Sassolas et al,[23] 2012	28	PCR-RFLP	7	No correlation with aggressive behavior
Ricarte-Filho et al,[21] 2013	26: radiation exposed	Mass spectrometry	3: radiation induced	Fusion genes are more common in radiation-exposed PTC (9 out of 27; 33%) and point mutations are more common in sporadic PTC (9 out of 27; 33%)
	27: sporadic		26: sporadic	No clinical correlation provided
Henke et al,[16] 2014	27	PCR-RFLP	61	No clinical correlation provided
Givens et al,[15] 2014	19	Pyrosequencing	37	No correlation with invasive behavior
Ballester et al,[14] 2016	27	PCR-RFLP	37	Similar % with lymph node metastasis compared with *RET-PTC*
Picarsic et al,[19] 2016	18	NGS (7-gene panel) and NGS (14-gene panel with 42 gene fusions)	17	Fusion genes (*RET-PTC1* and *NTRK3-ETV6*) more invasive than *BRAF*
Prasad et al,[20] 2016	27	NGS (14-gene panel with 42 gene fusions)	48	Fusion genes (*RET-PTC* 1 and 3, *NTRK1-TPR*, *NTRK3-ETV6*) more invasive than *BRAF*
Nikita et al,[18] 2016	28	PCR sequencing	32	No difference compared with tumors with *NRAS* or *RET-PTC*

Abbreviations: NGS, next-generation sequencing; PCR, polymerase chain reaction.

locoregional lymph node and distant (pulmonary) metastasis, as well as an increased risk for persistent and recurrent disease in patients with sporadic and radiation-induced PTC.[41–43] *RET-PTC* is found in approximately 15% of adult PTC, in 50% to 80% of patients with a history of radiation exposure, and in 40% to 70% of pediatric patients.[44–46] *RET/PTC1* and *RET/PTC3* are the most common of the rearrangements described to date, although variability in detection exists because of differences in detection methods and heterogeneity of expression within the tumor.[47,48]

RAS

Point mutations in the *RAS* genes, *H-RAS*, *N-RAS*, and *K-RAS*, have been reported in a wide range of thyroid tumors, including follicular adenoma (FA), FTC (40%–53%), PTC (0%–20%), fvPTC (17%–25%), and poorly differentiated and anaplastic thyroid carcinoma (20%–60%).[9,28,49–52] In an effort to clarify the role of the *RAS* oncogene, Vasko and colleagues[9] pooled data from 39 previous studies, and also examined 80 additional follicular tumors and found that codon 61 mutation of *NRAS* (N2) was more frequently identified in follicular tumors compared with papillary cancers (19% vs 5%, respectively) and that the N2 mutation was more frequently found in malignant compared with benign lesions (25% vs 14%, respectively). The more recently published TCGA data reported that *NRAS* was the second most common point mutation, with an incidence of 8.5%.[10] Data in pediatric DTC are limited, with most studies reporting less than 10% of tumors having a *RAS* mutation, most being limited to codon 61 (Q61) of the *NRAS* gene, and all associated with either FTC or fvPTC disorder (see **Table 1**).[12,17–19,23,53]

These data suggest that the presence of a *RAS* mutation is suggestive of a follicular tumor that is within the continuum from an atypical, preinvasive lesion to a true malignancy; either FTC, fvPTC, PTC, or poorly differentiated thyroid cancer (PDTC).[50,54]

The recently reclassified indolent (noninvasive) form of fvPTC to noninvasive follicular thyroid neoplasm with papillarylike nuclear features (NIFTP) highlights the potential impact of how an increase in the *RAS* mutation level detected by next-generation sequencing (NGS) may correlate with tumor progression with tumors displaying less than a 20% mutation level showing noninvasive behavior.[55] Additional data are needed to establish whether this correlation holds true with *RAS*-positive tumors displaying more invasive disease and how the increasing mutation level alters downstream signaling, including protein associated with maintenance of thyroid cell differentiation.

ADDITIONAL ONCOGENIC VARIANTS

Point mutation in *BRAF* and *RAS* as well as gene fusions in *RET*, *PPARG*, *NTRK1/3*, and *BRAF* were the most prevalent driver mutations identified for adult PTC samples in the TCGA. The *PAX8-PPARG* fusion is most commonly associated with FTC compared with FA and *PAX8-PPARG*–positive tumors typically show more extensive capsular and vascular invasion compared with *RAS*-positive tumors.[7,56] However, in contrast with *RAS* mutations, *PAX8-PPARG* fusions are not associated with poorly differentiated foci or PDTC.[7,57] Data on the role of *PAX8-PPARG* in pediatric DTC tumorigenesis are limited, but, within this cohort of patients, *PAX8-PPARG* and *RAS* are both more commonly associated with FTC and fvPTC,[17,19] with the exception of 2 patients with solid-variant PTC reported by Ricarte-Filho and colleagues.[21] A similar paucity of data exists within pediatrics for tumors with NTRK1/3 fusions and BRAF fusions; however, in contrast with *PAX8-PPARG* and *RAS*, both of these fusions seem to be associated with invasive forms of PTC (see **Table 1**).[19–21,58]

POTENTIAL APPLICATION OF ONCOGENE DATA INTO CLINICAL PRACTICE

Similar to adults, up to 35% of pediatric patients undergoing fine-needle aspiration (FNA) have indeterminate cytology within The Bethesda System for Reporting Thyroid Cytopathology (TBSRTC; categories 3 or 4) and within these categories the risk of malignancy for pediatric patients is higher compared with adults: 28% versus 5% to 15% for atypia of undetermined significance (category III) and 58% versus 15% to 30% for a follicular neoplasm (category IV), pediatrics versus adults.[17,59,60] Preoperative, adjunct testing with oncogene panels, gene expression classifiers, and miR have been incorporated into clinical practice in an effort to more accurately select and stratify adult patients with indeterminate cytology. Despite continued controversy over how and when to incorporate testing in adult patients,[61,62] several panels have received approval as medically necessary tests, increasing the likelihood of receiving insurance authorization. Thus, despite a higher prevalence of malignancy, with an associated increased likelihood of the test having improved positive predictive value to rule in disease, the incorporation of adjunct molecular testing into clinical practice for pediatric patients with indeterminate cytology remains limited.

Gene expression classifiers are not validated for use in patients less than 21 years of age and there are no data on miR expression in pediatric thyroid cancer. Thus, only oncogene panels should be considered. Although further data are needed, the following approach is based on the current available data (**Table 3**):

Table 3 Thyroid oncogene, risk of invasive disease, and anticipated surgical approach		
Point Mutation or Oncogene Fusion	**Increased Risk of DTC with Invasive Disease**	**Surgical Approach**
BRAF V600E	Adults (yes) Pediatrics (no)[a]	Total thyroidectomy with central neck dissection;
RET-PTC fusion	Yes	lateral neck lymph node
NTRK fusion	Yes	dissection based on
BRAF fusion	Yes (very limited data)	clinical findings and FNA
ALK fusion	No data in pediatrics	confirmation of
TERT plus additional mutation		metastasis
RAS (N)	No • Increasing risk of FTC and fvPTC if >20% of cells with mutation	Lobectomy • Consider completion thyroidectomy if invasive histology
PAX8-PPARG	No	Lobectomy • Consider completion thyroidectomy if invasive histology
TSHR	No	Surveillance or definitive
THADA	No	treatment if associated
GNAS	No	with autonomous function (*TSHR* or *GNAS*)
AKT1, CTNNB1, EIF1AX, and others	Unknown	No specific recommendation

Abbreviations: AKT1, v-akt murine thymoma viral oncogene homolog 1; EIF1AX, eukaryotic translation initiation factor 1A, X-chromosomal; GNAS, guanine nucleotide-binding protein (G protein) stimulatory alpha subunit; THADA, thyroid adenoma associated.
[a] Associated with PTC but limited data suggest that it is less invasive than in adults.

1. Oncogene panels are the only tests that have clinical utility to predict an increased risk for malignancy in patients younger than 19 years.
2. Oncogene panels should only be ordered on FNA samples with indeterminate cytology (TBSRTC categories III and IV). The addition of oncogene testing for solid nodules with indeterminate or high-risk US features but benign cytology (TBSRTC category II) should also be considered. High-risk US features include hypoechogenicity, solid composition, lobulated or irregular margins, taller than wide shape in transverse imaging, and/or the presence of microcalcifications.[63]
3. In pediatric patients, the presence of a *RET-PTC*, *NTRK1/3*, or *BRAF* gene fusion is associated with an increased risk of invasive disease. Total thyroidectomy with central neck lymph node dissection should be performed. For these patients, complete preoperative US screening for abnormal lymph nodes in the lateral neck must be ensured, with FNA of at least 1 lymph node per neck level, to stratify and optimize therapeutic lateral neck lymph node dissection. Although preliminary data suggest that nodules with point mutations in BRAF may not portend disease that is as invasive as in adult patients, because of the association with cPTC, until further data are available, it is prudent to consider a similar approach.
4. The presence of the other mutations (eg, RAS) or gene fusions (PAX8-PPARG) seems to be associated with an increased risk of malignancy but a higher likelihood of less invasive disease. Thus, as long as the preoperative US is suggestive of disease limited to the thyroid, until further data are available, lobectomy is the surgery of choice. A low mutation level in *RAS* detected by NGS (defined as <10% alleles, corresponding with <20% of cells with a mutation) may be associated with benign disease, including NIFTP. Thus, diagnostic lobectomy should also be considered as the initial surgical approach in these cases.

RADIATION-INDUCED THYROID CANCERS

Exposure to ionizing radiation, especially at young age, increases the risk for thyroid neoplasia (benign and malignant).[64] Radiation-induced thyroid malignancies seem to occur as early as 5 years after exposure, and to develop in younger patients compared with spontaneous thyroid cancers, for which the peak incidence occurs during adolescence.[65,66] In general, radiation-induced thyroid cancers are more likely to be multifocal,[67,68] there is a higher association with gene fusions compared with point mutations,[21] and they express higher levels of vascular endothelial growth factor than do other forms of childhood thyroid cancer.[21,69,70] A cellular model that likely explains the observed increase in gene fusions is the spatial geometry that allows *ELE-1* and *RET* (*RET-PTC3*), as well as *H4* and *RET* (*RET-PTC1L*), to recombine following chromosomal breaks that arise from radiation exposure.[71,72]

INHERITED CANCER SYNDROMES

Inheritable forms of thyroid cancer account for approximately 5% of thyroid malignancy within the pediatric population. DTC is most commonly associated with an inherited tumor syndrome, including PTEN (phosphate and tensin homologue deleted on chromosome 10) hamartoma tumor syndrome (PHTS or Cowden syndrome; OMIM [Online Mendelian Inheritance in Man data base] 601728 and GeneReviews), familial adenomatous polyposis (or Gardner syndrome; OMIM 175100 and GeneReviews), DICER1-pleuropulmonary blastoma familial tumor predisposition syndrome (OMIM 606241 and GeneReviews), and Carney complex (OMIM 160980 and GeneReviews), or as an isolated event in which DTC is diagnosed in 2 or more first-degree relatives, termed familial nonmedullary thyroid carcinoma (FNMTC; OMIM 188550 and several other OMIM entries). PHTS is caused by inactivating mutations in the *PTEN* or *SDHx* tumor suppressor genes, or hypermethylation of *KLLN* (the PTEN promotor) resulting in overactivation of protein kinase B (Akt).[73–75] Clinical features of PHTS include macrocephaly, freckling of the glans penis, development of multiple hamartomas, and an increased lifetime risk of breast (women only, 85% lifetime risk), endometrial, and renal carcinomas, as well as multinodular goiter and DTC, both FTC and PTC.[74,75] Thyroid cancer may be the earliest expression of malignancy, with a 9-fold risk for developing thyroid cancer before 18 years of age.[75] The youngest patient reported to have PHTS-associated thyroid cancer was 7 years of age.[76] Surveillance for associated malignancies is recommended beginning at age 30 years (female mammogram or MRI, transvaginal US, colonoscopy for men and women, and renal imaging) with initiation of annual thyroid US at the time of diagnosis.[77] Familial adenomatous polyposis is a colon cancer predisposition syndrome with onset of adenomatous polyps by age 18 years. Colon cancer typically develops by age 30 to 35 years. There is an increased risk of hepatoblastoma (risk increased >750×), adrenal tumors, and thyroid cancer (1%–2%).[78] The cribriform-morular variant of PTC is a uniquely associated with familial adenomatous polyposis (FAP) and thyroid tumorigenesis is associated with acquisition of a somatic mutation in *APC*, *CTNNB1* (beta-catenin), *RAS*, or a *RET-PTC*.[79] DICER-1 syndrome is associated with missense mutations within the RNase IIIb domain of *DICER 1* with somatic loss of function of the other allele associated with an increased risk for pleuropulmonary blastoma (PPB), Sertoli-Leydig cell tumors, and cystic nephroma.[80] Multinodular goiter is the most common clinical features of DICER-1 syndrome, with an increased risk for malignant transformation directly[81] or associated with previous treatment of PPB.[82] The Carney complex is caused by mutations in the protein kinase A regulatory subunit type Ia gene (*PRKAR1A*), and is associated with spotty skin pigmentation (lentigines), myxomas (heart, breast, and other locations), schwannomas, primary pigmented nodular adrenocortical disease, growth hormone–secreting pituitary adenomas or hyperplasia, large-cell calcifying Sertoli cell tumors of the testes (also found in Peutz-Jeghers syndrome), and thyroid cancer.[83] In FNMTC, approximately 11 chromosomal loci have been identified; however, only 4 of them have an identified susceptibility gene: *SRGAP1* (12q14), *TITF1/NKX2.1* (14q13), *FOXE1* (9q22.33), and *HABP2* (10q25.3), with only *FOXE1* and *HABP2* confirmed by independent investigators.[84,85]

MTC is a neuroendocrine malignancy that derives from the neural crest-originated parafollicular C cells of the thyroid gland.[86] Thus, in contrast with follicular cell–derived thyroid tumors (FTC and PTC), MTC cells are not responsive to TSH, do not express the sodium-iodide symporter, and do not produce Tg; they secrete calcitonin and carcinoembryonic antigen, both of which serve as tumor markers of MTC. In children, MTC is a monogenic disorder caused by a dominantly inherited or de novo gain-of-function mutation in the *RET* proto-oncogene associated with MEN type 2, either MEN 2A or 2B, depending on the specific mutation (**Table 4**).[86] In children with hereditary MEN 2B, macroscopic MTC may be detectable within the first year of life and nodal metastases may occur before 5 years of age. The recognition of mucosal neuromas, a history of alacrima, constipation (secondary to intestinal ganglioneuromatosis), and marfanoid facial features and body habitus is critical to early recognition and diagnosis because the RET mutation (codon 918) associated with MEN 2B is often de novo.[87] The timing for thyroidectomy based on the American Thyroid Association guidelines on the diagnosis and management of medullary thyroid cancer is listed in **Table 4**.[86] Approximately 50% of patients with MEN 2B develop a pheochromocytoma, with a varying degree of risk for developing pheochromocytoma and hyperparathyroidism in MEN 2A based on the specific RET mutation.[86]

Table 4
Risk levels and management based on common *RET* mutations detected on genetic screening

MTC Risk Level	*RET* Mutation	Age for Prophylactic Thyroidectomy
Highest (MEN2B)	M918T	Total thyroidectomy in the first year of life, ideally before 5 y of age. Risk of metastasis increases after 5 y of age
High (MEN2A)	A883F C634F/G/R/S/W/Y	Total thyroidectomy at or before 5 y of age based on serum calcitonin levels
Moderate (MEN2A)	G533C, C609F/G/R/S/Y C611F/G/S/Y/W, C618F/R/S, C620F/R/S, C630R/Y, D631Y, K666E, E768D, L790F, V804L, V804M, S891A, R912P	Total thyroidectomy to be performed when the serum calcitonin levels is above the normal range or at convenience if the parents do not wish to embark on a lengthy period of surveillance

Data from Wells SA Jr, Asa SL, Dralle H, et al. Revised American Thyroid Association guidelines for the management of medullary thyroid carcinoma. Thyroid 2015;25(6):567–610.

ADDITIONAL GENOMIC ASSAYS

As the TCGA has shown, comprehensive, multiplatform analysis is critical to improving the understanding of thyroid tumorigenesis to increase the accuracy of diagnosis as well as optimize stratification of care, both surgical and medical. Efforts must be made to expand knowledge of the genomic, epigenomic, and proteomic profile of pediatric DTC. The number of tumors that have been interrogated with NGS is limited (see **Table 1**) and there are no data on incorporating additional platforms, including, but not limited to, miR expression and whole-exome and gene expression profiles to determine whether pediatric PTC can be divided into a similar adult paradigm of *BRAF*-like versus *RAS*-like signaling and differentiation.[10] Advances in the molecular landscape of pediatric DTC have significant potential to improve the approach to diagnosis and care of pediatric patients and there is a high likelihood that a greater understanding of how tumors with similar oncogenic alterations can maintain differentiation will also positively affect the care provided to adult patients with refractory disease.

SUMMARY

All patients with DTC stand to benefit from the identification and incorporation of a reliable molecular profiling system, in both the preoperative and postoperative stages of evaluation and treatment. Ideally, the selective and appropriate incorporation of genomic data and tools into clinical care would allow for stratification of treatment, limiting aggressive therapy for patients at high risk for persistent or recurrent disease, for whom aggressive intervention and monitoring are warranted. The return in investment for deciphering the genomic landscape for pediatric thyroid cancer will be realized over the lifetimes of children or adolescents through decreased and potentially avoidable medical and surgical complications.

REFERENCES

1. Saji M, Ringel MD. The PI3K-Akt-mTOR pathway in initiation and progression of thyroid tumors. Mol Cell Endocrinol 2010;321(1):20–8.

2. Xing M. Genetic alterations in the phosphatidylinositol-3 kinase/Akt pathway in thyroid cancer. Thyroid 2010;20(7):697–706.
3. Fagin JA, Mitsiades N. Molecular pathology of thyroid cancer: diagnostic and clinical implications. Best Pract Res Clin Endocrinol Metab 2008;22(6):955–69.
4. Santoro M, Melillo RM, Carlomagno F, et al. Minireview: RET: normal and abnormal functions. Endocrinology 2004;145(12):5448–51.
5. Xing M. BRAF mutation in papillary thyroid cancer: pathogenic role, molecular bases, and clinical implications. Endocr Rev 2007;28(7):742–62.
6. Dwight T, Thoppe SR, Foukakis T, et al. Involvement of the PAX8/peroxisome proliferator-activated receptor gamma rearrangement in follicular thyroid tumors. J Clin Endocrinol Metab 2003;88(9):4440–5.
7. Nikiforova MN, Lynch RA, Biddinger PW, et al. RAS point mutations and PAX8-PPAR gamma rearrangement in thyroid tumors: evidence for distinct molecular pathways in thyroid follicular carcinoma. J Clin Endocrinol Metab 2003;88(5): 2318–26.
8. Nikiforova MN, Nikiforov YE. Molecular diagnostics and predictors in thyroid cancer. Thyroid 2009;19(12):1351–61.
9. Vasko V, Ferrand M, Di Cristofaro J, et al. Specific pattern of RAS oncogene mutations in follicular thyroid tumors. J Clin Endocrinol Metab 2003;88(6):2745–52.
10. Cancer Genome Atlas Research Network. Integrated genomic characterization of papillary thyroid carcinoma. Cell 2014;159(3):676–90.
11. Cordioli MI, Moraes L, Alves MT, et al. Thyroid-specific genes expression uncovered age-related differences in pediatric thyroid carcinomas. Int J Endocrinol 2016;2016:1956740.
12. Kumagai A, Namba H, Saenko VA, et al. Low frequency of BRAFT1796A mutations in childhood thyroid carcinomas. J Clin Endocrinol Metab 2004;89(9): 4280–4.
13. Penko K, Livezey J, Fenton C, et al. BRAF mutations are uncommon in papillary thyroid cancer of young patients. Thyroid 2005;15(4):320–5.
14. Ballester LY, Sarabia SF, Sayeed H, et al. Integrating molecular testing in the diagnosis and management of children with thyroid lesions. Pediatr Dev Pathol 2016; 19(2):94–100.
15. Givens DJ, Buchmann LO, Agarwal AM, et al. BRAF V600E does not predict aggressive features of pediatric papillary thyroid carcinoma. Laryngoscope 2014;124(9):E389–93.
16. Henke LE, Perkins SM, Pfeifer JD, et al. BRAF V600E mutational status in pediatric thyroid cancer. Pediatr Blood Cancer 2014;61(7):1168–72.
17. Monaco SE, Pantanowitz L, Khalbuss WE, et al. Cytomorphological and molecular genetic findings in pediatric thyroid fine-needle aspiration. Cancer Cytopathology 2012;120(5):342–50.
18. Nikita ME, Jiang W, Cheng SM, et al. Mutational analysis in pediatric thyroid cancer and correlations with age, ethnicity, and clinical presentation. Thyroid 2016; 26(2):227–34.
19. Picarsic JL, Buryk MA, Ozolek J, et al. Molecular characterization of sporadic pediatric thyroid carcinoma with the DNA/RNA THYROSeq v2 next-generation sequencing assay. Pediatr Dev Pathol 2016;19(2):115–22.
20. Prasad ML, Vyas M, Horne MJ, et al. NTRK fusion oncogenes in pediatric papillary thyroid carcinoma in northeast United States. Cancer 2016;122(7):1097–107.
21. Ricarte-Filho JC, Li S, Garcia-Rendueles ME, et al. Identification of kinase fusion oncogenes in post-Chernobyl radiation-induced thyroid cancers. J Clin Invest 2013;123(11):4935–44.

22. Rosenbaum E, Hosler G, Zahurak M, et al. Mutational activation of BRAF is not a major event in sporadic childhood papillary thyroid carcinoma. Mod Pathol 2005; 18(7):898–902.

23. Sassolas G, Hafdi-Nejjari Z, Ferraro A, et al. Oncogenic alterations in papillary thyroid cancers of young patients. Thyroid 2012;22(1):17–26.

24. Francis GL, Waguespack SG, Bauer AJ, et al. Management guidelines for children with thyroid nodules and differentiated thyroid cancer: the American Thyroid Association Guidelines Task Force on Pediatric Thyroid Cancer. Thyroid 2015; 25(7):716–59.

25. Handkiewicz-Junak D, Czarniecka A, Jarzab B. Molecular prognostic markers in papillary and follicular thyroid cancer: current status and future directions. Mol Cell Endocrinol 2010;322(1–2):8–28.

26. Xing M, Clark D, Guan H, et al. BRAF mutation testing of thyroid fine-needle aspiration biopsy specimens for preoperative risk stratification in papillary thyroid cancer. J Clin Oncol 2009;27(18):2977–82.

27. Xing M. BRAF mutation in thyroid cancer. Endocr Relat Cancer 2005;12(2): 245–62.

28. Kunstman JW, Juhlin CC, Goh G, et al. Characterization of the mutational landscape of anaplastic thyroid cancer via whole-exome sequencing. Hum Mol Genet 2015;24(8):2318–29.

29. Dhillon AS, Kolch W. Oncogenic B-Raf mutations: crystal clear at last. Cancer Cell 2004;5(4):303–4.

30. Wan PT, Garnett MJ, Roe SM, et al. Mechanism of activation of the RAF-ERK signaling pathway by oncogenic mutations of B-RAF. Cell 2004;116(6):855–67.

31. Mitsutake N, Miyagishi M, Mitsutake S, et al. BRAF mediates RET/PTC-induced mitogen-activated protein kinase activation in thyroid cells: functional support for requirement of the RET/PTC-RAS-BRAF pathway in papillary thyroid carcinogenesis. Endocrinology 2006;147(2):1014–9.

32. Liu D, Liu Z, Condouris S, et al. BRAF V600E maintains proliferation, transformation, and tumorigenicity of BRAF-mutant papillary thyroid cancer cells. J Clin Endocrinol Metab 2007;92(6):2264–71.

33. Mitsutake N, Knauf JA, Mitsutake S, et al. Conditional BRAFV600E expression induces DNA synthesis, apoptosis, dedifferentiation, and chromosomal instability in thyroid PCCL3 cells. Cancer Res 2005;65(6):2465–73.

34. Xing M, Westra WH, Tufano RP, et al. BRAF mutation predicts a poorer clinical prognosis for papillary thyroid cancer. J Clin Endocrinol Metab 2005;90(12): 6373–9.

35. Kebebew E, Weng J, Bauer J, et al. The prevalence and prognostic value of BRAF mutation in thyroid cancer. Ann Surg 2007;246(3):466–70 [discussion: 470–1].

36. Elisei R, Ugolini C, Viola D, et al. BRAF(V600E) mutation and outcome of patients with papillary thyroid carcinoma: a 15-year median follow-up study. J Clin Endocrinol Metab 2008;93(10):3943–9.

37. Riesco-Eizaguirre G, Rodriguez I, De la Vieja A, et al. The BRAFV600E oncogene induces transforming growth factor beta secretion leading to sodium iodide symporter repression and increased malignancy in thyroid cancer. Cancer Res 2009; 69(21):8317–25.

38. Edge SB, Byrd DR, Compton CC, et al. Thyroid. In: Edge SB, Byrd DR, Compton CC, et al, editors. American Joint Committee on Cancer (AJCC) Cancer Staging Manual. 7th edition. New York: Springer; 2010. p. 87–96.

39. Barollo S, Pennelli G, Vianello F, et al. BRAF in primary and recurrent papillary thyroid cancers: the relationship with (131)I and 2-[(18)F]fluoro-2-deoxy-D-glucose uptake ability. Eur J Endocrinol 2010;163(4):659–63.

40. Pillai S, Gopalan V, Smith RA, et al. Diffuse sclerosing variant of papillary thyroid carcinoma–an update of its clinicopathological features and molecular biology. Crit Rev Oncol Hematol 2015;94(1):64–73.

41. Adeniran AJ, Zhu Z, Gandhi M, et al. Correlation between genetic alterations and microscopic features, clinical manifestations, and prognostic characteristics of thyroid papillary carcinomas. Am J Surg Pathol 2006;30(2):216–22.

42. Malandrino P, Russo M, Regalbuto C, et al. The outcome of the diffuse sclerosing variant of papillary thyroid cancer: a meta-analysis. Thyroid 2016;26(9):1285–92.

43. Koo JS, Hong S, Park CS. Diffuse sclerosing variant is a major subtype of papillary thyroid carcinoma in the young. Thyroid 2009;19(11):1225–31.

44. Fenton CL, Lukes Y, Nicholson D, et al. The ret/PTC mutations are common in sporadic papillary thyroid carcinoma of children and young adults. J Clin Endocrinol Metab 2000;85(3):1170–5.

45. Nikiforov YE, Rowland JM, Bove KE, et al. Distinct pattern of ret oncogene rearrangements in morphological variants of radiation-induced and sporadic thyroid papillary carcinomas in children. Cancer Res 1997;57(9):1690–4.

46. Rabes HM, Demidchik EP, Sidorow JD, et al. Pattern of radiation-induced RET and NTRK1 rearrangements in 191 post-Chernobyl papillary thyroid carcinomas: biological, phenotypic, and clinical implications. Clin Cancer Res 2000;6(3): 1093–103.

47. Unger K, Zitzelsberger H, Salvatore G, et al. Heterogeneity in the distribution of RET/PTC rearrangements within individual post-Chernobyl papillary thyroid carcinomas. J Clin Endocrinol Metab 2004;89(9):4272–9.

48. Zhu Z, Ciampi R, Nikiforova MN, et al. Prevalence of RET/PTC rearrangements in thyroid papillary carcinomas: effects of the detection methods and genetic heterogeneity. J Clin Endocrinol Metab 2006;91(9):3603–10.

49. Esapa CT, Johnson SJ, Kendall-Taylor P, et al. Prevalence of Ras mutations in thyroid neoplasia. Clin Endocrinol 1999;50(4):529–35.

50. Kondo T, Ezzat S, Asa SL. Pathogenetic mechanisms in thyroid follicular-cell neoplasia. Nat Rev Cancer 2006;6(4):292–306.

51. Santarpia L, Myers JN, Sherman SI, et al. Genetic alterations in the RAS/RAF/mitogen-activated protein kinase and phosphatidylinositol 3-kinase/Akt signaling pathways in the follicular variant of papillary thyroid carcinoma. Cancer 2010; 116(12):2974–83.

52. Di Cristofaro J, Marcy M, Vasko V, et al. Molecular genetic study comparing follicular variant versus classic papillary thyroid carcinomas: association of N-ras mutation in codon 61 with follicular variant. Hum Pathol 2006;37(7):824–30.

53. Ricarte-Filho J, Ganly I, Rivera M, et al. Papillary thyroid carcinomas with cervical lymph node metastases can be stratified into clinically relevant prognostic categories using oncogenic BRAF, the number of nodal metastases, and extra-nodal extension. Thyroid 2012;22(6):575–84.

54. Vasko VV, Gaudart J, Allasia C, et al. Thyroid follicular adenomas may display features of follicular carcinoma and follicular variant of papillary carcinoma. Eur J Endocrinol 2004;151(6):779–86.

55. Nikiforov YE, Seethala RR, Tallini G, et al. Nomenclature revision for encapsulated follicular variant of papillary thyroid carcinoma: a paradigm shift to reduce overtreatment of indolent tumors. JAMA Oncol 2016;2(8):1023–9.

56. Freitas BC, Cerutti JM. Genetic markers differentiating follicular thyroid carcinoma from benign lesions. Mol Cell Endocrinol 2010;321(1):77–85.
57. Volante M, Rapa I, Gandhi M, et al. RAS mutations are the predominant molecular alteration in poorly differentiated thyroid carcinomas and bear prognostic impact. J Clin Endocrinol Metab 2009;94(12):4735–41.
58. Cordioli MI, Moraes L, Carvalheira G, et al. AGK-BRAF gene fusion is a recurrent event in sporadic pediatric thyroid carcinoma. Cancer Med 2016;5(7):1535–41.
59. Cibas ES, Ali SZ. The Bethesda System for reporting thyroid cytopathology. Am J Clin Pathol 2009;132(5):658–65.
60. Smith M, Pantanowitz L, Khalbuss WE, et al. Indeterminate pediatric thyroid fine needle aspirations: a study of 68 cases. Acta Cytol 2013;57(4):341–8.
61. Ferris RL, Baloch Z, Bernet V, et al. American Thyroid Association statement on surgical application of molecular profiling for thyroid nodules: current impact on perioperative decision making. Thyroid 2015;25(7):760–8.
62. Noureldine SI, Najafian A, Aragon Han P, et al. Evaluation of the effect of diagnostic molecular testing on the surgical decision-making process for patients with thyroid nodules. JAMA Otolaryngol Head Neck Surg 2016;142(7):676–82.
63. Grant EG, Tessler FN, Hoang JK, et al. Thyroid ultrasound reporting lexicon: white paper of the ACR Thyroid Imaging, Reporting and Data System (TIRADS) Committee. J Am Coll Radiol 2015;12(12 Pt A):1272–9.
64. Thompson DE, Mabuchi K, Ron E, et al. Cancer incidence in atomic bomb survivors. Part II: solid tumors, 1958-1987. Radiat Res 1994;137(2 Suppl):S17–67.
65. Astakhova LN, Anspaugh LR, Beebe GW, et al. Chernobyl-related thyroid cancer in children of Belarus: a case-control study. Radiat Res 1998;150(3):349–56.
66. Pacini F, Vorontsova T, Demidchik EP, et al. Post-Chernobyl thyroid carcinoma in Belarus children and adolescents: comparison with naturally occurring thyroid carcinoma in Italy and France. J Clin Endocrinol Metab 1997;82(11):3563–9.
67. Antonelli A, Miccoli P, Derzhitski VE, et al. Epidemiologic and clinical evaluation of thyroid cancer in children from the Gomel region (Belarus). World J Surg 1996;20(7):867–71.
68. Nikiforov Y, Gnepp DR. Pediatric thyroid cancer after the Chernobyl disaster. Pathomorphologic study of 84 cases (1991-1992) from the Republic of Belarus. Cancer 1994;74(2):748–66.
69. Beimfohr C, Klugbauer S, Demidchik EP, et al. NTRK1 re-arrangement in papillary thyroid carcinomas of children after the Chernobyl reactor accident. Int J Cancer 1999;80(6):842–7.
70. Rabes HM. Gene rearrangements in radiation-induced thyroid carcinogenesis. Med Pediatr Oncol 2001;36(5):574–82.
71. Nikiforov YE, Koshoffer A, Nikiforova M, et al. Chromosomal breakpoint positions suggest a direct role for radiation in inducing illegitimate recombination between the ELE1 and RET genes in radiation-induced thyroid carcinomas. Oncogene 1999;18(46):6330–4.
72. Nikiforov YE. Spatial positioning of RET and H4 following radiation exposure leads to tumor development. ScientificWorldJournal 2001;1(5):186–7.
73. Mahdi H, Mester JL, Nizialek EA, et al. Germline PTEN, SDHB-D, and KLLN alterations in endometrial cancer patients with Cowden and Cowden-like syndromes: an international, multicenter, prospective study. Cancer 2015;121(5):688–96.
74. Ngeow J, Eng C. PTEN hamartoma tumor syndrome: clinical risk assessment and management protocol. Methods 2015;77-78:11–9.
75. Ngeow J, Mester J, Rybicki LA, et al. Incidence and Clinical Characteristics of Thyroid Cancer in prospective series of individuals with Cowden and Cowden-

Like Syndrome characterized by germline PTEN, SDH, or KLLN alterations. J Clin Endocrinol Metab 2011;96(12):E2063–71.

76. Smith JR, Marqusee E, Webb S, et al. Thyroid nodules and cancer in children with PTEN hamartoma tumor syndrome. J Clin Endocrinol Metab 2011;96(1):34–7.

77. Eng C. PTEN hamartoma tumor syndrome (PHTS). In: Pagon RA, Adam MP, Ardinger HH, et al, editors. GeneReviews(R). Seattle (WA): University of Washington, Seattle; 1993.

78. Gruner BA, DeNapoli TS, Andrews W, et al. Hepatocellular carcinoma in children associated with Gardner syndrome or familial adenomatous polyposis. J Pediatr Hematol Oncol 1998;20(3):274–8.

79. Giannelli SM, McPhaul L, Nakamoto J, et al. Familial adenomatous polyposis-associated, cribriform morular variant of papillary thyroid carcinoma harboring a K-RAS mutation: case presentation and review of molecular mechanisms. Thyroid 2014;24(7):1184–9.

80. Cai S, Zhao W, Nie X, et al. Multimorbidity and genetic characteristics of DICER1 syndrome based on systematic review. J Pediatr Hematol Oncol 2016. [Epub ahead of print].

81. Rutter MM, Jha P, Schultz KA, et al. DICER1 mutations and differentiated thyroid carcinoma: evidence of a direct association. J Clin Endocrinol Metab 2016; 101(1):1–5.

82. de Kock L, Sabbaghian N, Soglio DB, et al. Exploring the association between DICER1 mutations and differentiated thyroid carcinoma. J Clin Endocrinol Metab 2014;99(6):E1072–7.

83. Stratakis CA. Carney complex: a familial lentiginosis predisposing to a variety of tumors. Rev Endocr Metab Disord 2016;17(3):367–71.

84. Bauer AJ. Clinical behavior and genetics of nonsyndromic, familial nonmedullary thyroid cancer. Front Horm Res 2013;41:141–8.

85. Peiling Yang S, Ngeow J. Familial non-medullary thyroid cancer: unraveling the genetic maze. Endocr Relat Cancer 2016;23(12):R577–95.

86. Wells SA Jr, Asa SL, Dralle H, et al. Revised American Thyroid Association guidelines for the management of medullary thyroid carcinoma. Thyroid 2015;25(6): 567–610.

87. Waguespack SG, Rich TA. Multiple endocrine neoplasia [corrected] syndrome type 2B in early childhood: long-term benefit of prophylactic thyroidectomy. Cancer 2010;116(9):2284.

Genetics of Hyperparathyroidism, Including Parathyroid Cancer

William F. Simonds, MD

KEYWORDS

- Tumor suppressor • Oncogene • Multiple endocrine neoplasia • MEN1 • MEN2A
- CDC73 • CCND1 • RET

KEY POINTS

- Primary hyperparathyroidism, caused by parathyroid tumors, is mostly sporadic.
- The molecular genetic investigation of rare syndromic forms of hyperparathyroidism has nevertheless led to significant advances in the understanding of both familial and sporadic parathyroid neoplasia.
- Both oncogenes and tumor suppressors have been implicated in the cause of parathyroid tumors.
- The discovery of novel parathyroid tumor susceptibility genes is likely to result from the application of next-generation sequencing methods to the analysis of sporadic parathyroid tumors and nonsyndromic familial cases of hyperparathyroidism.

INTRODUCTION

Primary hyperparathyroidism (HPT) is a disorder of mineral metabolism, typically manifesting in hypercalcemia, that results from the excessive secretion of parathyroid hormone from 1 or more neoplastic parathyroid glands.[1] Although HPT is mostly sporadic, familial forms of HPT represent some 2% to 5% of total cases, most of which are caused by germline mutation of known HPT-susceptibility genes (**Table 1**). Investigation of the molecular genetics underlying these rare familial syndromes has yielded significant insight into the pathophysiology of both sporadic and familial parathyroid neoplasms. Signaling involving the G

Disclosure Statement: The author has no commercial, financial, or personal conflict of interest that has inappropriately influenced the content of this article. The Intramural Research Program of the National Institute of Diabetes and Digestive and Kidney Diseases (DK043012-15) supported this research.
Metabolic Diseases Branch, National Institute of Diabetes and Digestive and Kidney Diseases, National Institutes of Health, Building 10, Room 8C-101, 10 Center Drive, MSC 1752, Bethesda, MD 20892, USA
E-mail address: wfs@helix.nih.gov

Table 1
Genes implicated in syndromic and sporadic parathyroid tumorigenesis, and related syndromes

Gene	Protein Encoded	Associated Hyperparathyroid Syndrome: Main Syndromic Manifestations	Features of Syndromic Parathyroid Tumors	Defect in Sporadic Parathyroid Tumors
MEN1	Menin	MEN1: anterior pituitary, parathyroid, enteropancreatic, foregut carcinoid tumors	Multiple, asymmetric tumors typical (>99% benign)	Inactivation in ~25%–35% of benign tumors; mutation exceedingly rare in cancer
CDC73/HRPT2	Parafibromin	HPT–jaw tumor syndrome: fibro-osseous jaw, parathyroid, uterine tumors; renal cysts	Single tumor common (~15% malignant)	Inactivation in ~70% of cancers; mutation rare in sporadic adenomas
CDKN1B	P27(Kip1)	MEN4: anterior pituitary, other involvement varies	Single to multiple glands (benign in reports to date); can be recurrent	Loss-of-function mutation in ~5% of sporadic adenomas; including germline mutation in sporadic presentation
CASR	Calcium-sensing receptor	FHH1 with heterozygous inactivation; NSHPT with homozygous inactivation	FHH1: near-normal size and surgical pathology; altered serum calcium set-point for PTH release NSHPT: marked enlargement of multiple glands by polyclonal (nonneoplastic) mechanism	Decreased expression common; mutation exceedingly rare
GNA11	G protein α11 subunit	FHH2	ND	ND
AP2S1	Adaptor protein-2 sigma subunit	FHH3: hypercalcemia more severe than in FHH1	ND	ND
RET	c-Ret	MEN2A: medullary thyroid cancer, pheochromocytoma, parathyroid tumors	Single tumor common (>99% benign)	Mutation exceedingly rare
CCND1/PRAD1	Cyclin D1	NA	NA	Overexpression results from DNA rearrangement involving PTH gene

Abbreviations: MEN1, multiple endocrine neoplasia type 1; MEN4, multiple endocrine neoplasia type 4; NA, not applicable; ND, not determined (lack of relevant published studies); NSHPT, neonatal severe hyperparathyroidism; PTH, parathyroid hormone.

protein–coupled calcium-sensing receptor (CaSR) affects the hormonal function of parathyroid cells, and the mutation of genes involved in CaSR signaling has also been implicated in familial syndromes of parathyroid hormone (PTH)–dependent hypercalcemia. This article reviews current knowledge of the genetics of HPT and PTH-dependent hypercalcemia caused by benign and malignant parathyroid disease.

PATHOPHYSIOLOGY OF PRIMARY HYPERPARATHYROIDISM

Maintenance of the serum calcium concentration within a narrow physiologic range is achieved by regulation of PTH secretion from parathyroid cells in response to changes in the circulating ionized calcium level. The G protein–coupled CaSR located on the surface membrane of the parathyroid chief cells negatively regulates the secretion of PTH.[2,3] In clinical medicine, HPT is typically defined by the conjunction of increased serum ionized calcium level with inappropriately increased PTH level.[1] Most parathyroid tumors are benign adenomas. Parathyroid carcinoma is a rare cause of HPT seen in less than 1% of cases.

Approximately 2% to 5% of cases of HPT are associated with familial disease. Study of this small subset has nevertheless provided great insight into the genetic changes and molecular pathways that promote parathyroid neoplasia (see **Table 1**). The most common genetic disorders associated with HPT are multiple endocrine neoplasia (MEN) type 1 (MEN1), MEN2A, HPT–jaw tumor (HPT-JT) syndrome, and familial isolated HPT (FIHP).[4–7] Familial hypocalciuric hypercalcemia (FHH) is a related, genetically heterogeneous, largely benign condition of PTH-dependent hypercalcemia often mimicking HPT that does not correct with partial or subtotal parathyroidectomy (PTX).[8] These genetic disorders and their relation to the underlying molecular and genetic alterations relevant to parathyroid neoplasia are discussed in detail later.

KNUDSON'S 2-HIT HYPOTHESIS AND TUMOR SUPPRESSOR GENES

Some 45 years ago, Alfred Knudson[9] proposed a model for tumor development based on his epidemiologic analysis of retinoblastoma. Familial retinoblastoma is much more rare than sporadic retinoblastoma, but the former has a much earlier age of onset and is more frequently binocular. According to the so-called 2-hit hypothesis of neoplasia proposed by Knudson,[9] 2 events (or hits) in an affected cell confer a selective growth advantage and result in its clonal expansion.[10]

In accordance with clinical and molecular genetic data accrued since his original proposal, Knudson's[9] concept can be updated. In many hereditary tumor syndromes, an inherited mutation in the germline DNA affecting 1 allele of a tumor suppressor gene represents the first event or hit that is present in all the cells of the affected offspring (**Fig. 1**). The tendency for bilateral and/or multifocal disease in hereditary tumor syndromes as well as the earlier age of onset are explained by the greater likelihood of any particular cell acquiring a second hit; that is, a somatic mutation in a second allele of the same tumor suppressor gene. The second hit, which inactivates the remaining wild-type allele, most often results from large subchromosomal or even chromosomal deletion or else DNA rearrangement (see **Fig. 1**). Biallelic inactivating mutation of the MEN1 and the CDC73/HRPT2 tumor suppressor genes can frequently be shown in DNA derived from parathyroid tumors, in the context of the familial syndromes MEN1 and HPT-JT, respectively. In most such patients, a germline loss-of-function mutation of the associated tumor suppressor gene can be shown, representing the first hit (see **Fig. 1**).

Patient *without* germline *CDC73/HRPT2* mutation

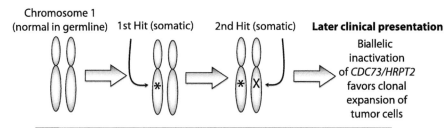

Patient *with* germline *CDC73/HRPT2* mutation

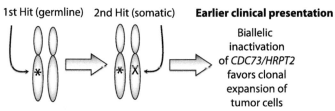

Fig. 1. Two-hit loss-of-function mutation of the *CDC73/HRPT2* tumor suppressor in parathy-roid neoplasia. Benign or malignant parathyroid tumors causing HPT can result from 2-hit loss of function of the *CDC73/HRPT2* tumor suppressor gene according to the Knudson hy-pothesis (see text). The human *CDC73/HRPT2* gene is on chromosome 1 at location 1q25. (*Top*) In a patient without germline *CDC73/HRPT2* mutation, both alleles of *CDC73/HRPT2* are initially normal in all parathyroid cells. Subsequent stepwise acquired or somatic inacti-vation of both alleles in the same parathyroid cell results in clonal expansion that may lead to a sporadic parathyroid tumor. (*Bottom*) In a patient with germline *CDC73/HRPT2* muta-tion in 1 allele, an acquired or somatic DNA mutation at the *CDC73/HRPT2* locus of the re-maining allele in a parathyroid cell results in clonal expansion of that cell that may lead to a benign or malignant parathyroid tumor. Patients with germline *CDC73/HRPT2* mutation who develop parathyroid adenomas or cancer can present sporadically (if lacking or un-aware of relevant family medical history), or belong to a kindred with familial isolated HPT or the HPT-JT syndrome. The presence of the first germline mutation at birth in all para-thyroid tissue accelerates the acquisition of 2 hits within a single parathyroid cell and ac-counts for the earlier age of disease presentation typical of familial forms of HPT such as HPT-JT.

CLINICAL FEATURES AND GENETICS OF MULTIPLE ENDOCRINE NEOPLASIA TYPE 1

MEN1 is the most common familial cause of primary HPT.[11] MEN1 is characterized by a tendency to develop tumors in the anterior pituitary, parathyroid glands, and enter-opancreatic endocrine cells, although tumors in several other endocrine organs and in nonendocrine tissues such as skin and smooth muscle can also be associated with the syndrome.[5,12] Some 10% of MEN1 is sporadic.

Familial MEN1 is inherited in an autosomal dominant fashion. Germline inactivation of 1 allele of the *MEN1* gene on chromosome 11q13 confers the tumor susceptibility.[13] More than 400 distinct germline mutations in *MEN1* have been described in patients and kindreds with MEN1. Most parathyroid and other syndromic tumors from patients with MEN1 can be shown to harbor a somatic mutation or deletion of the second wild-type *MEN1* allele.[5,14]

Molecular genetic analysis of sporadic parathyroid adenomas using conventional DNA sequencing methods identified somatic *MEN1* mutation involving at least 1 allele with a frequency of 3% to 35%.[15–19] The frequency ranged from 26% to 37% in studies that assessed loss of heterozygosity at 11q13 in sporadic parathyroid adenomas. Studies of sporadic benign parathyroid tumor DNA using whole-exome sequencing (WES) methodology identified somatic *MEN1* mutation in some 35% of tumors, similar to results using conventional DNA sequencing methods.[20,21] Because HPT is the most penetrant feature of MEN1 and is usually its initial manifestation, bona fide MEN1 kindreds may rarely be misassigned a provisional diagnosis of FIHP if only younger mutation carriers are evaluated at the time of initial family ascertainment.

The association of *MEN1* mutation with parathyroid carcinoma is rare. At least 2 cases of parathyroid cancer have been reported in patients with MEN1, one with associated parathyroid adenoma, and the other with bilateral parathyroid carcinoma.[22,23]

CLINICAL FEATURES AND GENETICS OF THE HYPERPARATHYROIDISM–JAW TUMOR SYNDROME

HPT-JT is a rare autosomal dominant familial cancer syndrome of variable and incomplete penetrance manifested by HPT, cemento-ossifying tumors of the maxilla and mandible, and less commonly uterine tumors and/or renal cysts.[24–26] HPT is the most penetrant feature and usually the presenting manifestation. In contrast with MEN1, parathyroid carcinoma is frequent in HPT-JT, affecting some 20% or more of those with HPT.[24–27] Approximately 10% of obligate or genetically confirmed carriers have no clinical manifestations.

A loss-of-function mutation of *CDC73/HRPT2* can be shown in the germlines of most HPT-JT kindreds.[28] Most such *CDC73/HRPT2* mutations are predicted to inactivate gene function via frameshift or nonsense mutation.[29] Patients with germline deletion of the *CDC73/HRPT2* gene have also been reported.[30–32] The *CDC73/HRPT2* gene encodes the protein parafibromin.[28] Parafibromin is a presumed tumor suppressor protein because germline-inactivating mutation of the *CDC73/HRPT2* gene predisposes to the full or partial expression of HPT-JT. Somatic mutation of *CDC73/HRPT2* is uncommon in sporadic parathyroid adenomas.[33] In contrast, mutations of *CDC73/HRPT2* are frequently seen in apparently sporadic cases of parathyroid carcinoma.[34–36] Exome sequence analysis of tumor DNA from parathyroid carcinoma revealed preferential amplification of the mutant *CDC73/HRPT2* allele.[37] Some 25% of patients with apparently sporadic parathyroid cancer may harbor germline *CDC73/HRPT2* mutations, suggesting that such cases may represent undiagnosed or incompletely penetrant HPT-JT.[35,36] Besides HPT-JT kindreds, a subset of patients with the FIHP phenotype also harbor germline mutation of *CDC73/HRPT2*, indicating that this familial disorder may represent an incomplete expression of HPT-JT.

CLINICAL FEATURES AND GENETICS OF MULTIPLE ENDOCRINE NEOPLASIA TYPE 4

MEN4 (sometimes called MENX) is a syndrome originally described by Pellegata and colleagues[38] in a multigenerational family with MEN1-like features, including a proband with acromegaly and HPT but lacking *MEN1* mutation. Several members of this kindred, including the proband, were shown to harbor a germline heterozygous nonsense mutation in *CDKN1B*, encoding the cyclin-dependent kinase inhibitor p27(Kip1).[38] Investigation of this locus followed from the genetic analysis of rats with the MenX phenotype, a recessively inherited condition characterized by the development of bilateral pheochromocytomas, paragangliomas, parathyroid adenomas, and thyroid C-cell hyperplasia.[38,39] Only a single member of the MEN4/MENX kindred described by Pellegata and colleagues[38] manifested HPT (the proband).

Since the original report by Pellegata and colleagues,[38] several groups have investigated a role for mutation of *CDKN1B* in parathyroid neoplasia. Apart from the demonstration of HPT linked to *CDKN1B* mutation in monozygotic twins,[40] none of the studies of *CDKN1B* mutation–positive kindreds expressing MEN1-like tumors but lacking *MEN1* germline mutation, and thus characterized by the MEN4 designation, has identified kindreds that include more than 1 genetically unique member with HPT proved to segregate with germline *CDKN1B* mutation.[38,40–45] At least 1 study of patients with features of genetic predisposition to HPT failed to identify any cases with germline *CDKN1B* mutation.[18] In contrast, nonfamilial presentation of primary HPT caused by parathyroid adenomas in association with somatic and germline mutation of *CDKN1B* has been documented.[46]

The characterization of *CDKN1B* as a low-penetrance susceptibility gene for the development of primary parathyroid tumors is supported by good evidence.[46,47] As such, *CDKN1B* remains a reasonable hypothetical candidate for which germline mutation may provide an cause for some cases of familial HPT. However, more research will be required to justify including germline-inactivating mutation of *CDKN1B*, associated with MEN4, in the differential diagnosis of familial HPT. At a minimum, such justification seems to require identification and characterization of at least 1 family that includes more than 1 genetically unique member with HPT linked to pathologic mutation of *CDKN1B* in the germline.

CLINICAL FEATURES AND GENETICS OF FAMILIAL ISOLATED HYPERPARATHYROIDISM

FIHP is a genetically heterogeneous, nonsyndromic, clinically defined diagnosis of exclusion in kindreds with 2 or more cases of HPT but lacking the specific features of MEN1, MEN2A, HPT-JT, or FHH. Although germline mutation of *MEN1*, *CDC73/HRPT2*, or *CASR* may account for a minority of kindreds with the FIHP phenotype on initial ascertainment,[7,48–50] most FIHP kindreds lack mutations in these known HPT-susceptibility genes.[7,48] A distinct genetic cause resulting in the FIHP phenotype has not yet been defined, although a genome-wide screen of 7 FIHP families has identified a 1.7-Mb region of suggestive linkage on the short arm of chromosome 2, at location 2p14-p13.3.[51]

CLINICAL FEATURES AND GENETICS OF FAMILIAL HYPOCALCIURIC HYPERCALCEMIA

FHH is a genetically heterogeneous, clinically benign condition of PTH-dependent hypercalcemia often mimicking HPT (see **Table 1**).[8] FHH cases almost always remain hypercalcemic following partial or subtotal PTX. FHH is a transmitted in an autosomal dominant fashion and usually causes mild HPT with relative hypocalciuria; hypercalcemia in FHH is highly penetrant at all ages, even in the perinatal period.[8] Most cases of FHH are type 1 (FHH1) and result from a heterozygous loss-of-function mutation of the *CASR* gene on chromosome 3 that encodes the CaSR.[2,3,52–54] The homozygous or compound heterozygous inheritance of 2 inactive *CASR* alleles typically results in the phenotype of neonatal severe HPT (NSHPT).[52–54] The nonneoplastic nature of the abnormal parathyroids associated with germline *CASR* loss-of-function mutation was underscored by a recent molecular genetic analysis of enlarged parathyroid glands from a patient with NSHPT that showed generalized polyclonal hyperplasia, rather than the monoclonality that is expected in bona fide parathyroid tumors.[55]

Somatic inactivation of *CASR* has not been found in sporadic parathyroid tumors studied to date,[56,57] even though significant loss of *CASR* expression, not caused by allelic loss, has been documented in parathyroid adenomas and likely contributes to their altered calcium set-point for PTH release.[58]

Type 2 FHH (FHH2) caused by germline loss-of-function mutation of *GNA11*, encoding the G protein α11 subunit,[59,60] and type 3 FHH (FHH3) caused by germline loss-of-function mutation in *AP2S1*, encoding the adaptor protein-2 sigma subunit involved in clathrin-mediated endocytosis,[61–64] have recently been described. Somatic mutation of neither *GNA11* nor *AP2S1* has been reported in sporadic parathyroid tumors.

ONCOGENES AND PROTO-ONCOGENES

Oncogenes derive from naturally occurring genes, referred to as proto-oncogenes, that positively regulate cell division and/or cell growth.[65] Oncogenes represent mutationally activated or overexpressed forms of proto-oncogenes that can induce tumor formation, often in a tissue-specific fashion. Proto-oncogenes frequently encode proteins that are involved in signal transduction, particularly in pathways mediating mitogenic signals. Among the causes of currently recognized familial cancer syndromes, germline mutational activation of proto-oncogenes is rare compared with the germline inactivation of tumor suppressor genes, presumably because of the disruptive effect that constitutive proliferative signaling created by the activation of most proto-oncogenes would likely have on embryonic and fetal development.

CLINICAL FEATURES AND GENETICS OF MULTIPLE ENDOCRINE NEOPLASIA TYPE 2A

Classic MEN2A is a familial syndrome characterized by medullary thyroid cancer (MTC), pheochromocytoma, and primary HPT. HPT in MEN2A resembles sporadic HPT in its clinical presentation, is usually mild, and is almost always caused by benign parathyroid tumors. MEN2A is transmitted in an autosomal dominant fashion. MEN2A is caused by germline gain-of-function mutation in the *RET* (rearranged during transfection) proto-oncogene. *RET* encodes a transmembrane receptor tyrosine kinase that, in conjunction with glial-derived neurotrophic factor (GDNF) family α coreceptors, binds GDNF family ligands.[66]

Germline gain-of-function mutations of *RET* are associated with 3 different endocrine tumor syndromes, all associated with MTC: MEN2A, MEN2B, and familial MTC (FMTC). Parathyroid tumors and HPT are not part of the MEN2B or FMTC disease pattern. Different germline *RET* mutations can result in the different disease phenotypes. In 95% of patients, MEN2A is associated with germline missense mutations that map to the receptor tyrosine kinase's extracellular cysteine-rich domain, involving *RET* codons 609, 611, 618, or 620 of exon 10 or codon 634 of exon 11.[67] About 85% of cases of MEN2A result from missense mutation of the cysteine residue present at codon 634.[68]

THE ROLE OF THE *CCND1* ONCOGENE IN THE PATHOPHYSIOLOGY OF PARATHYROID TUMORS

The *CCND1* (or *PRAD1* [parathyroid adenomatosis 1]) oncogene was discovered during the molecular genetic analysis of several large sporadic parathyroid adenomas that harbored DNA rearrangements involving the PTH gene locus on chromosome 11.[69–71] The *CCND1/PRAD1* oncogene in sporadic parathyroid tumors was identified downstream of a breakpoint caused by the pericentromeric inversion of chromosome 11 DNA.[71] The chromosomal inversion positions the 5′ PTH gene regulatory region (normally located at 11p15) just upstream of the *CCND1/PRAD1* proto-oncogene resident at 11q13.[69–71] The product encoded by the proto-oncogene was subsequently recognized to be a member of the cyclin family based on sequence homology[71] and the gene was renamed cyclin D1 (*CCND1*). It was subsequently shown that transgenic overexpression of *CCND1* in the parathyroid tissue of mice causes cell proliferation and recapitulates the metabolic abnormalities typical of HPT in humans.[72]

CCND1 is overexpressed in some 20% to 40% of sporadic benign parathyroid tumors and in an even higher percentage of parathyroid cancers.[73–76] Activating missense mutations in the CCND1 coding region have not been observed in sporadic parathyroid adenomas.[77] No somatic chromosomal rearrangements involving *CCND1* have been reported in parathyroid carcinoma. Neither germline activating missense mutations nor germline chromosomal translocations/rearrangements involving *CCND1* have been identified in any familial form of HPT.

THE ROLE OF OTHER ONCOGENES IN THE PATHOPHYSIOLOGY OF PARATHYROID TUMORS

Analysis of 8 sporadic parathyroid adenomas by WES and the subsequent targeted sequencing of DNA from an additional 185 parathyroid adenomas showed the Y641N missense mutation in *EZH2* (enhancer of zeste 2) in 2 out of 193 independent parathyroid tumors.[20] *EZH2* encodes the catalytic subunit of polycomb repressive complex 2 and somatic mutations of EZH2 residue Y641, including Y641N, had previously been reported in certain categories of lymphoma.[78] However, mutational analysis of a subsequent set of 80 sporadic benign and malignant parathyroid tumors by an independent group did not find any pathogenic *EZH2* variants, suggesting such somatic mutation may be rare.[79] In the context of lymphoma, *EZH2* is thought to function as a proto-oncogene.[78] Because *EZH2* Y641N mutation and gene overexpression have been reported in parathyroid tumors, *EZH2* may also be considered a candidate proto-oncogene in the parathyroid context if further investigation confirms these initial observations. No transgenic mouse models targeting *EZH2* mutation or overexpression to parathyroid tissue have yet been reported.

Somatic mutations in the candidate parathyroid proto-oncogene *ZFX*, a member of the Krüppel-associated box domain–containing zinc finger protein transcription factors, were first identified by WES analysis of DNA extracted from 19 parathyroid adenomas and matched germline DNA, with confirmation by direct sequencing of tumor DNA from an additional 111 parathyroid adenomas.[80] Several lines of evidence suggest that the somatically acquired mutant *ZFX* alleles detected in parathyroid tumors may act as oncogenes.[81] Development of a transgenic mouse model targeting mutant ZFX protein expression to parathyroid tissue and/or in vitro functional characterization of the mutant ZFX protein will help to clarify the potential significance of *ZFX* as a parathyroid proto-oncogene.

FUTURE CONSIDERATIONS

It is likely that the dysregulation of other genes, besides those discussed earlier, predispose to parathyroid neoplasia. As previously noted, the susceptibility to parathyroid neoplasia in most FIHP kindreds seems to result from the germline mutation of genes not currently recognized for a role in parathyroid disease: 53 among 76 families initially considered as having FIHP in 5 clinical studies that investigated for germline

MEN1, *CASR*, and *CDC73/HRPT2* gene mutation, or nearly 70%, had no currently recognized syndromic cause.[7,48–50]

The existence of currently unidentified parathyroid tumor suppressors and oncogenes is also suggested by the analysis of parathyroid tumors for the loss or gain of specific regions of chromosomal DNA using techniques such as comparative genomic hybridization. Several investigators have found recurrent loss of chromosomal DNA at the 1p, 6q, 9p, and 13q loci in parathyroid tumors, indicating the potential presence there of novel parathyroid tumor suppressor genes.[82–85] The possible presence of novel oncogenes at 9q, 16p, 19p, and Xq is suggested by a convergence of results from several laboratories that show specific chromosomal gain at these loci in benign or malignant parathyroid tumors.[82,84–86]

WES analysis of benign and malignant parathyroid tumors shows great promise for the identification of somatic and germline gene mutations predisposing to parathyroid neoplasia. The success of this method in the identification of the candidate parathyroid oncogenes *EXH2*[20] and *ZFX*[80] has been discussed earlier. Similarly, exome sequence analysis of DNA from parathyroid carcinomas has highlighted the potential significance of recurrent germline and somatic inactivating mutations of *PRUNE2* in this context.[37] The sensitivity and comprehensive quality of WES and other emerging next-generation sequencing modalities will undoubtedly accelerate the understanding of the pathophysiology of familial and sporadic parathyroid neoplasia in the years ahead.

ACKNOWLEDGMENTS

The author thanks his colleagues Drs Stephen J. Marx, Lee S. Weinstein, Michael T. Collins, Monica C. Skarulis, Sunita K. Agarwal, and Electron Kebebew for their ongoing support and encouragement.

REFERENCES

1. Bilezikian JP, Cusano NE, Khan AA, et al. Primary hyperparathyroidism. Nat Rev Dis Primers 2016;2:16033.
2. Brown EM, Pollak M, Seidman CE, et al. Calcium-ion-sensing cell-surface receptors. N Engl J Med 1995;333(4):234–40.
3. Brown EM. Role of the calcium-sensing receptor in extracellular calcium homeostasis. Best Pract Res Clin Endocrinol Metab 2013;27(3):333–43.
4. Fraser WD. Hyperparathyroidism. Lancet 2009;374(9684):145–58.
5. Marx SJ. Molecular genetics of multiple endocrine neoplasia types 1 and 2. Nat Rev Cancer 2005;5(5):367–75.
6. Jackson MA, Rich TA, Hu MI, et al. CDC73-Related disorders. GeneReviews® [Internet]. Seattle (WA): University of Washington, Seattle; 2015. p. 1993–2015.
7. Simonds WF, James-Newton LA, Agarwal SK, et al. Familial isolated hyperparathyroidism: clinical and genetic characteristics of thirty-six kindreds. Medicine (Baltimore) 2002;81:1–26.
8. Marx SJ, Attie MF, Levine MA, et al. The hypocalciuric or benign variant of familial hypercalcemia: clinical and biochemical features in fifteen kindreds. Medicine (Baltimore) 1981;60:397–412.
9. Knudson AG Jr. Mutation and cancer: statistical study of retinoblastoma. Proc Natl Acad Sci U S A 1971;68(4):820–3.
10. Knudson AG. Two genetic hits (more or less) to cancer. Nat Rev Cancer 2001;1(2):157–62.

11. Arnold A, Marx SJ. Familial hyperparathyroidism (including MEN, FHH, and HPT-JT). Primer on the metabolic bone diseases and disorders of mineral metabolism. 7th edition. Washington, DC: American Society for Bone and Mineral Research; 2008. p. 361–6.

12. Schussheim DH, Skarulis MC, Agarwal SK, et al. Multiple endocrine neoplasia type 1: new clinical and basic findings. Trends Endocrinol Metab 2001;12:173–8.

13. Chandrasekharappa SC, Guru SC, Manickam P, et al. Positional cloning of the gene for multiple endocrine neoplasia-type 1. Science 1997;276:404–7.

14. Lemos MC, Thakker RV. Multiple endocrine neoplasia type 1 (MEN1): analysis of 1336 mutations reported in the first decade following identification of the gene. Hum Mutat 2008;29(1):22–32.

15. Miedlich S, Krohn K, Lamesch P, et al. Frequency of somatic MEN1 gene mutations in monoclonal parathyroid tumours of patients with primary hyperparathyroidism. Eur J Endocrinol 2000;143(1):47–54.

16. Uchino S, Noguchi S, Sato M, et al. Screening of the Men1 gene and discovery of germ-line and somatic mutations in apparently sporadic parathyroid tumors. Cancer Res 2000;60(19):5553–7.

17. Scarpelli D, D'Aloiso L, Arturi F, et al. Novel somatic MEN1 gene alterations in sporadic primary hyperparathyroidism and correlation with clinical characteristics. J Endocrinol Invest 2004;27(11):1015–21.

18. Vierimaa O, Villablanca A, Alimov A, et al. Mutation analysis of MEN1, HRPT2, CASR, CDKN1B, and AIP genes in primary hyperparathyroidism patients with features of genetic predisposition. J Endocrinol Invest 2009;32(6):512–8.

19. Heppner C, Kester MB, Agarwal SK, et al. Somatic mutation of the MEN1 gene in parathyroid tumours. Nat Genet. 1997;16:375–8.

20. Cromer MK, Starker LF, Choi M, et al. Identification of somatic mutations in parathyroid tumors using whole-exome sequencing. J Clin Endocrinol Metab 2012; 97(9):E1774–81.

21. Newey PJ, Nesbit MA, Rimmer AJ, et al. Whole-exome sequencing studies of nonhereditary (sporadic) parathyroid adenomas. J Clin Endocrinol Metab 2012; 97(10):E1995–2005.

22. Dionisi S, Minisola S, Pepe J, et al. Concurrent parathyroid adenomas and carcinoma in the setting of multiple endocrine neoplasia type 1: presentation as hypercalcemic crisis. Mayo Clin Proc 2002;77(8):866–9.

23. Shih RY, Fackler S, Maturo S, et al. Parathyroid carcinoma in multiple endocrine neoplasia type 1 with a classic germline mutation. Endocr Pract 2009;15(6): 567–72.

24. Jackson CE, Norum RA, Boyd SB, et al. Hereditary hyperparathyroidism and multiple ossifying jaw fibromas: a clinically and genetically distinct syndrome. Surgery 1990;108:1006–12.

25. Bradley KJ, Hobbs MR, Buley ID, et al. Uterine tumours are a phenotypic manifestation of the hyperparathyroidism-jaw tumour syndrome. J Intern Med 2005; 257(1):18–26.

26. Chen JD, Morrison C, Zhang C, et al. Hyperparathyroidism-jaw tumour syndrome. J Intern Med 2003;253(6):634–42.

27. Mehta A, Patel D, Rosenberg A, et al. Hyperparathyroidism-jaw tumor syndrome: results of operative management. Surgery 2014;156(6):1315–24 [discussion: 1324–5].

28. Carpten JD, Robbins CM, Villablanca A, et al. HRPT2, encoding parafibromin, is mutated in hyperparathyroidism-jaw tumor syndrome. Nat Genet 2002;32(4): 676–80.

29. Newey PJ, Bowl MR, Thakker RV. Parafibromin–functional insights. J Intern Med 2009;266(1):84–98.

30. Domingues R, Tomaz RA, Martins C, et al. Identification of the first germline HRPT2 whole-gene deletion in a patient with primary hyperparathyroidism. Clin Endocrinol 2012;76(1):33–8.

31. Cascon A, Huarte-Mendicoa CV, Javier Leandro-Garcia L, et al. Detection of the first gross CDC73 germline deletion in an HPT-JT syndrome family. Genes Chromosomes Cancer 2011;50(11):922–9.

32. Bricaire L, Odou MF, Cardot-Bauters C, et al. Frequent large germline HRPT2 deletions in a French national cohort of patients with primary hyperparathyroidism. J Clin Endocrinol Metab 2013;98(2):E403–8.

33. Krebs LJ, Shattuck TM, Arnold A. HRPT2 mutational analysis of typical sporadic parathyroid adenomas. J Clin Endocrinol Metab 2005;90(9):5015–7.

34. Howell VM, Haven CJ, Kahnoski K, et al. HRPT2 mutations are associated with malignancy in sporadic parathyroid tumours. J Med Genet 2003;40(9):657–63.

35. Cetani F, Pardi E, Borsari S, et al. Genetic analyses of the HRPT2 gene in primary hyperparathyroidism: germline and somatic mutations in familial and sporadic parathyroid tumors. J Clin Endocrinol Metab 2004;89(11):5583–91.

36. Shattuck TM, Valimaki S, Obara T, et al. Somatic and germ-line mutations of the HRPT2 gene in sporadic parathyroid carcinoma. N Engl J Med 2003;349(18): 1722–9.

37. Yu W, McPherson JR, Stevenson M, et al. Whole-exome sequencing studies of parathyroid carcinomas reveal novel PRUNE2 mutations, distinctive mutational spectra related to APOBEC-catalyzed DNA mutagenesis and mutational enrichment in kinases associated with cell migration and invasion. J Clin Endocrinol Metab 2015;100(2):E360–4.

38. Pellegata NS, Quintanilla-Martinez L, Siggelkow H, et al. Germ-line mutations in p27Kip1 cause a multiple endocrine neoplasia syndrome in rats and humans. Proc Natl Acad Sci U S A 2006;103(42):15558–63.

39. Fritz A, Walch A, Piotrowska K, et al. Recessive transmission of a multiple endocrine neoplasia syndrome in the rat. Cancer Res 2002;62(11):3048–51.

40. Agarwal SK, Mateo CM, Marx SJ. Rare germline mutations in cyclin-dependent kinase inhibitor genes in multiple endocrine neoplasia type 1 and related states. J Clin Endocrinol Metab 2009;94(5):1826–34.

41. Georgitsi M, Raitila A, Karhu A, et al. Germline CDKN1B/p27Kip1 mutation in multiple endocrine neoplasia. J Clin Endocrinol Metab 2007;92(8):3321–5.

42. Molatore S, Marinoni I, Lee M, et al. A novel germline CDKN1B mutation causing multiple endocrine tumors: clinical, genetic and functional characterization. Hum Mutat 2010;31(11):E1825–35.

43. Malanga D, De Gisi S, Riccardi M, et al. Functional characterization of a rare germline mutation in the gene encoding the cyclin-dependent kinase inhibitor p27Kip1 (CDKN1B) in a Spanish patient with multiple endocrine neoplasia-like phenotype. Eur J Endocrinol 2012;166(3):551–60.

44. Occhi G, Regazzo D, Trivellin G, et al. A novel mutation in the upstream open reading frame of the CDKN1B gene causes a MEN4 phenotype. PLoS Genet 2013;9(3):e1003350.

45. Tonelli F, Giudici F, Giusti F, et al. A heterozygous frameshift mutation in exon 1 of CDKN1B gene in a patient affected by MEN4 syndrome. Eur J Endocrinol 2014; 171(2):K7–17.

46. Costa-Guda J, Marinoni I, Molatore S, et al. Somatic mutation and germline sequence abnormalities in CDKN1B, encoding p27Kip1, in sporadic parathyroid adenomas. J Clin Endocrinol Metab 2011;96(4):E701–6.

47. Costa-Guda J, Arnold A. Genetic and epigenetic changes in sporadic endocrine tumors: parathyroid tumors. Mol Cell Endocrinol 2014;386(1–2):46–54.

48. Simonds WF, Robbins CM, Agarwal SK, et al. Familial isolated hyperparathyroidism is rarely caused by germline mutation in HRPT2, the gene for the hyperparathyroidism-jaw tumor syndrome. J Clin Endocrinol Metab 2004;89(1): 96–102.

49. Warner J, Epstein M, Sweet A, et al. Genetic testing in familial isolated hyperparathyroidism: unexpected results and their implications. J Med Genet 2004;41(3): 155–60.

50. Cetani F, Pardi E, Ambrogini E, et al. Genetic analyses in familial isolated hyperparathyroidism: implication for clinical assessment and surgical management. Clin Endocrinol 2006;64(2):146–52.

51. Warner JV, Nyholt DR, Busfield F, et al. Familial isolated hyperparathyroidism is linked to a 1.7 Mb region on chromosome 2p13.3-14. J Med Genet 2006;43(3): e12.

52. Brown EM. Familial hypocalciuric hypercalcemia and other disorders with resistance to extracellular calcium. Endocrinol Metab Clin North Am 2000;29(3): 503–22.

53. Pollak MR, Brown EM, Chou Y-HW, et al. Mutations in the human Ca2+-sensing receptor gene cause familial hypocalciuric hypercalcemia and neonatal severe hyperparathyroidism. Cell 1993;75:1297–303.

54. Hendy GN, D'Souza-Li L, Yang B, et al. Mutations of the calcium-sensing receptor (CASR) in familial hypocalciuric hypercalcemia, neonatal severe hyperparathyroidism, and autosomal dominant hypocalcemia. Hum Mutat 2000;16:281–96.

55. Corrado KR, Andrade SC, Bellizzi J, et al. Polyclonality of parathyroid tumors in neonatal severe hyperparathyroidism. J Bone Miner Res 2015;30(10):1797–802.

56. Hosokawa Y, Pollak MR, Brown EM, et al. Mutational analysis of the extracellular Ca(2+)-sensing receptor gene in human parathyroid tumors. J Clin Endocrinol Metab 1995;80(11):3107–10.

57. Cetani F, Pinchera A, Pardi E, et al. No evidence for mutations in the calcium-sensing receptor gene in sporadic parathyroid adenomas. J Bone Miner Res 1999;14(6):878–82.

58. Farnebo F, Enberg U, Grimelius L, et al. Tumor-specific decreased expression of calcium sensing receptor messenger ribonucleic acid in sporadic primary hyperparathyroidism. J Clin Endocrinol Metab 1997;82(10):3481–6.

59. Nesbit MA, Hannan FM, Howles SA, et al. Mutations affecting G-protein subunit alpha11 in hypercalcemia and hypocalcemia. N Engl J Med 2013;368(26): 2476–86.

60. Gorvin CM, Cranston T, Hannan FM, et al. A G-protein subunit-alpha11 loss-of-function mutation, Thr54Met, causes familial hypocalciuric hypercalcemia type 2 (FHH2). J Bone Miner Res 2016;31(6):1200–6.

61. Nesbit MA, Hannan FM, Howles SA, et al. Mutations in AP2S1 cause familial hypocalciuric hypercalcemia type 3. Nat Genet 2013;45(1):93–7.

62. Hendy GN, Canaff L, Newfield RS, et al. Codon Arg15 mutations of the AP2S1 gene: common occurrence in familial hypocalciuric hypercalcemia cases negative for calcium-sensing receptor (CASR) mutations. J Clin Endocrinol Metab 2014;99(7):E1311–5.

63. Hannan FM, Howles SA, Rogers A, et al. Adaptor protein-2 sigma subunit mutations causing familial hypocalciuric hypercalcaemia type 3 (FHH3) demonstrate genotype-phenotype correlations, codon bias and dominant-negative effects. Hum Mol Genet 2015;24(18):5079–92.

64. Vargas-Poussou R, Mansour-Hendili L, Baron S, et al. Familial hypocalciuric hypercalcemia types 1 and 3 and primary hyperparathyroidism: similarities and differences. J Clin Endocrinol Metab 2016;101(5):2185–95.

65. Harris TJ, McCormick F. The molecular pathology of cancer. Nat Rev Clin Oncol 2010;7(5):251–65.

66. Wells SA Jr, Santoro M. Targeting the RET pathway in thyroid cancer. Clin Cancer Res 2009;15(23):7119–23.

67. Frank-Raue K, Raue F. Hereditary medullary thyroid cancer genotype-phenotype correlation. Recent Results Cancer Res 2015;204:139–56.

68. Eng C, Clayton D, Schuffenecker I, et al. The relationship between specific RET proto-oncogene mutations and disease phenotype in multiple endocrine neoplasia type 2. International RET mutation consortium analysis. JAMA 1996; 276(19):1575–9.

69. Arnold A, Kim HG, Gaz RD, et al. Molecular cloning and chromosomal mapping of DNA rearranged with the parathyroid hormone gene in a parathyroid adenoma. J Clin Invest 1989;83(6):2034–40.

70. Rosenberg CL, Kim HG, Shows TB, et al. Rearrangement and overexpression of D11S287E, a candidate oncogene on chromosome 11q13 in benign parathyroid tumors. Oncogene 1991;6(3):449–53.

71. Motokura T, Bloom T, Kim HG, et al. A novel cyclin encoded by a bcl1-linked candidate oncogene. Nature 1991;350(6318):512–5.

72. Imanishi Y, Hosokawa Y, Yoshimoto K, et al. Primary hyperparathyroidism caused by parathyroid-targeted overexpression of cyclin D1 in transgenic mice. J Clin Invest 2001;107(9):1093–102.

73. Hsi ED, Zukerberg LR, Yang WI, et al. Cyclin D1/PRAD1 expression in parathyroid adenomas: an immunohistochemical study. J Clin Endocrinol Metab 1996;81(5): 1736–9.

74. Hemmer S, Wasenius VM, Haglund C, et al. Deletion of 11q23 and cyclin D1 overexpression are frequent aberrations in parathyroid adenomas. Am J Pathol 2001; 158(4):1355–62.

75. Tominaga Y, Tsuzuki T, Uchida K, et al. Expression of PRAD1/cyclin D1, retinoblastoma gene products, and Ki67 in parathyroid hyperplasia caused by chronic renal failure versus primary adenoma. Kidney Int 1999;55(4):1375–83.

76. Vasef MA, Brynes RK, Sturm M, et al. Expression of cyclin D1 in parathyroid carcinomas, adenomas, and hyperplasias: a paraffin immunohistochemical study. Mod Pathol 1999;12(4):412–6.

77. Hosokawa Y, Tu T, Tahara H, et al. Absence of cyclin D1/PRAD1 point mutations in human breast cancers and parathyroid adenomas and identification of a new cyclin D1 gene polymorphism. Cancer Lett 1995;93(2):165–70.

78. Yap DB, Chu J, Berg T, et al. Somatic mutations at EZH2 Y641 act dominantly through a mechanism of selectively altered PRC2 catalytic activity, to increase H3K27 trimethylation. Blood 2011;117(8):2451–9.

79. Sanpaolo E, Miroballo M, Corbetta S, et al. EZH2 and ZFX oncogenes in malignant behaviour of parathyroid neoplasms. Endocrine 2016;54(1):55–9.

80. Soong CP, Arnold A. Recurrent ZFX mutations in human sporadic parathyroid adenomas. Oncoscience 2014;1(5):360–6.

81. Arnold A, Soong CP. New role for ZFX in oncogenesis. Cell Cycle 2014;13(22): 3465–6.
82. Palanisamy N, Imanishi Y, Rao PH, et al. Novel chromosomal abnormalities identified by comparative genomic hybridization in parathyroid adenomas. J Clin Endocrinol Metab 1998;83(5):1766–70.
83. Agarwal SK, Schrock E, Kester MB, et al. Comparative genomic hybridization analysis of human parathyroid tumors. Cancer Genet Cytogenet 1998;106:30–6.
84. Farnebo F, Kytölä S, Teh BT, et al. Alternative genetic pathways in parathyroid tumorigenesis. J Clin Endocrinol Metab 1999;84:3775–80.
85. Kytölä S, Farnebo F, Obara T, et al. Patterns of chromosomal imbalances in parathyroid carcinomas. Am J Pathol 2000;157:579–86.
86. Garcia JL, Tardio JC, Gutierrez NC, et al. Chromosomal imbalances identified by comparative genomic hybridization in sporadic parathyroid adenomas. Eur J Endocrinol 2002;146(2):209–13.

Genetics of Adrenocortical Development and Tumors

 CrossMark

Maya Lodish, MD, MHSc

KEYWORDS

- Adrenal development • Adrenocortical carcinoma • Ontogenesis • Zonation
- Signaling • Pathway • Genetic • Driver mutation

KEY POINTS

- Current understanding of normal adrenocortical development sheds light on the molecular pathways that, when altered, may stimulate abnormal proliferation and drive adrenocortical tumor formation.
- Knowledge obtained from inherited syndromes that are characterized by adrenocortical tumors and next-generation sequencing of adrenocortical tumors have helped find causative mutations for these lesions.
- Recent studies have identified cyclic AMP-dependent protein kinase A (PKA) signaling as a key mediator of cortisol secretion by the normal adrenal cortex. It therefore follows that mutations in genes that involve dysregulated cAMP/PKA pathway components are implicated in adrenocortical pathology.
- ARMC5 is a recently discovered gene that is associated with bilateral macronodular adrenocortical hyperplasia.

INTRODUCTION

This article links the understanding of the developmental physiology of the adrenal cortex to adrenocortical tumor formation. Many molecular mechanisms that lead to the formation of adrenocortical tumors have been discovered via next-generation sequencing approaches. The most frequently mutated genes in adrenocortical tumors are also factors in normal adrenal development and homeostasis, including those that alter the p53 and Wnt/β-catenin pathways. In addition, dysregulated protein kinase A (PKA) signaling and *ARMC5* mutations have been identified as key mediators of

Disclosure Statement: The author has nothing to disclose.
Funding: This work was supported by the Intramural Research Program of the *Eunice Kennedy Shriver* National Institute of Child Health and Human Development, National Institutes of Health.
Pediatric Endocrinology Fellowship, Eunice Kennedy Shriver National Institute of Child Health and Human Development, National Institutes of Health, Building 10, Room 9D42, 10 Center Drive, MSC 1830, Bethesda, MD 20892-1830, USA
E-mail address: lodishma@mail.nih.gov

adrenocortical tumorigenesis. The growing understanding of the genetic changes that orchestrate adrenocortical development and disease pave the way for potential targeted treatment strategies.

Adrenocortical carcinoma (ACC) has a bimodal age distribution with a peak in early childhood with a mean age of diagnosis at 3.2 years, and a peak in adulthood in the fourth and fifth decades.[1,2] ACC has an annual incidence of 0.7 to 2 per million.[3,4] The understanding of the pathophysiology of ACC is limited, and the disease carries a poor prognosis.[5] Recent identification of genetic characteristics of ACC may lead to the development of novel therapeutic interventions. Several genes have been implicated as tumor drivers in sporadic ACC, including mutations in insulin-like growth factor 2 (IGF2), β-catenin (CTNNB1 or ZNRF3), and TP53.[6,7] Importantly, germline variants of some of the same genes identified to be drivers of sporadic ACC are also associated with familial tumor syndromes characterized by ACC, including Beckwith-Wiedemann syndrome (BWS), familial adenomatous polyposis (FAP), and Li-Fraumeni syndrome.

Elevated cAMP signaling is related to most benign cortisol-producing tumors of the adrenal gland. The first human disease that directly linked cAMP signaling to cortisol-producing lesions was with the discovery more than 25 years ago that activating mutations in GNAS1 caused adrenocortical tumors in infants with McCune-Albright syndrome (MAS). Mutations in the regulatory subunit type 1 α (R1α) of the cAMP-dependent protein kinase or PKA were then identified as the cause of another form of cortisol-producing hyperplasia, primary pigmented nodular adrenocortical disease (PPNAD). Inactivating mutations in inhibitors of the cAMP-signaling pathway (phosphodiesterases [PDEs]) were later identified as another cause of adrenocortical hyperplasia. Most recently, somatic activating mutations in the main catalytic subunit of PKA have been discovered in cortisol-producing adenomas. Put together, these findings provide convincing proof that increased cAMP signaling is key to adrenal tumor development. The implications of this finding lead to the search for targeted treatment strategies for adrenal tumors and hypercortisolism that act on the cAMP/PKA cascade.

A novel gene was recently identified that provides evidence that bilateral macronodular adrenal hyperplasia is frequently a genetic disorder. Germline mutations in the tumor suppressor gene ARMC-5 lead to the development of an autosomal dominantly inherited form of Cushing syndrome (CS). Because this type of CS may present in a cyclical manner that may take many years to diagnose, the potential to identify individuals at risk for the development of CS based on genetic findings has the potential to lead to more timely diagnosis of CS. Recent advances in the understanding of adrenocortical signaling have taught that cortisol secretion within the adrenal gland is more complex than previously thought. It is now known that paracrine signaling via intra-adrenal secretion of corticotrophin is a factor in adrenal hyperplasia.

OVERVIEW OF ADRENOCORTICAL DEVELOPMENT

The adrenal cortex derives from components of the urogenital ridge, sharing a common origin with the kidney and gonads.[8] The human adult adrenal cortex is separated into three distinct zones that may be characterized by their functionality and histology. The outermost layer, the zona glomerulosa, secretes aldosterone; the middle zona fasiculata secretes glucocorticoids; and the innermost zona reticularis produces sex steroid hormone precursors androstenedione and dehydroepiandrosterone (**Fig. 1**).

Adrenocortical cell precursors originate from the coelomic epithelium that, together with the gonadal cell precursors, forms the adrenogonadal primordium. The

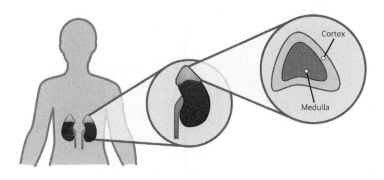

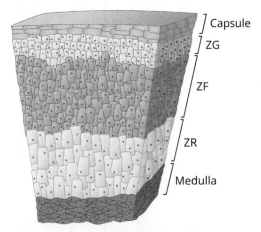

Fig. 1. The anatomy and structure of the adrenal glands. The adrenal glands are located at the upper poles of the kidneys. In humans, the adrenal gland has three distinct cortical zones (1) the zona glomerulosa, (2) the zona fasiculata, and (3) the zona reticularis. The inner part of the adrenal gland is the medulla, responsible for catecholamine synthesis. ZF, zona fasiculata; ZG, zona glomerulosa; ZR, zona reticularis.

encapsulation of the adrenal primordium, creating the fetal adrenal gland, occurs by 9 weeks postconception.[9,10] By midgestation, the fetal adrenals are composed of two distinct cortical zones: the predominant fetal zone and the surrounding definitive zone. Shortly after birth, the adrenal cortex is remodeled and the fetal zone recedes. The establishment of the adrenal zona glomerulosa and zona fasiculata occurs in late fetal development; however, the zona reticularis is not completely established until adrenarche (**Fig. 2**). Corticotrophin is the primary regulator of development of the human fetal adrenal mediated through locally expressed growth factors including epidermal growth factor (EGF), basic fibroblast growth factor (bFGF), and insulin-like growth factor (IGF)-I and -II.[10] As the definitive cortex grows and the fetal cortex regresses, capsular cells give rise to steroid-producing adrenocortical cells.[11]

ADRENOCORTICAL TUMORS: OVERVIEW OF GENETIC BASIS

Current understanding of normal adrenocortical development sheds light on the molecular pathways that, when altered, may stimulate abnormal proliferation and drive adrenocortical tumor formation. Adrenal tumors may be functional and lead to

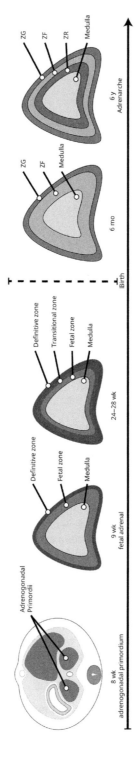

Fig. 2. Early adrenal development. The adrenal cortex develops from a thickening of the coelomic epithelium at the intersection of the urogenital ridge and the dorsal mesentery. This group of cells is called the adrenogonadal primordium, and these cells express the transcription factors SF-1 and NR5A1. The chromaffin cells form the medulla, and the adrenal primordium cells form the fetal adrenal gland, which is surrounded by the definitive adrenal gland. The fetal adrenal cortex differentiates into a definitive zone and a fetal zone after 9 weeks' gestation. The transitional zone appears after 24 weeks' gestation. After birth the fetal adrenals involute, and the adult adrenals form. By 6 months of age the adult adrenal cortex consists of the zona glomerulosa and the zona fasciculata. During adrenarche (age 6–7) the zona reticularis is formed. ZF, zona fasiculata; ZG, zona glomerulosa; ZR, zona reticularis.

syndromes of hormone excess, hypercortisolism (CS), hyperaldosteronism (Conn syndrome), hyperandrogenism (virilizing syndrome), or mixed. CS may be caused by oversecretion of cortisol from adrenocortical hyperplasia, tumors, or cancer. Most (75%–90%) of these tumors are benign unilateral adenomas. ACC is infrequent, making up less than 5% of all ACTs. The remainder of the adrenal lesions (10%) are related to bilateral hyperplasia: PPNAD and primary bilateral macronodular adrenal disease (PBMAD). Knowledge of the molecular pathways involved in adrenocortical tumorigenesis arises from the genetic basis of inherited syndromes that include adrenocortical tumors (**Table 1**), and from next-generation sequencing approaches of tumor and germline DNA (**Table 2**).

Several paracrine and endocrine signals are key players in adrenocortical development. Steroidogenic factor-1 (*SF-1, NR5A1*) and nuclear receptor subfamily 0 group B member 1 (*DAX-1, NR0B1*) are key transcription factors critical for adrenocortical development.[12] The sonic hedgehog pathway is central to adrenocortical development and has been implicated in ACC with up-regulation in adult ACCs, and down-regulation in pediatric ACCs.[13] The maintenance of the adrenal cortex involves the central migration of sonic hedgehog: positive progenitor cells where they differentiate into the cells making up the zona glomerulosa that later transition to zona fasiculata.[14] The fibroblast growth factor (FGF) signaling pathway is integral to adrenal proliferation and differentiation. The four main signaling pathways downstream of FGF receptor activation are (1) Janus kinase/signal transducer and activator of transcription (Jak/Stat), (2) phosphoinositide phospholipase C (PLCγ), (3) phosphatidylinositol 3-kinase (PI3K), and (4) mitogen-activated protein kinase/extracellular signal-regulated kinase (MAPK/Erk).[15] FGFR1 and FGFR4 overexpression has been found in 65% of adrenocortical tumors and is associated with worse prognosis.[16]

INSULIN-LIKE GROWTH FACTOR SIGNALING PATHWAY

The IGF signaling pathway is involved in differentiation and growth of the adrenal cortex. IGF-2 is highly expressed in human fetal adrenal glands. The chromosomal location of IGF-2 is within an imprinted locus on 11p15.5 that also includes the cyclin-dependent kinase inhibitor 1 C (*CDKN1C*) and *H19*.[17] The importance of IGF2 in adrenocortical development is illustrated by BWS, a pediatric overgrowth disorder with a predisposition to tumor development characterized by macroglossia and hemihypertrophy. BWS is caused by mutation, deletion, or hypermethylation of imprinted genes within the chromosome 11p15.5 region, encompassing *CDKN1C, H19, IGF2*, and *P57*.[18,19] Adrenal cytomegaly with cysts is the predominant adrenal phenotype in BWS; however, ACC occurs with increased frequency in patients with BWS as ACC occurs in 7% of patients.[20,21] Structural and functional abnormalities at 11p15 are also associated with sporadic adrenocortical tumors.[22] Whole-genome, whole-exome, and/or transcriptome sequencing of 37 ACCs found that 91% show loss of heterozygosity of chromosome 11p; IGF2 on chromosome 11p was overexpressed in all tumors.[23]

WNT SIGNALING PATHWAY

The mammalian wingless-type MMTV integration site (Wnt) pathway is a central developmental regulator.[24] In the absence of Wnt signaling, ß-catenin is in a complex with axin, APC, and GSK3-ß. Within this complex, ß-catenin is then phosphorylated and targeted for degradation. When Wnt signaling is activated, ß-catenin is uncoupled from the degradation complex and translocates to the nucleus, where it activates target genes.[25] Constitutive activation of ß-catenin drives adrenocortical tumorigenesis. Defects in Wnt pathway activation, including genetic loss of APC or gain-of-function mutations in

Table 1
Genetic syndromes associated with adrenal hyperplasia/neoplasia

Syndrome	Gene	Locus	Function of the WT Protein	Associated Manifestations
Primary bilateral macronodular adrenocortical disease	ARMCS	16p11	Potential role in regulation of apoptosis and steroidogenesis	Meningioma?
Multiple endocrine neoplasia type 1	Menin	11q13	Regulator of gene transcription, cell proliferation, apoptosis, and genome stability	Multiple endocrine neoplasia type 1 hyperparathyroidism, pituitary adenomas, pancreatic neuroendocrine tumors
Hereditary leiomyomatosis and renal cell cancer	FH	1q42	Krebs cycle, amino acid metabolism	Hereditary leiomyomatosis and renal cell carcinoma
Li-Fraumeni syndrome	TP53	17p13.1	Cell cycle regulator	Breast cancer and soft tissue sarcomas, brain tumors, osteosarcoma, leukemia, and adrenocortical carcinoma
McCune-Albright syndrome	GNAS1	20q13	Stimulation of adenyl cyclase, activation of the cAMP/protein kinase A pathway	Fibrous bone dysplasia, cafe-au-lait spots, precocious puberty, acromegaly, toxic multinodular goiter
Gardner syndrome	APC	5q12-22	Prevent β-catenin accumulation, inhibition of the Wnt/β-catenin pathway	Familial adenomatous polyposis: colon adenomas and carcinomas, pigmented retinal lesions, desmoid tumors, other malignant tumors as adrenocortical carcinomas
Beckwith-Wiedemann syndrome	IGF2	11p15 imprinting	Growth factor	Hemihypertrophy, macroglossia, ear pits, hypoglycemia, aisceromegaly, abdominal wall defects, Wilms tumor, hepatoblastoma, adrenocortical carcinoma
Carney complex	PRKAR1A	17q22-24	Activation of the cAMP/protein kinase A pathway	Lentigines, pituitary adenomas, cardiac myxomas

Table 2
Driver genes in adrenocortical carcinomas

Gene	Cytogenetic Location	Gene Name	OMIM
TERF2	16q22.1	TELOMERIC REPEAT-BINDING FACTOR 2	602027
ZNRF3	22q12.1	ZINC FINGER AND RING FINGER PROTEIN 3	612062
TP53	17p13.1	TUMOR PROTEIN p53	191170
CTNNB1	3p22.1	CATENIN, BETA-1	116806
PRKAR1A	17q24.2	PROTEIN KINASE, cAMP-DEPENDENT, REGULATORY, TYPE 1, ALPHA	188830
CCNE1	19q12	CYCLIN E1	123837
IGF2	11p15.5	INSULIN-LIKE GROWTH FACTOR II	147470
FGFR1	8p11.23	FIBROBLAST GROWTH FACTOR RECEPTOR 1	136350
FGFR4	5q35.2	FIBROBLAST GROWTH FACTOR RECEPTOR 4	134935
RB1	13q14.2	RB1 GENE	614041

CTNNB1, are known driver mutations of ACC.[7,26] In fact, Wnt signaling has been found to be the most frequently mutated pathway in ACCs.[27] CTNNB1 mediates cell-cell adhesion and anchors the actin cytoskeleton, thereby regulating cell growth.[28] CCNE1 encodes cyclin E, a regulatory subunit of cyclin-dependent kinase. Cyclin E is a key regulator of the cell cycle and is overexpressed in many human tumors.[29] Whole-exome sequencing of 41 matched ACC and normal tissues identified somatic mutations in CTNNB1 in 10% of tumors.[27]

The role of the Wnt/ß-catenin pathway in adrenocortical tumors is illustrated in the autosomal dominantly inherited syndrome FAP. Germline inactivating mutations of the tumor suppressor gene APC characterize FAP, leading to multiple colonic polyps, colon cancer, and adrenocortical tumors caused by dysregulated Wnt/ß-catenin signaling.[26] Gain-of-function mutations in β-catenin have been found in roughly 25% of benign and malignant adrenocortical tumors, highlighting the importance of activation of the Wnt signaling pathway.[7] Exome sequencing of ACCs identified ZNRF3, encoding a cell surface E3 ubiquitin ligase, as a potential new tumor suppressor gene related to the ß-catenin and Wnt signaling pathway.[30] A total of 19.3% of ACC samples out of 91 ACCs recently analyzed through the Cancer Genome Atlas were found to have alterations of ZNRF3.[31,32] Another large whole exome sequencing analysis of 41 tumors and matched normal samples found homozygous deletion at 22q12.1 including the Wnt repressors ZNRF3 and KREMEN1 in 9.8% and 7.3% of tumors, respectively.[27]

CELL CYCLE REGULATORS

The transcription factor p53 on chromosome 17p13 is a tumor suppressor that regulates cell cycle arrest, apoptosis, senescence, metabolism, and DNA repair. In many cancers, activity of p53 is lost.[33] Whole-exome sequencing of 41 matched ACC and normal tissues identified somatic mutations in TP53 in 20% of ACC tumors.[27] Pediatric ACC is exceedingly rare and carries a poor prognosis; the most common germline alteration in pediatric ACC is caused by p53. Whole-genome, whole-exome, and/or transcriptome sequencing of 37 ACCs found TP53 mutations and chromosome 17 loss of heterozygosity in 76% of pediatric ACCs.[23] Li-Fraumeni syndrome is an autosomal-dominant cancer syndrome caused by heterozygous germline mutations in the p53 gene, and is associated with an increased risk of malignancies. Children with Li-Fraumeni syndrome are at an especially high risk of developing ACC.[34] The median age of ACC diagnosis among TP53 mutation carriers is 4.8 years of age.[35] Multiple endocrine neoplasia type 1 (MEN1) is another autosomal-dominant cancer syndrome involving dysregulation of the cell cycle. MEN1 is characterized by the "three Ps" of primary hyperparathyroidism, pancreatic endocrine tumors, and pituitary adenomas; adrenal lesions may also occur. Loss of function mutations in MENIN disrupt cell cycle regulation and lead to cell proliferation. In approximately 20% to 40% of patients with MEN1, enlarged adrenals are found, with bilateral adrenal tumors in 1.3%.[36] In two recent studies reporting exome sequencing in ACC, between 4% and 7% of tumors had inactivating mutations in MENIN.[30] Finally, in the cell cycle during chromosome replication, telomeres are critical for maintaining genomic integrity. TERF2, a protein that plays a key role in the protective activity of telomeres, has also been found to be amplified in ACC.[31,37]

cAMP-DEPENDENT PROTEIN KINASE PATHWAY

The cAMP-dependent PKA pathway plays a central role in controlling the development, function, and proliferation of adrenocortical cells. Breaking down the components of the cAMP/PKA pathway, first corticotrophin binds the MC2R G protein-coupled receptor, leading to the stimulation of adenylyl cyclase and release of cyclic-AMP. Next, cAMP activates PKA, a heterotetramer of two regulatory and two catalytic subunits; the PKA catalytic subunit (a serine-threonine kinase) then goes on to phosphorylate several targets, including those leading to cortisol synthesis. Four different genes encode four distinct isoforms of the regulatory subunits (R1α, R1β, R2α, and R2β).[38] In addition, four unique catalytic subunits of PKA are known (Cα, Cβ, Cγ, and PRKX). Following the binding of cAMP to PKA, the catalytic subunits dissociate from the regulatory subunits, allowing for the phosphorylation of PKA targets in the cytoplasm and the nucleus. Modifications in specific subunits of PKA, including, PRKAR1α and PRKACα, play a major role in adrenal physiology and pathophysiology (**Fig. 3**).[39,40]

MAS is the first disorder identified to connect cAMP/PKA pathway alterations to the growth of adrenal tumors. MAS is caused by postzygotic gain-of-function mutations in the alpha subunit of the gene for the stimulatory guanine-nucleotide-binding protein (Gsa) leading to constitutive activation of adenylate cyclase.[40–42] Clinically, patients present with the classic triad of fibrous dysplasia, cafe-au-lait skin pigmentation, and precocious puberty. CS is present in a subset of patients with MAS caused by activating mutations of Gsa.[43,44] Multiple nodules that develop from adrenocortical cells with fetal features characterize the adrenals in MAS affected by CS. In a small number of sporadic cortisol-producing adenomas, somatic mutations of GNAS have been identified.[3]

Carney complex (CNC) is an autosomal-dominant MEN syndrome, including myxomas, endocrine tumors, and endocrine gland involvement.[45,46] Endocrine tumors associated with CNC include testicular large cell, calcifying Sertoli cell tumors, growth hormone–producing pituitary adenomas, thyroid nodules, and PPNAD. Germline inactivating mutations of the PRKAR1A gene coding for the regulatory 1-α (R1α) subunit of PKA are the cause of for CNC in most patients.[47,48] PPNAD is found in 60% of patients with CNC.[49,50] A series of 212 patients with PPNAD found that in 20% of the cases adrenal tumors were isolated without any other manifestations of CNC, with a

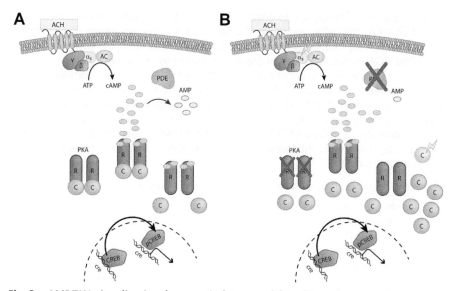

Fig. 3. cAMP/PKA signaling in adrenocortical tumors. (*A*) In the resting state, PKA exists as an inactive tetramer comprising a dimer of regulatory subunits bound to catalytic subunits. PDEs act as inhibitors of the pathway by degrading cAMP to regulate signal transduction. Adenylyl cyclase catalyzes the conversion of ATP to cAMP, and elevation in cellular cAMP levels leads to activation of PKA, release of the catalytic subunits, and phosphorylation of downstream targets, including the transcription factor cAMP response-element binding protein (CREB). (*B*) In McCune-Albright syndrome, activating mutations in the GNAS gene, which encodes the stimulatory guanine nucleotide-binding protein (Gsα) subunit, lead to constitutive activation of the Gsα protein subunit that couples hormone receptors to intracellular generation of cAMP. Mutations in Gsα lead to prolonged activation of Gsα and its downstream effectors. In Carney complex, inactivating mutations in the regulatory subunit 1α of PKA (R1α) subunit of PKA lead to suppression of its inhibitory action, release of the catalytic subunits, and transcription of downstream targets. Inactivating mutations in PDEs lead to accumulation of cAMP and dysregulated activation of the cAMP-PKA pathway. Activating mutations in the catalytic subunit of PKA result in up-regulation of the PKA pathway and phosphorylation of downstream targets. AC, adenylyl cyclase; Cα, catalytic subunit of PKA.

preponderance of females.[49] Somatic mutations in PRKAR1A and chromosomal loss of the region encompassing PRKAR1A have been identified in sporadic cortisol-secreting adenomas. One study of 44 sporadic adrenocortical tumors found somatic 17q22 to 24 losses were seen in 23% of adenomas and 53% of adrenal cancers. In three tumors, somatic, PRKAR1A-inactivating mutations were identified, leading to protein truncation.[51,52] More recently, in whole exome sequencing from 84 ACCs, seven (8%) cases were found to have inactivating PRKAR1A mutations, and three additional cases had homozygous deletions of PRKAR1A, increasing the role of PKA signaling in ACC.[31] In addition, this finding leads to a potential relationship between benign and malignant adrenocortical tumors.[53] PPNAD and micronodular adrenocortical hyperplasia have both been associated with genetic defects in cAMP-binding PDEs. The role of PDEs is to lower cAMP levels after stimulation of the cAMP/PKA pathway; inactivating mutations of PDE cause buildup of cAMP and stimulation of the PKA signaling cascade. PDE11 A and PDE8B mutations have been found in patients with PPNAD and iMAD, and PDE8B have also been shown to be associated with predisposition to iMAD.[47,54,55] Constitutive activation of the catalytic subunit of PKA, PRKACA, has been found to be a common cause of CS.[40,56–59] PRKACA-activating mutations are responsible for 42% of sporadic CS.[40,56–59] Activating PRKACA mutations obstruct the interaction of the regulatory subunit with the catalytic subunit, leading to constitutive activation of PKA, increased cortisol production, and altered tumor growth.[59] Genetic copy number gains encompassing PRKACA on chromosome 19p13.2p13.12 locus are another described cause of CS related to activation of the PKA pathway.[40,60] Most recently, ACC has been found to be associated with somatic mutations of PRKAR1A.[31] All of these findings have led to a search for novel targeted treatment strategies with PRKACA inhibitors for management of adrenocortical tumors.[56,58]

Genetics of Primary Bilateral Macronodular Adrenal Disease

PBMAD may be seen in multiple tumor syndromes MEN-1 and FAP and also include hereditary leiomyomatosis and renal cell carcinoma (HLRCC, caused by fumarate hydratase gene [FH] mutations). In HLRCC, inactivating mutations of FH lead predominantly to hereditary leiomyomatosis and renal cancer; however, in approximately 8% of patients adrenal lesions are found.[61] A single case of clinical CS associated with PBMAD in the context of HLRCC has been described, in which loss of heterozygosity for FH was found in the adrenal lesion.[62]

ARMC5 is another armadillo-containing protein with homology to β-catenin and APC that is involved in adrenocortical pathophysiology. Inactivating ARMC5 mutations have been found in more than half of cases of primary bilateral macronodular adrenal hyperplasia.[42] Additional studies have confirmed the high frequency of ARMC5 mutations in this disorder.[63–66] ARMC5 is a putative tumor suppressor that regulates apoptosis. ARMC5 has also been shown in vitro to directly interact with PKA subunits, linking ARMC5 to the PKA/cAMP pathway.[67] Intra-adrenal corticotrophin secretion by clusters of adrenocortical cells is a paracrine signaling pathway found to occur in PBMAD.[68] Abnormal G-protein-coupled receptors expressed by adrenocortical cells themselves, including receptors for vasopressin, catecholamines, luteinizing hormone, serotonin, and glucose-dependent insulinotropic peptide, may also serve to regulate cortisol secretion.[69–72] Intra-adrenal production of corticotrophin may offer a potential therapeutic target for CS in certain types of adrenal hyperplasia through the application of corticotrophin receptor inhibitors (melanocorticon type 2 receptor antagonists).[73]

Genetics of aldosterone producing adenomas

Aldosterone-producing adenomas may be caused by somatic mutations in genes that regulate intracellular calcium concentration. Somatic mutation of two ATPases, ATPA1A (encoding the alpha subunit of the sodium/potassium ATPase) and ATP2B3 (encoding the plasma membrane calcium-transporting ATPase3) have been found in aldosterone-producing adenomas.[74] KCNJ5 mutations, a gene that encodes a potassium channel, have also been found in 40% of aldosterone-producing adenomas.[75,76] Mutations in KCNJ5 alter the channel's permeability to potassium ultimately leading to activation of the calcium-calmodulin-dependent protein kinase II.[77] Germline ARMC5 variants may also be associated with primary aldosteronism.[78]

SUMMARY AND FUTURE CONSIDERATIONS

The most frequently mutated genes in adrenocortical tumors are also factors involved in normal adrenal development and homeostasis. A better understanding is being gained of the molecular genetics of adrenocortical tumor development. The most common somatic alterations in ACC are mutations or deletions of *TP53* and ZNRF3 or *CTNNB1*, altering either the p53 or the Wnt/β-catenin pathway. The PKA/cAMP signaling pathway plays a crucial role in adrenocortical physiology and pathophysiology; activating mutations of pathway regulators and inactivating mutations of pathway inhibitors both lead to cortisol excess. Germline mutations of *PRKAR1A* lead to PPNAD and CS in adolescence or early adulthood. Somatic *PRKACA*-activating, *PRKAR1A*-inactivating, or *GNAS*-activating mutations may cause cortisol-secreting adenomas. Recently, whole-genome expression profile of normal adrenals was compared with *PRKAR1A* and *GNAS*-mutant adrenal glands, and it was shown that although activation of certain oncogenic signals were shared between these two lesions, others including Wnt signaling were differentially expressed depending on the lesion.[79] These discoveries offer the possibility to target molecular alterations in this pathway with novel mechanisms to treat cortisol excess in CS, and highlight the importance of genetic testing in adrenocortical tumors.

ACKNOWLEDGMENTS

Figure design was performed by Jeremy Swan and Nicole Jonas.

REFERENCES

1. Michalkiewicz E, Sandrini R, Figueiredo B, et al. Clinical and outcome characteristics of children with adrenocortical tumors: a report from the International Pediatric Adrenocortical Tumor Registry. J Clin Oncol 2004;22(5):838–45.
2. Ng L, Libertino JM. Adrenocortical carcinoma: diagnosis, evaluation and treatment. J Urol 2003;169(1):5–11.
3. Bilimoria KY, Shen WT, Elaraj D, et al. Adrenocortical carcinoma in the United States: treatment utilization and prognostic factors. Cancer 2008;113(11):3130–6.
4. Else T, Kim AC, Sabolch A, et al. Adrenocortical carcinoma. Endocr Rev 2014; 35(2):282–326.
5. Fassnacht M, Allolio B. Clinical management of adrenocortical carcinoma. Best Pract Res Clin Endocrinol Metab 2009;23(2):273–89.
6. Giordano TJ, Thomas DG, Kuick R, et al. Distinct transcriptional profiles of adrenocortical tumors uncovered by DNA microarray analysis. Am J Pathol 2003; 162(2):521–31.
7. Tissier F, Cavard C, Groussin L, et al. Mutations of beta-catenin in adrenocortical tumors: activation of the Wnt signaling pathway is a frequent event in both benign and malignant adrenocortical tumors. Cancer Res 2005;65(17):7622–7.
8. Else T, Hammer GD. Genetic analysis of adrenal absence: agenesis and aplasia. Trends Endocrinol Metab 2005;16(10):458–68.
9. Mesiano S, Jaffe RB. Developmental and functional biology of the primate fetal adrenal cortex. Endocr Rev 1997;18(3):378–403.
10. Mesiano S, Jaffe RB. Role of growth factors in the developmental regulation of the human fetal adrenal cortex. Steroids 1997;62(1):62–72.
11. Wood MA, Acharya A, Finco I, et al. Fetal adrenal capsular cells serve as progenitor cells for steroidogenic and stromal adrenocortical cell lineages in M. musculus. Development 2013;140(22):4522–32.
12. Walczak EM, Hammer GD. Regulation of the adrenocortical stem cell niche: implications for disease. Nat Rev Endocrinol 2015;11(1):14–28.
13. Gomes DC, Leal LF, Mermejo LM, et al. Sonic hedgehog signaling is active in human adrenal cortex development and deregulated in adrenocortical tumors. J Clin Endocrinol Metab 2014;99(7):E1209–16.

14. Xing Y, Lerario AM, Rainey W, et al. Development of adrenal cortex zonation. Endocrinol Metab Clin North Am 2015;44(2):243–74.

15. Lanner F, Rossant J. The role of FGF/Erk signaling in pluripotent cells. Development 2010;137(20):3351–60.

16. Brito LP, Ribeiro TC, Almeida MQ, et al. The role of fibroblast growth factor receptor 4 overexpression and gene amplification as prognostic markers in pediatric and adult adrenocortical tumors. Endocr Relat Cancer 2012;19(3):L11–3.

17. Weksberg R, Shuman C, Smith AC. Beckwith-Wiedemann syndrome. Am J Med Genet C Semin Med Genet 2005;137C(1):12–23.

18. Mussa A, Molinatto C, Baldassarre G, et al. Cancer risk in Beckwith-Wiedemann syndrome: a systematic review and meta-analysis outlining a novel (Epi)genotype specific histotype targeted screening protocol. J Pediatr 2016;176:142–9.e1.

19. Mussa A, Russo S, De Crescenzo A, et al. (Epi)genotype-phenotype correlations in Beckwith-Wiedemann syndrome. Eur J Hum Genet 2016;24(2):183–90.

20. Henry I, Jeanpierre M, Couillin P, et al. Molecular definition of the 11p15.5 region involved in Beckwith-Wiedemann syndrome and probably in predisposition to adrenocortical carcinoma. Hum Genet 1989;81(3):273–7.

21. Lapunzina P. Risk of tumorigenesis in overgrowth syndromes: a comprehensive review. Am J Med Genet C Semin Med Genet 2005;137C(1):53–71.

22. Gicquel C, Raffin Sanson ML, Gaston V, et al. Structural and functional abnormalities at 11p15 are associated with the malignant phenotype in sporadic adrenocortical tumors: study on a series of 82 tumors. J Clin Endocrinol Metab 1997; 82(8):2559–65.

23. Pinto EM, Chen X, Easton J, et al. Genomic landscape of paediatric adrenocortical tumours. Nat Commun 2015;6:6302.

24. Reya T, Clevers H. Wnt signalling in stem cells and cancer. Nature 2005; 434(7035):843–50.

25. Rattis FM, Voermans C, Reya T. Wnt signaling in the stem cell niche. Curr Opin Hematol 2004;11(2):88–94.

26. Gaujoux S, Pinson S, Gimenez-Roqueplo AP, et al. Inactivation of the APC gene is constant in adrenocortical tumors from patients with familial adenomatous polyposis but not frequent in sporadic adrenocortical cancers. Clin Cancer Res 2010; 16(21):5133–41.

27. Juhlin CC, Goh G, Healy JM, et al. Whole-exome sequencing characterizes the landscape of somatic mutations and copy number alterations in adrenocortical carcinoma. J Clin Endocrinol Metab 2015;100(3):E493–502.

28. Peifer M. Cancer, catenins, and cuticle pattern: a complex connection. Science 1993;262(5140):1667–8.

29. Spruck CH, Won KA, Reed SI. Deregulated cyclin E induces chromosome instability. Nature 1999;401(6750):297–300.

30. Assie G, Letouze E, Fassnacht M, et al. Integrated genomic characterization of adrenocortical carcinoma. Nat Genet 2014;46(6):607–12.

31. Zheng S, Cherniack AD, Dewal N, et al. Comprehensive pan-genomic characterization of adrenocortical carcinoma. Cancer cell 2016;29(5):723–36.

32. Hao HX, Xie Y, Zhang Y, et al. ZNRF3 promotes Wnt receptor turnover in an R-spondin-sensitive manner. Nature 2012;485(7397):195–200.

33. Toledo F, Wahl GM. Regulating the p53 pathway: in vitro hypotheses, in vivo veritas. Nat Rev Cancer 2006;6(12):909–23.

34. Gonzalez KD, Noltner KA, Buzin CH, et al. Beyond Li Fraumeni syndrome: clinical characteristics of families with p53 germline mutations. J Clin Oncol 2009;27(8): 1250–6.

35. Palmero EI, Achatz MI, Ashton-Prolla P, et al. Tumor protein 53 mutations and inherited cancer: beyond Li-Fraumeni syndrome. Curr Opin Oncol 2010;22(1): 64–9.

36. Gatta-Cherifi B, Chabre O, Murat A, et al. Adrenal involvement in MEN1. Analysis of 715 cases from the Groupe d'etude des Tumeurs Endocrines database. Eur J Endocrinol 2012;166(2):269–79.

37. van Steensel B, Smogorzewska A, de Lange T. TRF2 protects human telomeres from end-to-end fusions. Cell 1998;92(3):401–13.

38. Taylor SS, Ilouz R, Zhang P, et al. Assembly of allosteric macromolecular switches: lessons from PKA. Nat Rev Mol Cell Biol 2012;13(10):646–58.

39. Bourdeau I, Stratakis CA. Cyclic AMP-dependent signaling aberrations in macronodular adrenal disease. Ann N Y Acad Sci 2002;968:240–55.

40. Beuschlein F, Fassnacht M, Assie G, et al. Constitutive activation of PKA catalytic subunit in adrenal Cushing's syndrome. N Engl J Med 2014;370(11):1019–28.

41. Horvath A, Mericq V, Stratakis CA. Mutation in PDE8B, a cyclic AMP-specific phosphodiesterase in adrenal hyperplasia. N Engl J Med 2008;358(7):750–2.

42. Assie G, Libe R, Espiard S, et al. ARMC5 mutations in macronodular adrenal hyperplasia with Cushing's syndrome. N Engl J Med 2013;369(22):2105–14.

43. Carney JA, Young WF, Stratakis CA. Primary bimorphic adrenocortical disease: cause of hypercortisolism in McCune-Albright syndrome. Am J Surg Pathol 2011;35(9):1311–26.

44. Brown RJ, Kelly MH, Collins MT. Cushing syndrome in the McCune-Albright syndrome. J Clin Endocrinol Metab 2010;95(4):1508–15.

45. Weinstein LS, Shenker A, Gejman PV, et al. Activating mutations of the stimulatory G protein in the McCune-Albright syndrome. N Engl J Med 1991;325(24): 1688–95.

46. Groussin L, Kirschner LS, Vincent-Dejean C, et al. Molecular analysis of the cyclic AMP-dependent protein kinase A (PKA) regulatory subunit 1A (PRKAR1A) gene in patients with Carney complex and primary pigmented nodular adrenocortical disease (PPNAD) reveals novel mutations and clues for pathophysiology: augmented PKA signaling is associated with adrenal tumorigenesis in PPNAD. Am J Hum Genet 2002;71(6):1433–42.

47. Horvath A, Boikos S, Giatzakis C, et al. A genome-wide scan identifies mutations in the gene encoding phosphodiesterase 11A4 (PDE11A) in individuals with adrenocortical hyperplasia. Nat Genet 2006;38(7):794–800.

48. Kirschner LS, Carney JA, Pack SD, et al. Mutations of the gene encoding the protein kinase A type I-alpha regulatory subunit in patients with the Carney complex. Nat Genet 2000;26(1):89–92.

49. Bertherat J, Horvath A, Groussin L, et al. Mutations in regulatory subunit type 1A of cyclic adenosine 5′-monophosphate-dependent protein kinase (PRKAR1A): phenotype analysis in 353 patients and 80 different genotypes. J Clin Endocrinol Metab 2009;94(6):2085–91.

50. Aqil M, Deliu Z, Elseth KM, et al. Part II-mechanism of adaptation: A549 cells adapt to high concentration of nitric oxide through bypass of cell cycle checkpoints. Tumour Biol 2014;35(3):2417–25.

51. Bertherat J, Groussin L, Sandrini F, et al. Molecular and functional analysis of PRKAR1A and its locus (17q22-24) in sporadic adrenocortical tumors: 17q losses, somatic mutations, and protein kinase A expression and activity. Cancer Res 2003;63(17):5308–19.

52. Gaujoux S, Tissier F, Groussin L, et al. Wnt/beta-catenin and 3′,5′-cyclic adenosine 5′-monophosphate/protein kinase A signaling pathways alterations and

somatic beta-catenin gene mutations in the progression of adrenocortical tumors. J Clin Endocrinol Metab 2008;93(10):4135–40.

53. Greenhill C. Adrenal gland: the genetics of adrenocortical carcinoma revealed. Nat Rev Endocrinol 2016;12(8):433.

54. Rothenbuhler A, Horvath A, Libe R, et al. Identification of novel genetic variants in phosphodiesterase 8B (PDE8B), a cAMP-specific phosphodiesterase highly expressed in the adrenal cortex, in a cohort of patients with adrenal tumours. Clin Endocrinol 2012;77(2):195–9.

55. Horvath A, Giatzakis C, Tsang K, et al. A cAMP-specific phosphodiesterase (PDE8B) that is mutated in adrenal hyperplasia is expressed widely in human and mouse tissues: a novel PDE8B isoform in human adrenal cortex. Eur J Hum Genet 2008;16(10):1245–53.

56. Cao Y, He M, Gao Z, et al. Activating hotspot L205R mutation in PRKACA and adrenal Cushing's syndrome. Science 2014;344(6186):913–7.

57. Goh G, Scholl UI, Healy JM, et al. Recurrent activating mutation in PRKACA in cortisol-producing adrenal tumors. Nat Genet 2014;46(6):613–7.

58. Sato Y, Maekawa S, Ishii R, et al. Recurrent somatic mutations underlie corticotropin-independent Cushing's syndrome. Science 2014;344(6186): 917–20.

59. Di Dalmazi G, Kisker C, Calebiro D, et al. Novel somatic mutations in the catalytic subunit of the protein kinase A as a cause of adrenal Cushing's syndrome: a European multicentric study. J Clin Endocrinol Metab 2014;99(10):E2093–100.

60. Lodish MB, Yuan B, Levy I, et al. Germline PRKACA amplification causes variable phenotypes that may depend on the extent of the genomic defect: molecular mechanisms and clinical presentations. Eur J Endocrinol 2015;172(6):803–11.

61. Shuch B, Ricketts CJ, Vocke CD, et al. Adrenal nodular hyperplasia in hereditary leiomyomatosis and renal cell cancer. J Urol 2013;189(2):430–5.

62. Matyakhina L, Freedman RJ, Bourdeau I, et al. Hereditary leiomyomatosis associated with bilateral, massive, macronodular adrenocortical disease and atypical Cushing syndrome: a clinical and molecular genetic investigation. J Clin Endocrinol Metab 2005;90(6):3773–9.

63. Alencar GA, Lerario AM, Nishi MY, et al. ARMC5 mutations are a frequent cause of primary macronodular adrenal hyperplasia. J Clin Endocrinol Metab 2014; 99(8):E1501–9.

64. Gagliardi L, Schreiber AW, Hahn CN, et al. ARMC5 mutations are common in familial bilateral macronodular adrenal hyperplasia. J Clin Endocrinol Metab 2014; 99(9):E1784–92.

65. Faucz FR, Zilbermint M, Lodish MB, et al. Macronodular adrenal hyperplasia due to mutations in an armadillo repeat containing 5 (ARMC5) gene: a clinical and genetic investigation. J Clin Endocrinol Metab 2014;99(6):E1113–9.

66. Espiard S, Drougat L, Libe R, et al. ARMC5 mutations in a large cohort of primary macronodular adrenal hyperplasia: clinical and functional consequences. J Clin Endocrinol Metab 2015;100(6):E926–35.

67. Drougat L. Functional study of ARMC5, a new tumour suppressor gene involved in primary bilateral macronodular adrenal hyperplasia. 17th European Congress of Endocrinology. Dublin (Ireland), May 16-20, 2015.

68. Louiset E, Duparc C, Young J, et al. Intraadrenal corticotropin in bilateral macronodular adrenal hyperplasia. N Engl J Med 2013;369(22):2115–25.

69. Lacroix A. ACTH-independent macronodular adrenal hyperplasia. Best Pract Res Clin Endocrinol Metab 2009;23(2):245–59.

70. Lacroix A, Bourdeau I, Lampron A, et al. Aberrant G-protein coupled receptor expression in relation to adrenocortical overfunction. Clin Endocrinol 2010; 73(1):1–15.
71. Libe R, Coste J, Guignat L, et al. Aberrant cortisol regulations in bilateral macronodular adrenal hyperplasia: a frequent finding in a prospective study of 32 patients with overt or subclinical Cushing's syndrome. Eur J Endocrinol 2010;163(1): 129–38.
72. Hsiao HP, Kirschner LS, Bourdeau I, et al. Clinical and genetic heterogeneity, overlap with other tumor syndromes, and atypical glucocorticoid hormone secretion in adrenocorticotropin-independent macronodular adrenal hyperplasia compared with other adrenocortical tumors. J Clin Endocrinol Metab 2009; 94(8):2930–7.
73. Lacroix A. Heredity and cortisol regulation in bilateral macronodular adrenal hyperplasia. N Engl J Med 2013;369(22):2147–9.
74. Beuschlein F, Boulkroun S, Osswald A, et al. Somatic mutations in ATP1A1 and ATP2B3 lead to aldosterone-producing adenomas and secondary hypertension. Nat Genet 2013;45(4):440–4, 444e1–2.
75. Boulkroun S, Golib Dzib JF, Samson-Couterie B, et al. KCNJ5 mutations in aldosterone producing adenoma and relationship with adrenal cortex remodeling. Mol Cell Endocrinol 2013;371(1–2):221–7.
76. Fernandes-Rosa FL, Williams TA, Riester A, et al. Genetic spectrum and clinical correlates of somatic mutations in aldosterone-producing adenoma. Hypertension 2014;64(2):354–61.
77. Monticone S, Hattangady NG, Nishimoto K, et al. Effect of KCNJ5 mutations on gene expression in aldosterone-producing adenomas and adrenocortical cells. J Clin Endocrinol Metab 2012;97(8):E1567–72.
78. Zilbermint M, Xekouki P, Faucz FR, et al. Primary aldosteronism and ARMC5 variants. J Clin Endocrinol Metab 2015;100(6):E900–9.
79. Almeida MQ, Azevedo MF, Xekouki P, et al. Activation of cyclic AMP signaling leads to different pathway alterations in lesions of the adrenal cortex caused by germline PRKAR1A defects versus those due to somatic GNAS mutations. J Clin Endocrinol Metab 2012;97(4):E687–93.

Genetics of Congenital Adrenal Hyperplasia

Fady Hannah-Shmouni, MD[a], Wuyan Chen, PhD[b], Deborah P. Merke, MD, MS[a,c,*]

KEYWORDS

- Congenital adrenal hyperplasia • Genetics • Adrenal insufficiency
- 21-hydroxylase deficiency • Pseudogene • Genetic counseling

KEY POINTS

- Congenital adrenal hyperplasia (CAH) refers to a group of autosomal recessive disorders due to single-gene defects in the various enzymes required for cortisol biosynthesis.
- CAH represents a continuous phenotypic spectrum with more than 95% of all cases caused by 21-hydroxylase deficiency. Genotyping is an important tool in confirming the diagnosis or carrier state, provides prognostic information on disease severity, and is essential for genetic counseling.
- The genes for the various variants of CAH are well characterized, and mutation analysis is widely available.
- Certain ethnic groups have a predilection to certain genotypes, which may have resulted from an ancient founder effect, a hot spot in the gene, unequal crossing-over during meiosis, or gene conversion of point mutations from a pseudogene.
- Several pitfalls in the genetic diagnosis of patients with CAH exist.

INTRODUCTION

Congenital adrenal hyperplasia (CAH) refers to a group of autosomal recessive disorders that impair cortisol biosynthesis. Consequently, overproduction of corticotropin-releasing hormone (CRH) and adrenocorticotropic hormone (ACTH)

Disclosure Statement: The authors report no conflict of interest. This work was supported in part by the Intramural Research Programs of the National Institutes of Health Clinical Center and The Eunice Kennedy Shriver National Institutes of Child Health and Human Development (NICHD). All authors have contributed equally to the article. Dr D.P. Merke ensured the scientific integrity of this work.
[a] Section on Endocrinology and Genetics, The Eunice Kennedy Shriver National Institute of Child Health and Human Development, National Institutes of Health, Building 10, CRC, Room 1-2740, 10 Center Drive, MSC 1932, Bethesda, MD 20892-1932, USA; [b] Clinical DNA Testing and DNA Banking, PreventionGenetics, 3800 South Business Park Avenue, Marshfield, WI 54449, USA; [c] Department of Pediatrics, The National Institutes of Health Clinical Center, 10 Center Drive, Bethesda, MD 20892-1932, USA
* Corresponding author. National Institutes of Health, Building 10, CRC, Room 1-2740, 10 Center Drive, MSC 1932, Bethesda, MD 20892-1932, USA
E-mail address: dmerke@cc.nih.gov

from the hypothalamus and pituitary glands, respectively, results in an increase and accumulation of various steroid precursors proximal to the block. This accumulation leads to defective cortisol synthesis, shunting of the accumulated steroid precursors through alternative pathways, and often adrenal gland hyperplasia. The biochemical defects in CAH translate to a spectrum of clinical consequences, which include adrenal insufficiency, genital ambiguity or disordered sex development, infertility, short stature, hypertension, and an increased risk of metabolic syndrome during adolescence and adulthood. The severity and clinical features of CAH vary depending on the enzymatic defect, its residual activity, age of presentation, and genotype.

CAH represents a continuous phenotypic spectrum (**Table 1**). More than 95% of all cases of CAH are caused by 21-hydroxylase deficiency (21-OHD); 21-OHD is classified into 3 subtypes according to clinical severity: classic salt wasting (SW), classic simple virilizing (SV), and nonclassic CAH (NCCAH; mild or late onset).[1] The classic

Table 1
Types of congenital adrenal hyperplasia

CAH Type	Causative Gene	Clinical Manifestation
21-Hydroxylase deficiency	CYP21A2	Classic: 46,XX ambiguous genitalia, adrenal insufficiency, salt-wasting, postnatal virilization Nonclassic: hyperandrogenism during childhood or early adulthood; may be asymptomatic
	CYP21A2 and TNXB	CAH-X: in addition to the above, joint hypermobility, joint pain, multiple joint dislocations, midline defects including possible cardiac structural abnormalities
11β-Hydroxylase deficiency	CYP11B1	Classic: 46,XX ambiguous genitalia, postnatal virilization, hypertension Nonclassic: hyperandrogenism during childhood or early adulthood; may be asymptomatic
17α-Hydroxylase deficiency	CYP17A1	Classic: female phenotype (46,XX or 46,XY sex reversal), hypertension, pubertal delay with absence of secondary sexual characteristics Partial: 46,XY variable degrees of genital ambiguity; 46, XX variable development of secondary sexual characteristics
3β-Hydroxysteroid dehydrogenase type 2 deficiency	HSD3B2	Classic: 46,XX and 46,XY ambiguous genitalia, adrenal insufficiency, salt wasting
POR deficiency	POR	46,XX and 46,XY ambiguous genitalia, adrenal insufficiency, severe salt wasting, possible maternal virilization during pregnancy; possible skeletal malformations (Antley-Bixler syndrome); no postnatal virilization
Lipoid CAH	StAR	Classic: phenotypic female (46,XX or 46,XY sex reversal), adrenal insufficiency, severe salt wasting Nonclassic: 46,XY variable degrees of genital ambiguity, adrenal insufficiency
Cholesterol side-chain cleavage enzyme deficiency	CYP11A1	Classic: phenotypic female (46,XX or 46,XY sex reversal), adrenal insufficiency, salt wasting Nonclassic: 46,XY variable degrees of genital ambiguity, adrenal insufficiency

Abbreviations: CAH-X, congenital adrenal hyperplasia with tenascin-X impairment; POR, P450 oxidoreductase; StAR, steroidogenic acute regulatory protein.

type affects approximately 1 in 16,000 live births.[2] NCCAH is one of the most common autosomal recessive disorders in humans and affects approximately 1 in 1000 individuals.[3] The second most common form of CAH, 11β-hydroxylase deficiency (11-OHD), occurs in 1 in 100,000 live births in the general population and accounts for approximately 5% of cases.[4] Other less common forms of CAH include 3β-hydroxysteroid dehydrogenase type 2 deficiency, 17α-hydroxylase deficiency that is more commonly seen in Brazil and Mennonite descendants from Dutch Friesland; congenital lipoid adrenal hyperplasia that is more commonly seen in the Japanese and Korean populations; side-chain cleavage (SCC) enzyme deficiency that is most commonly found in Turkey; and cytochrome P450 oxidoreductase deficiency, the only variant that can manifest with skeletal malformation.

Measurement of 17-hydroxyprogesterone (17-OHP) with or without ACTH stimulation establishes the diagnosis of CAH due to 21-OHD.[5] Similarly, the rarer forms of CAH are diagnosed based on hormonal testing. Biochemical methods are typically unable to discriminate heterozygotes from the normal population and disease severity. Thus, genotyping is essential in confirming the carrier state and is useful for genetic counseling.[6] Moreover, studies of the genetics of CAH have provided insight into the pathophysiology and subtle clinical aspects of the disease and may provide prognostic information on disease severity. The genes for the various variants of CAH are well characterized, and mutation analysis is widely available. However, several pitfalls in the genetic diagnosis of individuals with CAH exist. In this article, the authors provide an in-depth discussion on the genetics of CAH, including genetic diagnosis, molecular analysis, genotype-phenotype relationships, and counseling of patients and their families.

GENETIC FORMS OF CONGENITAL ADRENAL HYPERPLASIA
21-Hydroxylase Deficiency

21-OHD (Online Mendelian Inheritance in Man [OMIM] 201910) is the most common form of CAH, classified into classic (SW and SV) and NCCAH.[1] The classic or severe form is characterized by virilization of the external genitalia in newborn girls and by adrenal insufficiency and precocious pseudopuberty due to androgen overproduction in both sexes. Approximately 75% of patients with classic CAH have the SW form. Without neonatal screening, the SW form in boys presents with a severe life-threatening SW crisis in the neonatal period, whereas patients with the SV form may escape this because of small amounts of aldosterone production. Thus, boys with SV CAH, if not detected through neonatal screening, present as toddlers with signs and symptoms of hyperandrogenism. Girls with classic CAH are born with ambiguous genitalia; but without proper diagnosis, most girls would also experience a life-threatening SW crisis. NCCAH, the mild form, may manifest in childhood or early adulthood with precocious pubarche or a clinical picture resembling polycystic ovary syndrome and may be asymptomatic.[3]

CYP21A2 (previously called *P450c21B*, *CYP21B*, or *CYP21*) encodes 21-hydroxylase, a cytochrome P450 type II enzyme of 495 amino acids.[7,8] The *CYP21A2* gene and its duplicated pseudogene (*CYP21A1P*), a nonfunctional byproduct of the functional gene that was formed from selective pressure during evolution, are located 30-kb apart in the human leukocyte antigen (HLA) class III region in the major histocompatibility (MHC) locus on the short arm of chromosome 6 (band 6p21.3) and share approximately 98% sequence homology (**Figs. 1** and **2**).[9] The *CYP21A1P* gene is inactive because of the presence of approximately 11 deleterious mutations in its coding region (see **Fig. 2**). Both genes are arranged in tandem repeat with the *C4* (*C4A* and

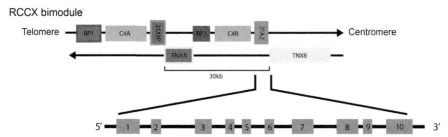

Fig. 1. The *CYP21A2* gene and its duplicated pseudogene (*CYP21A1P*) are located 30-kb apart in the HLA class III region in the MHC locus on the short arm of chromosome 6 (band 6p21.3) and share approximately 98% sequence homology. Both genes are arranged in tandem repeat with the *C4* (*C4A* and *C4B*) genes. *C4/CYP21A* is flanked by telomeric *RP* (*RP1* and *RP2*) and centromeric tenascin (*TNXA* and *TNXB*) genes. *RP1* encodes a serine/threonine nuclear protein kinase; *C4* encodes for the immune effector protein complement component; *TNX* encodes an extracellular matrix protein. With the exception of *C4*, each of the other functional genes (*RP1*, *CYP21A2*, and *TNXB*) has a corresponding highly homologous pseudogene (*RP2*, *CYP21A1P*, and *TNXA*). The *RP, TNX, C4,* and *CYP21* genes together compose the RCCX bimodule (*RP1-C4-CYP21A1P-TNXA-RP2-C4-CYP21A2-TNXB*). Enlarged area represents the 10 exons of *CYP21A2*. Active genes are solid colors. Pseudogenes are gray, outlined with the color of the corresponding active gene.

C4B) genes encoding the fourth component of complement; *C4/CYP212A* is flanked by telomeric *RP* (*RP1* and *RP2*) and centromeric *tenascin* (*TNXA* and *TNXB*) genes. This odd arrangement was probably caused by an ancestral duplication of 30-kb encompassing the *CYP21A2* and *C4* genes and represents a region with a high frequency of genomic recombination. *RP1* encodes a serine/threonine nuclear protein kinase; *C4* encodes for the immune effector protein complement component; *TNXB* encodes tenascin-X, an extracellular matrix protein. With the exception of *C4*, each of the other functional genes (*RP1*, *CYP21A2*, and *TNXB*) has a corresponding highly

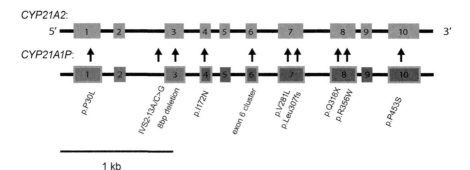

Fig. 2. The high degree of sequence homology between *CYP21A2* and its pseudogene *CYP21A1P* allows for recombination events. Unequal crossing-over through intergenic recombination results in large deletions and the transfer of deleterious pseudogene sequence to the active gene. Most mutations found in CAH due to 21-OHD are pseudogene derived or large 30-kb deletions resulting in chimeric genes. The most common pseudogene-derived mutations found in the *CYP21A2* are shown: p.P30L; IVS2-13A/C>G; 8bp deletion; p.I172N; exon 6 cluster (p.I236N, p.V237E, p.M239K); p.V281L; p.Leu307fs; p.Q318X; p.R356W; p.P453S.

homologous pseudogene (RP2, CYP21A1P, and TNXA). Together with the RP and TNX genes, the C4 and CYP21 genes compose the RCCX (RP, C4, CYP21, TNX) module; most chromosomes are bimodular (RP1-C4-CYP21A1P-TNXA-RP2-C4-CYP21A2-TNXB)[10] (see **Fig. 1**) with a CYP21A1P gene in the telomeric position and the CYP21A2 gene in the centromeric position. Mono-modular and trimodular haplotypes are also found in most populations.[10–12] These modules are characterized by modular duplication or deletion events in which each duplicated or deleted module usually covers a CYP21A1P-TNXA-RP2-C4 unit. Copy number variation (CNV) of C4, CYP21, and TNX is widely found in humans; in patients with CAH, a greater C4 CNV with mutation-specific associations has been shown to possibly confer protection for autoimmune disease.[13]

Because of the high degree of sequence homology between CYP21A2 and its pseudogene, recombination occurs. Approximately 70% of CYP21A2 disease-causing mutations are pseudogene-derived variants due to gene conversion, the transfer of deleterious pseudogene mutations to the active CYP21A2 gene[14]; approximately 25% to 30% are chimeric genes due to large deletions.[15,16] Misalignment during meiosis can result in a 30-kb gene deletion, which produces a nonfunctioning chimeric CYP21A1P/CYP21A2 gene.[17–19] Depending on the break points, such genetic alterations result in different types of chimeras between the homologous genes in the RCCX modules; 9 different CYP21A1P/CYP21A2 chimeras (CH) have been reported, which have a CH-1 through 9 designation.[20] These chimeras are numbered chronologically, based on when the junction sites were reported (**Fig. 3**). Approximately 1% to 2% of cases are caused by de novo mutations not carried by either parent due to the high variability of the CYP21A2 locus.[9] These de novo mutations result in complex genetic variation and unusual haplotypes, which can be detected in one in 10^3 to 10^5 sperm cells.[21] Uniparental disomy of chromosome 6 as a cause of CAH is a rare occurrence with an unknown prevalence.[22]

Genotype-phenotype correlation

CAH due to 21-OHD represents a spectrum of phenotypic heterogeneity, with a direct genotype-phenotype correlation seen in approximately 90% of cases.[23–26] Because most patients with CAH are compound heterozygotes carrying 2 different disease-causing mutations, the phenotype is defined by the mutation retaining the most enzyme activity.[6] Generally, the disease severity in childhood can be accurately predicted by genotypes predicted to result in the SW and NCCAH forms, whereas the most phenotypic variability is observed with the SV type.[6,17,23,25,26] Females are readily diagnosed clinically with classic CAH because of the genital ambiguity. However, with neonatal screening, classic CAH cases ascertained are equal between males and females.[27] Moreover, females are more likely to be found to have the p.V281L mutation and NCCAH because males may be asymptomatic.[28] Genotype is not a good predictor of the development of long-term health outcomes in adults with classic CAH, such as cardiovascular disease or osteoporosis, possibly due to treatment-related effects on comorbidities.[28,29]

Based on in vitro data, CYP21A2 mutations can be classified into 4 groups (null, A, B, C) according to their severity (**Table 2**).[9] Deletions or nonsense mutations that affect critical enzyme functions, such as membrane anchoring, heme binding, or altered enzyme stability, result in a complete loss of functionality and SW. Missense mutations with 1% to 2% of normal enzyme activity are found in patients with the SV form and affect the transmembrane region or conserved hydrophobic patches.[30–32] Mutations in p.V281L, p.P453S, and p.P30L cause an interference in oxidoreductase interactions, salt-bridge and hydrogen bonding networks, and produce

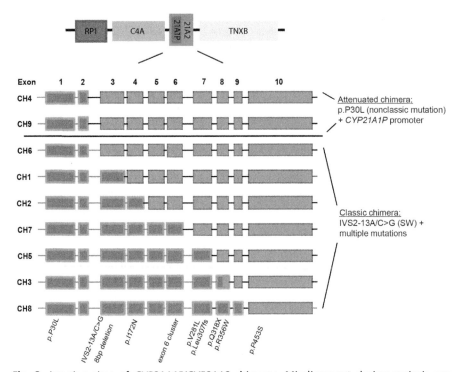

Fig. 3. Junction sites of *CYP21A1P/CYP21A2* chimeras. Misalignment during meiosis can result in a 30-kb gene deletion, which produces a chimeric *CYP21A1P/CYP21A2* gene. Nine different *CYP21A1P/CYP21A2* chimeras have been reported with unique junction sites. These chimeras are numbered chronologically, CH-1 through CH-9, based on when the junction sites were reported. The location of the junction site is clinically meaningful. Seven chimeras are nonfunctional and are associated with a classic SW phenotype. Two chimeras, CH-4 and CH-9, carry the p.P30L mutation and, along with a weak *CYP21A1P* promoter, only partially impair the gene. These chimera are referred to as attenuated and are associated with a milder phenotype.

enzymes retaining 20% to 60% of normal activity as seen in NCCAH (group C).[21,33,34] In general, there is good genotype-phenotype correlation for the NCCAH p.V281L and p.P453S mutations; but phenotypic variability has been described for p.P30L.[6,24]

Uncommon chimeric genes also account for some genotype-phenotype discrepancy, and the junction site of the chimeras that develop as a consequence of genetic rearrangements can be clinically meaningful (see **Fig. 3**).[20] Most commonly, the large deletions that are associated with *CYP21A1P/CYP21A2* chimeric genes totally inactivate the *CYP21A2* gene and, therefore, are associated with a classic SW phenotype. This type of *CYP21A1P/CYP21A2* chimera is referred to as a classic chimera. The classic *CYP21A1P/CYP21A2* chimeras contain the IVS2-13A/C>G mutation and often multiple other pseudogene mutations. The 21-hydroxylase enzyme activity is less severely impaired if the junction site occurs upstream of the pseudogene mutation IVS2-13A/C>G within intron 2. This chimera is referred to as an attenuated chimera.

Table 2
The classification of common *CYP21A2* and *CYP11B1* mutations based on in vitro data

Group	Null	A	B	C
21-OHD[23–25]				
Phenotype	SW	SW	SV	NC
In vitro activity of *CYP21A2* (%)	0	<1	1–2	20–60
Mutations[a]	30-kb deletion[b] 8bp deletion exon 6 cluster[c] p.Q318X p.R356W p.Leu307fs	IVS2-13A/C>G	p.I172N p.I77T	p.V281L p.R339H p.P453S p.P30L
11β-hydroxylase deficiency[66,67,70,76]				
Phenotype	Classic[70]			Nonclassic[76]
Mutations[a]	p.R448H p.R448C p.W247X p.W116G p.W116X p.W116C p.V129M p.L158P p.A165D p.K254_A259del p.R383Q p.P94L p.L299P p.T318M p.A331V p.R374Q p.F438del p.L464dup p.V441G			p.P42S p.P42L p.R43Q p.H125R p.P135S p.F139L p.P159L p.A297V p.R332Q p.R383Q p.N133H p.M88I p.R366C p.T401A p.T319M p.F79I p.R138C p.R143W p.T196A

Abbreviation: NC, nonclassic.
[a] Nomenclature at the protein level is based on conventional codon numbering.
[b] About 4% are attenuated chimeras in group C.
[c] p.I236N, p.V237E, p.M239K.

To date, 2 attenuated chimeras have been described: CH-4 and CH-9 (see **Fig. 3**). Both have junction sites upstream of the common pseudogene mutation IVS2-13A/C>G, carry a weak but active *CYP21A1P* promoter and a nonclassic mutation, p.P30L (c.92C_ T) in exon 1, and result in an SV or NCCAH phenotype.[20] In a large cohort study of patients with CAH, 96% of large deletions were classic chimeras and 4% were attenuated chimeras.[20]

Genotype-phenotype discordance or concordance may exist across all mutation groups. As a general rule, there is a high genotype-phenotype concordance in p.V281L, deletions, 8 bp deletion, p.Q318X, and p.R356W mutations (see **Table 2**). SV disease occurs in approximately 76% of patients with CAH who carry the p.I172N mutation on one allele and a severe mutation on the other, whereas 23% of these patients present with SW CAH, likely due to subtle variations in transcriptional regulation or downstream protein translation.[6] Moreover, the intron 2 IVS2-13A/C>G splicing mutation results primarily in SW CAH; however, approximately 20% of patients have an SV phenotype.[6]

Erroneous reporting may occur in the presence of gene duplication. For example, the p.Q318X mutation is sometimes associated with *CYP21A2* gene duplication. In this situation, the p.Q318X-mutated allele coexists with a normal *CYP21A2*-like gene within the RCCX module on the same chromosome.[6] This duplicate allele does not represent a mutated allele because the normal gene is expressed.

Several factors may be responsible for the genotype-phenotype variability in patients with CAH. Apart from the *CYP21A2* mutations, other genes that may impact phenotype by modifying steroid action or salt balance include the length of the CAG repeats of the androgen receptor,[35,36] the highly polymorphic enzyme P450 oxidoreductase, splice mutations variants in RNA splicing factors,[37,38] and other genes encoding proteins other than cytochrome P450 type II enzyme that have 21-hydroxylase activity.[39,40] A wide spectrum of phenotypes occurs, and genotype-phenotype discordance requires further research.

Congenital adrenal hyperplasia–tenascin-X syndrome

Some deletions that cause CAH due to 21-OHD also cause hypermobility-type Ehlers-Danlos syndrome due to the monoallelic presence of a chimera extending into the *TNXB* gene, encoding *tenascin*-X, an extracellular matrix protein. This contiguous gene deletion syndrome, involving both the *CYP21A2* and *TNXB* genes, is termed CAH-X syndrome.[41,42] The first study of the genetic spectrum of CAH-X in a mixed population of patients with CAH showed a contiguous *CYP21A2* deletion that extended into *TNXB* in 13% of patients (n = 12 of 91) carrying a *CYP21A2* deletion and a *TNXB* premature stop codon in a single patient, with an overall 7% prevalence of CAH-X among patients with CAH.[41] Additional chimeric genes have subsequently been identified; overall 9% of patients with CAH due to 21-OHD are estimated to have CAH-X, a connective tissue dysplasia, in addition to having CAH.[43]

The deletions associated with CAH-X are *TNXA/TNXB* chimeras (**Fig. 4**) and 3 types of chimeric genes have been identified to date, designated CAH-X CH-1, CAH-X CH-2, and CAH-X CH-3.[41,43,44] CAH-X CH-1 involves the 120 bp deletion in the exon 35 region of *TNXB* and leads to haploinsufficiency with reduced *tenascin*-X;

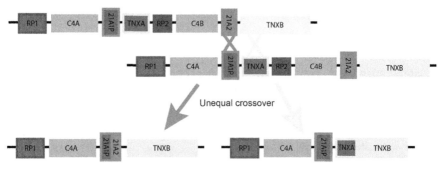

CYP21A1P/CYP21A2 chimera   TNXA/TNXB chimera

Fig. 4. Formation of *CYP21A1P/CYP21A2* and *TNXA/TNXB* chimeras. Because of the high degree of sequence homology between *CYP21A2* and *CYP21A1P*, recombination events occur. The deletions associated with CAH-X syndrome, a condition characterized by having a combination of CAH and a connective tissue dysplasia, are *TNXA/TNXB* chimeras. The formation of a *TNXA/TNXB* chimera results in deletion of the *CYP21A2* gene.

CAH-X CH-2 involves the c.12174 C>G (p.Cys4058Trp) variant in exon 40 of *TNXB*, which does not alter *tenascin*-X expression but rather causes a dominant-negative effect due to the loss of a critical disulfide bond in the *tenascin*-X fibrinogenlike domain; and CAH-X CH-3 involves a cluster of 3 variants and also causes a dominant-negative effect.

Patients with CAH-X may present with CAH and joint hypermobility, joint pain, and multiple joint dislocations.[41] Other clinical features include midline defects and major cardiac structural abnormalities.[42] Thus, clinicians involved in the care of patients with CAH, particularly those harboring a *CYP21A2* deletion, should provide a comprehensive evaluation for a connective tissue dysplasia.

Population genetics and ethnic diversity of CYP21A2 genotypes

Millions of newborns screened in the general population for the classic form of CAH have demonstrated an overall incidence of 1:13,000 to 1:16,000 live births.[45,46] The prevalence in specific populations varies, including 1:10,000 to 1:23,000 in the United States and Europe,[47] 1:21,000 in Japan,[48] 1:27,000 in New Zealand,[49] and 1:6000 in China[50] and India.[51] NCCAH is one of the most common autosomal recessive disorders in humans and affects approximately 1 in 1000 individuals.[3] Certain ethnic groups have a predilection to certain genotypes (**Table 3**),[9,23,24,52–58] which may have resulted from an ancient founder effect, unequal crossing over during meiosis, or gene conversion of point mutations in the pseudogene.[59]

In the United States, the allele frequency of the most common mutations might vary considerably between different ethnicities. For instance, the exon 7 p.V281L (c.1685G>T) mutation associated with NCCAH is very frequent in the Ashkenazi Jewish (AJ) population of New York (estimated in one study to be 1 in 27, with 1 in 3 being heterozygous), which has not been observed in the Asian and Native American populations.[6] However, this mutation also occurs in other populations. Among compound heterozygotes in the AJ population, the prevalent mutations are large deletion/p.V281L (c.1685G>T) and IVS2-13A/C>G (c.293–13 A/C>G)/p.V281L (c.1685 G>T).[59]

CAH is rare in Asian, African American, and East Indian populations of New York, whereas a large gene deletion is observed in Native Americans.[6] Conversely, the IVS2-13 A/C>G genotype and p.V281L are more prevalent in the Middle Eastern population; the common p.Q318X mutation is by far the most frequently found in the Tunisian population.[60] In the Yupik-speaking Eskimos of Western Alaska and Iranians, the IVS2-13A/C>G (c.293-13A/C>G) mutation predominates.[59] One study found at least half of all patients with 21-OHD in Finland were due to 3 most common founder mutation-haplotypes, and only one-sixth of the haplotypes represented single cases.[61] Of the chimeras, CH-7 was first identified in a Czech population and represents the most frequent allele.[20] Thus, knowledge about the ethnic diversity and specificity of the *CYP21A2* mutations might help guide clinicians toward a diagnosis of 21-OHD before molecular testing.

Molecular analysis of CYP21A2 mutations

The genetic diagnosis of CAH is complex because of the high variability of its genomic region. This variabilty includes the coexistence of 2 or more mutations on the same allele or the presence of more than one CYP21/C4 repeat unit on the same chromosome. Molecular analysis of *CYP21A2* should be extensive and performed in a certified laboratory with adequate quality controls and experience in the analysis of CAH genotypes. Care should be taken to prevent genotyping the pseudogene because genetic results can be complicated by the duplication, deletion, and recombination of *CYP21A2* in the chromosome 6q21.3 region. Moreover, mutant alleles must be

Table 3
Frequency of CYP21A2 mutations across various populations

Country	p.P30L	IVS2-13A/C>G	8bp del	p.I172 N	Exon 6 Cluster[a]	p.V281L	p.Leu307fs	p.Q318X	p.R356W	p.P453S	Del/Conv
United States[23]	0.8	23.4	0.5	12.6	1.0	12.6	0.3	3.3	3.6	0.5	30.5
Argentina[55]	0.7	20.6	0.8	8.2	2.0	26.2	ND	6.7	4.2	1.4	11.2
Netherlands[25]	0.3	28.1	4.3	ND	3.0	2.2	0.3	3.5	8.4	0.5	31.9
Sweden[52]	1.6	27.7	1.2	20.8	0.5	5.4	0.5	0.5	3.8	0.5	29.8
Brazil[56]	0.6	21.1	1.8	7.5	1.2	26.6	2.2	6.1	5.4	1.4	9.0
Germany[24]	2.6	30.3	1.6	19.7	1.0	2.9	0.3	4.8	4.5	0.3	27.4
Italy[54]	2.7	19.9	0.0	6.2	0.0	11.0	ND	8.2	0.0	ND	ND
France[57]	ND	20.5	2.7	8.9	5.0	16.7	1.2	3.9	ND	0	22.9
Spain[58]	2.6	22.4	3.9	1.3	0.0	15.8	2.0	3.9	3.9	ND	19.7
Mexico[113]	8.5	47.9	2.1	11.7	0.0	8.5	1.0	4.2	7.4	2.1	1.0

Nomenclature at the protein level is based on conventional codon numbering.
Abbreviations: Conv, conversions; Del, deletions; ND, not detected.
[a] p.I236N, p.V237E, p.M239K.

segregated in the parents to investigate their presence in different alleles, to determine if they are in the *cis* or *trans* configuration, and to verify de novo mutations. Targeted site-directed mutation analysis of the 12 most common mutations fails to identify mutations in approximately 10% of patients, and rare mutations are identified more often than expected with whole coding region sequencing.[23] Thus, *CYP21A2* sequencing is important in determining an accurate genotype, especially if genotype does not correspond to phenotype or if only one mutation is present in a patient with clinical and hormonal evidence of CAH.

The *CYP21A2* gene consists of 10 exons and relatively short introns, which allows for the amplification of the entire exon-intron region. Traditionally, the complete characterization of the locus regarding number of RCCX modules and their specific gene content required Southern blotting with probes for the different genes and using different combinations of restriction endonucleases.[62] However, given its labor intensity, the need for radioactivity, and the requirement for relatively large amounts of good-quality DNA, Southern blotting has been largely replaced by real-time quantitative polymerase chain reaction (PCR)[62] and multiplex ligation-depended probe amplification (MLPA)[63,64] methods for detecting large gene deletions and duplications. A well-established protocol for sequencing the *CYP21A2* gene is the use of long-range PCR that amplifies an 8.5-kb fragment (the CYP779f/Tena32 F amplicon) encompassing the full *CYP21A2* gene and part of the *TNXB* gene.[20] Because the forward primer is common for both *CYP21A2* and *CYP21A1P*, whereas the reverse primer anneals the unique (nonhomologous) sequence of the *TNXB* gene, an accurate analysis of the *CYP21A2* gene is guaranteed even when the *CYP21A2* gene is replaced by the pseudogene, either partially or totally. Therefore, the junction site of chimera genes can be automatically determined and MLPA is not needed for detecting large deletions.[20] Compared with the targeted common mutation analysis approaches, whole-gene (coding regions and canonical splicing sites) sequencing can reveal both common and rare mutations. This 8.5-kb CYP779f/Tena32 F amplicon is able to reveal *TNXA/TNXB* chimeras and has been used to study patients with CAH-X.[41,43,44]

Both the PCR- and MLPA-based strategies have limitations. First, allele dropout (ie, only one allele is amplified and sequenced) is a general limitation of PCR-based Sanger sequencing. If no heterozygotes are found, parental study should be performed to rule out the possibility of allele dropout. Second, the long-range PCR amplicon for sequencing the *CYP21A2* gene alone is not able to detect the *CYP21A2* duplication allele simultaneously. Another well-designed long-range PCR amplicon is required to detect *CYP21A2* duplication specifically. Third, MLPA is unable to distinguish attenuated chimeras CH-4 and CH-9 from classic chimera CH-6, owing to the lack of a probe for IVS2-13A/C>G, which is the crucial site for classifying chimeric *CYP21A1P/CYP21A2* genes into the classic and attenuated types.[20] Thus, an experienced laboratory in dealing with the *CYP21A2* gene analysis is highly advised for the correct molecular diagnosis of CAH due to 21-OHD. Genotyping for the presence of *TNXA/TNXB* chimeras should be performed in patients clinically suspicious for CAH-X.

11β-Hydroxylase Deficiency

11β-Hydroxylase deficiency (11-OHD) (OMIM 202010) is the second most common variant of CAH (approximately 5%–8% of all cases) with an incidence of 1 in 100,000 to 200,000 live births.[65] 11-OHD is caused by mutations in the 11β-hydroxylase gene (*CYP11B1*), with the highest prevalence among Moroccan Jews (approximately 1 in 5000–7000 live births), an association that is partially explained by the founder mutation p.R448H.[66,67] The CYP11B1 enzyme is a P450 type I mitochondrial enzyme, responsible for the conversion of 11-deoxycortisol to cortisol and 11-deoxy-corticosterone (DOC) to corticosterone; its defect results in hypertension from elevated DOC and possibly other steroid precursors and hyperandrogenism from shunted pre-cursors into the androgen synthesis pathway. Patients do not present with adrenal insufficiency due to the glucocorticoid effects of excess corticosterone. 11-OHD is divided into the classic form, which presents as virilization of the external genitalia in 46,XX newborn girls, and precocious pseudopuberty in both sexes. The nonclassic form is extremely rare and presents with hyperandrogenism during childhood.[68]

The CYP11B1 gene is located on chromosome 8q24.3 and consists of 9 exons that are approximately 40-kb from the highly homologous aldosterone synthase gene (CYP11B2).[69] More than 50 CYP11B1-inactivatig mutations that are distributed over the entire coding region exist, with the majority being missense and nonsense; but splice-site mutations, small deletions, small insertions, and complex rearrangements exist and result in absent or very little 11β-hydroxylase activity.[70] These mutations (see **Table 2**) cause the classic form and tend to cluster in exons 2, 6, 7, and 8.[71] Rarely, unequal crossing-over between the CYP11B2 and the CYP11B1 genes produces a chimera that is under the control of angiotensin II and potassium, rather than ACTH,[72] resulting in glucocorticoid-remediable aldosteronism (familial hyperaldosteronism type 1), which is not considered a type of CAH. Rare chimeric CYP11B2/CYP11B1 genes can also result in CAH due to 11-OHD.[73] A variety of milder mutations that result in nonclassic 11-OHD exist (see **Table 2**).[70,74] Novel mutations for both subtypes are being discovered routinely.[70,75,76]

17α-Hydroxylase Deficiency

17α-hydroxylase deficiency (17-OHD) (OMIM 202110) results from a defective CYP17A1 and accounts for approximately 1% of all CAH cases.[77] The CYP17A1 enzyme is a microsomal P450 type II enzyme that catalyzes 2 different enzymatic re-actions: 17-α hydroxylation of pregnenolone and progesterone and the conversion of 17-hydroxypregnenolone to dehydroepiandrosterone and, with lesser efficiency, of 17-OHP to androstenedione through the 17,20 lyase reaction. Thus, 17-OHD results in glucocorticoid and sex steroid deficiency and impairs both adrenal and gonadal function.[78] The accumulation of the mineralocorticoid precursors corticosterone and DOC exert glucocorticoid and mineralocorticoid activity respectively and lead to hy-pertension with hypokalemia. Thus, adrenal insufficiency is not a characteristic feature of 17-OHD. Patients present with hypertension, hypokalemia, and sexual infantilism. The classic presentation of severe 17-OHD is a phenotypic female (46,XX or 46,XY) with hypertension and absence of secondary sexual characteristics. In partial 17-OHD, patients with 46,XY may present with undervirilization and present as infants with ambiguous genitalia. Isolated 17,20 lyase deficiency that results in amino acid substitutions located within the area of the CYP17A1 molecule that interacts with the electron-donating redox partner, P450 oxidoreductase (POR), is a rare disorder that manifests with impaired sex steroid biosynthesis only.[79] These patients may pre-sent as a male with undervirilization and gynecomastia or a female with delayed pubarche and oligomenorrhea. Isolated 17,20 lyase deficiency is not considered a type of CAH.

The CYP17A1 gene consists of 8 exons encoding a 508-amino-acid protein and is located on chromosome 10 (10q24.32).[80] More than 70 CYP17A1-inactivating muta-tions exist, with no evidence of a hot spot in most large populations. Therefore, sequencing of the entire coding region is usually necessary for molecular genetic di-agnostics. However, certain ethnicities are at higher risk of 17-OHD, including

Canadian Mennonites and Dutch Frieslanders,[81] Japanese,[82] East Asians, and the Brazilian population,[83] whereby 82% of mutant alleles are due to 2 mutations, suggesting a founder effect.

3β-Hydroxysteroid Dehydrogenase Type 2 Deficiency

3β-hydroxysteroid dehydrogenase type 2 (HSD3B2) deficiency (OMIM 201810) is a rare autosomal recessive variant of CAH with an unknown incidence. 3β-hydroxysteroid dehydrogenase exists in 2 isoforms, type 1 and type 2, each encoded by genes (4 exons, of which exons 2–4 are translated) on chromosome 1 (1p12), *HSD3B1* and *HSD3B2*, respectively.[84] *HSD3B2* is highly expressed in the adrenal glands and gonads, whereas *HSD3B1* is expressed in the placenta and peripheral tissues. HSD3B2 is responsible for the conversion of the pregnenolone, 17-hydroxypregnenolone and dehydroepiandrosterone to progesterone, 17-OHP and androstenedione, respectively. Similar to 17-OHD, both gonadal and adrenal hormone synthesis is affected. Paradoxically, both male and female infants can be born with genital ambiguity, depending on the severity of the enzyme deficiency. A nonclassic form of HSD3B2 deficiency that causes hirsutism and menstrual irregularity in young adult women was previously suggested,[85] based on exaggerated 17-hydroxypregnenolone production after ACTH stimulation.[86] However, the *HSD3B2* gene was subsequently found to be normal in these patients, and they most likely have a form of polycystic ovary syndrome.[87] Thus, the diagnosis of a mild or nonclassic form is questionable and should not be considered unless the diagnostic laboratory parameters are at least 6 standard deviations greater than normal.[88] The genetics of HSD3B2 deficiency was first ascertained in a patient with 46,XY with ambiguous genitalia and a homozygous combined missense/frameshift mutation in exon 4.[89]

P450 Oxidoreductase Deficiency

POR deficiency (OMIM 613571) is a rare variant of CAH of unknown incidence and manifests as apparent combined CYP17A1 and CYP21A2 deficiency.[90] The POR gene is located on the long arm of chromosome 7 (7q11.23), consists of 15 translated exons spanning a region of approximately 32.9-kb, and serves as an electron donor enzyme for CYP17A1, CYP19A1 (aromatase), and CYP21A2.[90] Both sexes present clinically with severe sexual ambiguity; boys present with severe undervirilization and girls present with severe virilization. Reduced CYP19A1 activity induces androgen accumulation in the placenta, leading to virilization of the female fetus and sometimes the pregnant mother. Adrenal insufficiency is present in most patients.[91]

Craniofacial malformations may also be present and overlap with the Antley-Bixler syndrome (OMIM 201750), a rare craniosynostosis syndrome characterized by radiohumeral synostosis presenting in the perinatal period.[90] Most patients with mild to moderate skeletal malformations are compound heterozygous for missense mutations, whereas nearly all patients with severe malformations carried a major loss-of-function defect on one of the affected alleles.[91] Postnatally, females with POR deficiency have low androgens and virilization does not progress. POR-inactivating mutations, including missense, frameshift, and splice site mutations, are scattered throughout the gene with no apparent hot spots.[92,93] The most frequent mutation in Caucasians is p.A287P,[92] whereas p.R457H is the most frequent mutation in Japanese populations.[94,95] In one study of 30 patients with POR deficiency from 11 countries, 23 POR mutations including a deletion and a partial duplication were detected by MLPA and only 22% of unrelated patients carried homozygous POR mutations.[91] POR deficiency may present as a form of apparent 17,20 lyase deficiency due to mutations in the POR gene rather than the *CYP17A1* gene.[82]

Lipoid Congenital Adrenal Hyperplasia

Lipoid CAH (OMIM 201710) is the most severe disorder of adrenal and gonadal steroidogenesis and is due to a defect in a transport protein, steroidogenic acute regulatory protein (StAR) that regulates cholesterol transfer within the mitochondria. This step is the rate-limiting step in the production of steroid hormones. In classic congenital lipoid CAH, there is complete or near-complete absence of all steroid hormones. Lipoid CAH is caused by homozygous or compound heterozygous mutations in the gene encoding StAR on chromosome 8p11.23.[96] The pathophysiology involves an initial genetic loss of steroidogenesis that is StAR dependent and a subsequent loss of steroidogenesis that is StAR independent, due to cellular damage from accumulated cholesterol esters in the adrenal and gonadal glands.[97] Affected patients are phenotypic females with severe SW that is fatal if not treated in early infancy because of glucocorticoid and mineralocorticoid deficiency. This rare disease is most common among Japanese, Korean, and Palestinian Arab populations.[98] Several mutations in the StAR gene have been described and are mostly located in exons 5, 6, or 7: p.Q258X in Asians and p.R182L in Palestinian Arabs.[97]

A milder, nonclassic form of lipoid CAH was first described in 2006[99] and is caused by mutations that retain about 20% to 30% of normal StAR activity. Most of these patients carry the StAR mutation p.R188C, which has been found in patients from Canada, Jordan, India, Pakistan, and Thailand; however, other StAR mutations causing nonclassic lipoid CAH have also been described.

Cholesterol Side-Chain Cleavage Enzyme Deficiency

For years, it was thought that deficiency of cholesterol SCC enzyme was incompatible with life. This idea was reinforced with the discovery that StAR mutations cause lipoid CAH. However, 28 patients have now been described with *CYP11A1* mutations causing SCC deficiency (OMIM 118485).[100,101] Most of the reported cases are from Eastern Turkey and are homozygous for the missense mutation p.R451W.[102] Variable phenotype has been described, presumably due to mutation-specific variable effects on enzyme activity.[101]

GENETIC COUNSELING OF PATIENTS WITH CONGENITAL ADRENAL HYPERPLASIA

All forms of CAH are transmitted as autosomal recessive and the determination of disease risk depends on the carrier status of patients' parents. Genetic counseling should focus on the future risks of having an affected child. Having one normal gene and one gene carrying a CAH mutation results in a carrier state and carriers for CAH do not show symptoms. If both parents are carriers, then the risk of having an affected child, a child who is a carrier, and an unaffected child is 25%, 50%, and 25%, respectively (**Fig. 5**). However, if one parent is a heterozygous carrier and the other is affected with CAH, each child has a 50% chance of inheriting one mutation and a 50% chance of being affected. The risk is the same for males and females.

For CAH due to 21-OHD, the incidence of classic CAH is approximately 1:10,000 to 1:20,000, with a carrier rate in the general population of approximately 1:50 to 1:71 (median 1:60).[3,45,103] The chance that a patient with classic CAH will have a child with classic CAH is 1 in 120 (chance of partner being a carrier [0.016] $\times$ 0.5) if the carrier status of the partner is unknown. For NCCAH, about two-thirds of patients are compound heterozygotes, carrying one allele that causes classic CAH and one that causes NCCAH. The chance that a patient with NCCAH will have a child affected with classic CAH is 1 in 360 (chance of partner being a carrier $\times$ chance of nonclassic patient being a carrier of classic mutation $\times$ 0.25 = 0.016 $\times$ 0.666 $\times$ 0.25) if the carrier

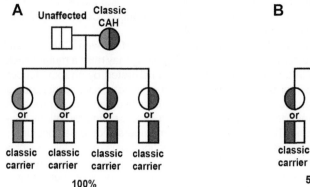
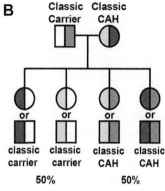

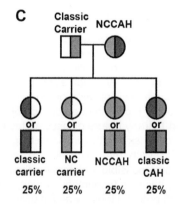

Fig. 5. Genetic risk in the offspring of a patient with CAH. (A) If the partner of a patient with classic CAH is unaffected, then all of the children will be carriers of classic CAH. (B) If the partner of a patient with classic CAH is a carrier of a classic mutation, then there is a 50% chance that a pregnancy will result in a child affected with classic CAH. Phenotype is determined by the most functional allele. (C) If the patient has NCCAH but carries a classic gene and the partner is a carrier of a classic mutation, then there is a 25% chance of having a child with classic CAH.

status of the partner is unknown.[28] This risk in reality may be higher; a retrospective study of women with NCCAH reported a 2.5% risk of a woman with NCCAH having a child with classic CAH.[104] When compared with an individual with 2 normal *CYP21A2* alleles, a heterozygote carrier may have slightly elevated 17-OHP levels when stimulated with ACTH; but hormonal testing does not accurately predict the carrier state. Thus, genetic testing is essential to determine the presence of mutations.

A successful patient counseling model for CAH would incorporate patients' values and attitudes toward their disease, underscoring the risks and benefits of genetic screening and counseling, psychosocial interventions, and service delivery. Other aspects of a successful counseling model include a thorough personal medical and family history (with a detailed family pedigree), education regarding the genetics of the condition, and discussions on preventing and screening options. Counseling should be carried out by an experienced genetic counselor.

When offering genetic counseling to individuals at risk of or with CAH, several important factors should be considered. First, genetic testing may miss a mutant allele and should be carried out in a reliable laboratory and interpreted by an experienced individual. Second, the optimal time for determination of genetic risk, carrier status, or treatment is before pregnancy. Third, testing of reproductive partners of probands for carrier status is recommended when one or both disease-causing mutations have been identified in the proband. Testing of other family members should be considered before reproduction but is not recommended on a routine basis, especially for children. Fourth, certainties and uncertainties about treatment, prognosis, morbidity, mortality, or the impact of a positive genetic screen on the individual or their families should be discussed in detail with patients or their surrogate before testing.

PRENATAL DIAGNOSIS OF CONGENITAL ADRENAL HYPERPLASIA

Prenatal diagnosis is an invasive approach that uses fetal DNA, obtained by amniocentesis or chorionic villus sampling, to establish a diagnosis based on genotype.[65] Determination of the fetal sex could allow for prenatal therapeutic decisions of 46,XX fetuses with virilizing CAH, although administration of dexamethasone to the pregnant mother to reduce masculinization of the genitalia in a fetus at risk for CAH is controversial and no longer recommended outside of a research setting.[1] Concerns include the need to start therapy before disease status is known, thus, exposing unaffected fetuses to unknown risk and the unknown long-term effects of in utero glucocorticoid exposure.[105,106] With the discovery of cell-free fetal DNA in maternal circulation,[107] it has become possible to determine the sex of the fetus by the seventh week of gestation. Thus, this new technology partially addresses some of the ethical concerns associated with prenatal therapy and, if used, would potentially avoid treatment of male fetuses and unaffected female fetuses.

FUTURE THERAPIES: GENE THERAPY AND STEM CELL TRANSPLANTATION

Conventional therapy for CAH includes glucocorticoid and mineralocorticoid replacement. However, because CAH is a disorder caused by a single-gene defect, and given the rapid molecular understanding of its pathogenesis, investigations into the use of gene therapy or stem cell approaches for the treatment of CAH are ongoing. The first gene therapy approach for CAH was reported in H–2aw18 mice with 21-OHD.[108] Other studies have examined the selective adrenotropism for adenoviruses using a single intra-adrenal injection of adenoviral vector encoding *CYP212A*.[109,110] These approaches restore the impaired adrenocortical function in 21-hydroxylase knockout mice and bovine adrenocortical cells.[110–112] Gene or stem cell transplantation therapies could be a feasible option for treatment of CAH in the future.

SUMMARY

CAH is a common disorder with genetic and clinical heterogeneity and is life-threatening in its most severe form. Lifesaving neonatal screening programs exist in the United States and many other countries based on hormonal testing; genetic diagnosis of neonates is not being used in screening programs because of deficiencies in accuracy, speed, and cost-effectiveness. However, the molecular analysis of CAH is useful in confirming the diagnosis and provides a powerful tool in genetic counseling.

Over the years, the development of comprehensive methodologic approaches has improved our ability to genotype patients. However, several pitfalls and challenges remain in the molecular diagnosis of CAH across its many genotypes. Although the various forms of CAH are monogenic disorders, the large number of possible mutations and the presence of duplicated genes make the development of inexpensive, fast, and accurate genetic tools particularly challenging. Future research is needed to assist in the molecular pathogenesis of CAH that will assist in the management of affected patients and their family members across all age groups. Advances in genetics are transforming medicine; one day, personalized genetic information that includes CAH genotyping may help guide individualized therapy.

List of Laboratories for Congenital Adrenal Hyperplasia Molecular Analysis in the United States

Esoterix Molecular Endocrinology, Calabasas Hills, California
www.esoterix.com

Molecular Genetics Laboratory, Emory, Atlanta, Georgia
www.geneticslab.emory.edu

Molecular Genetics Laboratory, Mayo Clinic, Rochester, Minnesota
www.mayoclinic.org

PreventionGenetics, Marshfield, Wisconsin
www.preventiongenetics.com

Quest Diagnostics, Nichols Institute, San Juan Capistrano, California
www.education.questdiagnostics.com

REFERENCES

1. Speiser PW, Azziz R, Baskin LS, et al. Congenital adrenal hyperplasia due to steroid 21-hydroxylase deficiency: an Endocrine Society clinical practice guideline. J Clin Endocrinol Metab 2010;95:4133–60.

2. Therrell BL Jr, Berenbaum SA, Manter-Kapanke V, et al. Results of screening 1.9 million Texas newborns for 21-hydroxylase-deficient congenital adrenal hyperplasia. Pediatrics 1998;101:583–90.

3. Speiser PW, Dupont B, Rubinstein P, et al. High frequency of nonclassical steroid 21-hydroxylase deficiency. Am J Hum Genet 1985;37:650–67.

4. White PC, Curnow KM, Pascoe L. Disorders of steroid 11 beta-hydroxylase isozymes. Endocr Rev 1994;15:421–38.

5. New MI, Lorenzen F, Lerner AJ, et al. Genotyping steroid 21-hydroxylase deficiency: hormonal reference data. J Clin Endocrinol Metab 1983;57:320–6.

6. New MI, Abraham M, Gonzalez B, et al. Genotype-phenotype correlation in 1,507 families with congenital adrenal hyperplasia owing to 21-hydroxylase deficiency. Proc Natl Acad Sci U S A 2013;110:2611–6.

7. Nebert DW, Nelson DR, Coon MJ, et al. The P450 superfamily: update on new sequences, gene mapping, and recommended nomenclature. DNA Cell Biol 1991;10:1–14.

8. Higashi Y, Yoshioka H, Yamane M, et al. Complete nucleotide sequence of two steroid 21-hydroxylase genes tandemly arranged in human chromosome: a pseudogene and a genuine gene. Proc Natl Acad Sci U S A 1986;83:2841–5.

9. Speiser PW, Dupont J, Zhu D, et al. Disease expression and molecular genotype in congenital adrenal hyperplasia due to 21-hydroxylase deficiency. J Clin Invest 1992;90:584–95.

10. Yang Z, Mendoza AR, Welch TR, et al. Modular variations of the human major histocompatibility complex class III genes for serine/threonine kinase RP, complement component C4, steroid 21-hydroxylase CYP21, and tenascin TNX (the RCCX module). A mechanism for gene deletions and disease associations. J Biol Chem 1999;274:12147–56.

11. Saxena K, Kitzmiller KJ, Wu YL, et al. Great genotypic and phenotypic diversities associated with copy-number variations of complement C4 and RP-C4-CYP21-TNX (RCCX) modules: a comparison of Asian-Indian and European American populations. Mol Immunol 2009;46:1289–303.

12. Blanchong CA, Zhou B, Rupert KL, et al. Deficiencies of human complement component C4A and C4B and heterozygosity in length variants of RP-C4-CYP21-TNX (RCCX) modules in Caucasians. The load of RCCX genetic diversity on major histocompatibility complex-associated disease. J Exp Med 2000;191: 2183–96.

13. Chen W, Xu Z, Nishitani M, et al. Complement component 4 copy number variation and CYP21A2 genotype associations in patients with congenital adrenal hyperplasia due to 21-hydroxylase deficiency. Hum Genet 2012;131:1889–94.

14. Speiser PW, White PC. Congenital adrenal hyperplasia. N Engl J Med 2003;349: 776–88.

15. Concolino P, Mello E, Minucci A, et al. A new CYP21A1P/CYP21A2 chimeric gene identified in an Italian woman suffering from classical congenital adrenal hyperplasia form. BMC Med Genet 2009;10:72.

16. Vrzalova Z, Hruba Z, Hrabincova ES, et al. Chimeric CYP21A1P/CYP21A2 genes identified in Czech patients with congenital adrenal hyperplasia. Eur J Med Genet 2011;54:112–7.

17. Lee HH, Chao HT, Ng HT, et al. Direct molecular diagnosis of CYP21 mutations in congenital adrenal hyperplasia. J Med Genet 1996;33:371–5.

18. White PC, Vitek A, Dupont B, et al. Characterization of frequent deletions causing steroid 21-hydroxylase deficiency. Proc Natl Acad Sci U S A 1988;85: 4436–40.

19. White PC, New MI, Dupont B. HLA-linked congenital adrenal hyperplasia results from a defective gene encoding a cytochrome P-450 specific for steroid 21-hydroxylation. Proc Natl Acad Sci U S A 1984;81:7505–9.

20. Chen W, Xu Z, Sullivan A, et al. Junction site analysis of chimeric CYP21A1P/CYP21A2 genes in 21-hydroxylase deficiency. Clin Chem 2012;58:421–30.

21. Tusie-Luna MT, White PC. Gene conversions and unequal crossovers between CYP21 (steroid 21-hydroxylase gene) and CYP21P involve different mechanisms. Proc Natl Acad Sci U S A 1995;92:10796–800.

22. Parker EA, Hovanes K, Germak J, et al. Maternal 21-hydroxylase deficiency and uniparental isodisomy of chromosome 6 and X results in a child with 21-hydroxylase deficiency and Klinefelter syndrome. Am J Med Genet A 2006;140: 2236–40.

23. Finkielstain GP, Chen W, Mehta SP, et al. Comprehensive genetic analysis of 182 unrelated families with congenital adrenal hyperplasia due to 21-hydroxylase deficiency. J Clin Endocrinol Metab 2011;96:E161–72.

24. Krone N, Braun A, Roscher AA, et al. Predicting phenotype in steroid 21-hydroxylase deficiency? Comprehensive genotyping in 155 unrelated, well defined patients from southern Germany. J Clin Endocrinol Metab 2000;85:1059–65.

25. Stikkelbroeck NM, Hoefsloot LH, de Wijs IJ, et al. CYP21 gene mutation analysis in 198 patients with 21-hydroxylase deficiency in The Netherlands: six novel

mutations and a specific cluster of four mutations. J Clin Endocrinol Metab 2003; 88:3852–9.

26. Jaaskelainen J, Levo A, Voutilainen R, et al. Population-wide evaluation of disease manifestation in relation to molecular genotype in steroid 21-hydroxylase (CYP21) deficiency: good correlation in a well defined population. J Clin Endocrinol Metab 1997;82:3293–7.

27. Brosnan PG, Brosnan CA, Kemp SF, et al. Effect of newborn screening for congenital adrenal hyperplasia. Arch Pediatr Adolesc Med 1999;153:1272–8.

28. Merke DP, Poppas DP. Management of adolescents with congenital adrenal hyperplasia. Lancet Diabetes Endocrinol 2013;1:341–52.

29. Krone N, Rose IT, Willis DS, et al. Genotype-phenotype correlation in 153 adult patients with congenital adrenal hyperplasia due to 21-hydroxylase deficiency: analysis of the United Kingdom Congenital Adrenal Hyperplasia Adult Study Executive (CaHASE) cohort. J Clin Endocrinol Metab 2013;98:E346–54.

30. Higashi Y, Tanae A, Inoue H, et al. Aberrant splicing and missense mutations cause steroid 21-hydroxylase [P-450(C21)] deficiency in humans: possible gene conversion products. Proc Natl Acad Sci U S A 1988;85:7486–90.

31. Amor M, Parker KL, Globerman H, et al. Mutation in the CYP21B gene (Ile-172—Asn) causes steroid 21-hydroxylase deficiency. Proc Natl Acad Sci U S A 1988; 85:1600–4.

32. Tusie-Luna MT, Traktman P, White PC. Determination of functional effects of mutations in the steroid 21-hydroxylase gene (CYP21) using recombinant vaccinia virus. The J Biol Chem 1990;265:20916–22.

33. Helmberg A, Tusie-Luna MT, Tabarelli M, et al. R339H and P453S: CYP21 mutations associated with nonclassic steroid 21-hydroxylase deficiency that are not apparent gene conversions. Mol Endocrinol 1992;6:1318–22.

34. Tusie-Luna MT, Speiser PW, Dumic M, et al. A mutation (Pro-30 to Leu) in CYP21 represents a potential nonclassic steroid 21-hydroxylase deficiency allele. Mol Endocrinol 1991;5:685–92.

35. Kaupert LC, Lemos-Marini SH, De Mello MP, et al. The effect of fetal androgen metabolism-related gene variants on external genitalia virilization in congenital adrenal hyperplasia. Clin Genet 2013;84:482–8.

36. Moura-Massari VO, Cunha FS, Gomes LG, et al. The presence of clitoromegaly in the nonclassical form of 21-hydroxylase deficiency could be partially modulated by the CAG polymorphic tract of the androgen receptor gene. PLoS One 2016;11:e0148548.

37. Buchner DA, Trudeau M, Meisler MH. SCNM1, a putative RNA splicing factor that modifies disease severity in mice. Science 2003;301:967–9.

38. L'Allemand D, Tardy V, Gruters A, et al. How a patient homozygous for a 30-kb deletion of the C4-CYP 21 genomic region can have a nonclassic form of 21-hydroxylase deficiency. J Clin Endocrinol Metab 2000;85:4562–7.

39. Witchel SF, Bhamidipati DK, Hoffman EP, et al. Phenotypic heterogeneity associated with the splicing mutation in congenital adrenal hyperplasia due to 21-hydroxylase deficiency. J Clin Endocrinol Metab 1996;81:4081–8.

40. Miller WL. Phenotypic heterogeneity associated with the splicing mutation in congenital adrenal hyperplasia due to 21-hydroxylase deficiency. J Clin Endocrinol Metab 1997;82:1304.

41. Merke DP, Chen W, Morissette R, et al. Tenascin-X haploinsufficiency associated with Ehlers-Danlos syndrome in patients with congenital adrenal hyperplasia. J Clin Endocrinol Metab 2013;98:E379–87.

42. Chen W, Kim MS, Shanbhag S, et al. The phenotypic spectrum of contiguous deletion of CYP21A2 and tenascin XB: quadricuspid aortic valve and other midline defects. Am J Med Genet A 2009;149A:2803–8.

43. Morissette R, Chen W, Perritt AF, et al. Broadening the spectrum of Ehlers Danlos syndrome in patients with congenital adrenal hyperplasia. J Clin Endocrinol Metab 2015;100:E1143–52.

44. Chen W, Perritt AF, Morissette R, et al. Ehlers-Danlos syndrome caused by biallelic TNXB variants in patients with congenital adrenal hyperplasia. Hum Mutat 2016;37(9):893–7.

45. Pang SY, Wallace MA, Hofman L, et al. Worldwide experience in newborn screening for classical congenital adrenal hyperplasia due to 21-hydroxylase deficiency. Pediatrics 1988;81:866–74.

46. Pang S, Clark A. Newborn screening, prenatal diagnosis, and prenatal treatment of congenital adrenal hyperplasia due to 21-hydroxylase deficiency. Trends Endocrinology Metabolism 1990;1:300–7.

47. van der Kamp HJ, Wit JM. Neonatal screening for congenital adrenal hyperplasia. Eur J Endocrinol 2004;151(Suppl 3):U71–5.

48. Mikami A, Fukushi M, Oda H, et al. Newborn screening for congenital adrenal hyperplasia in Sapporo City: sixteen years experience. Southeast Asian J Trop Med Public Health 1999;30(Suppl 2):100–2.

49. Heather NL, Seneviratne SN, Webster D, et al. Newborn screening for congenital adrenal hyperplasia in New Zealand, 1994-2013. J Clin Endocrinol Metab 2015;100:1002–8.

50. Zhong K, Wang W, He F, et al. The status of neonatal screening in China, 2013. J Med Screen 2016;23:59–61.

51. Kaur G, Thakur K, Kataria S, et al. Current and future perspective of newborn screening: an Indian scenario. J Pediatr Endocrinol Metab 2016;29:5–13.

52. Wedell A, Thilen A, Ritzen EM, et al. Mutational spectrum of the steroid 21-hydroxylase gene in Sweden: implications for genetic diagnosis and association with disease manifestation. J Clin Endocrinol Metab 1994;78:1145–52.

53. Ezquieta B, Oliver A, Gracia R, et al. Analysis of steroid 21-hydroxylase gene mutations in the Spanish population. Hum Genet 1995;96:198–204.

54. Carrera P, Bordone L, Azzani T, et al. Point mutations in Italian patients with classic, non-classic, and cryptic forms of steroid 21-hydroxylase deficiency. Hum Genet 1996;98:662–5.

55. Dardis A, Bergada I, Bergada C, et al. Mutations of the steroid 21-hydroxylase gene in an Argentinian population of 36 patients with classical congenital adrenal hyperplasia. J Pediatr Endocrinol Metab 1997;10:55–61.

56. de Carvalho DF, Miranda MC, Gomes LG, et al. Molecular CYP21A2 diagnosis in 480 Brazilian patients with congenital adrenal hyperplasia before newborn screening introduction. Eur J Endocrinol 2016;175:107–16.

57. Barbat B, Bogyo A, Raux-Demay MC, et al. Screening of CYP21 gene mutations in 129 French patients affected by steroid 21-hydroxylase deficiency. Hum Mutat 1995;5:126–30.

58. Ezquieta B, Cueva E, Oyarzabal M, et al. Gene conversion (655G splicing mutation) and the founder effect (Gln318Stop) contribute to the most frequent severe point mutations in congenital adrenal hyperplasia (21-hydroxylase deficiency) in the Spanish population. Clin Genet 2002;62:181–8.

59. Wilson RC, Nimkarn S, Dumic M, et al. Ethnic-specific distribution of mutations in 716 patients with congenital adrenal hyperplasia owing to 21-hydroxylase deficiency. Mol Genet Metab 2007;90:414–21.

60. Romdhane L, Kefi R, Azaiez H, et al. Founder mutations in Tunisia: implications for diagnosis in North Africa and Middle East. Orphanet J Rare Dis 2012;7:52.

61. Levo A, Partanen J. Mutation-haplotype analysis of steroid 21-hydroxylase (CYP21) deficiency in Finland. Implications for the population history of defective alleles. Hum Genet 1997;99:488–97.

62. Lee HH, Lee YJ, Chan P, et al. Use of PCR-based amplification analysis as a substitute for the southern blot method for CYP21 deletion detection in congenital adrenal hyperplasia. Clin Chem 2004;50:1074–6.

63. Jang JH, Jin DK, Kim JH, et al. Multiplex ligation-dependent probe amplification assay for diagnosis of congenital adrenal hyperplasia. Ann Clin Lab Sci 2011; 41:44–7.

64. Concolino P, Mello E, Toscano V, et al. Multiplex ligation-dependent probe amplification (MLPA) assay for the detection of CYP21A2 gene deletions/duplications in congenital adrenal hyperplasia: first technical report. Clin Chim Acta 2009; 402:164–70.

65. Speiser PW, White PC, Dupont J, et al. Prenatal diagnosis of congenital adrenal hyperplasia due to 21-hydroxylase deficiency by allele-specific hybridization and Southern blot. Hum Genet 1994;93:424–8.

66. Paperna T, Gershoni-Baruch R, Badarneh K, et al. Mutations in CYP11B1 and congenital adrenal hyperplasia in Moroccan Jews. J Clin Endocrinol Metab 2005;90:5463–5.

67. Rosler A, Leiberman E, Cohen T. High frequency of congenital adrenal hyperplasia (classic 11 beta-hydroxylase deficiency) among Jews from Morocco. Am J Med Genet 1992;42:827–34.

68. Reisch N, Hogler W, Parajes S, et al. A diagnosis not to be missed: nonclassic steroid 11beta-hydroxylase deficiency presenting with premature adrenarche and hirsutism. J Clin Endocrinol Metab 2013;98:E1620–5.

69. Geley S, Kapelari K, Johrer K, et al. CYP11B1 mutations causing congenital adrenal hyperplasia due to 11 beta-hydroxylase deficiency. J Clin Endocrinol Metab 1996;81:2896–901.

70. Parajes S, Loidi L, Reisch N, et al. Functional consequences of seven novel mutations in the CYP11B1 gene: four mutations associated with nonclassic and three mutations causing classic 11{beta}-hydroxylase deficiency. J Clin Endocrinol Metab 2010;95:779–88.

71. Curnow KM, Slutsker L, Vitek J, et al. Mutations in the CYP11B1 gene causing congenital adrenal hyperplasia and hypertension cluster in exons 6, 7, and 8. Proc Natl Acad Sci U S A 1993;90:4552–6.

72. Lifton RP, Dluhy RG, Powers M, et al. A chimaeric 11 beta-hydroxylase/aldosterone synthase gene causes glucocorticoid-remediable aldosteronism and human hypertension. Nature 1992;355:262–5.

73. Hampf M, Dao NT, Hoan NT, et al. Unequal crossing-over between aldosterone synthase and 11beta-hydroxylase genes causes congenital adrenal hyperplasia. J Clin Endocrinol Metab 2001;86:4445–52.

74. Joehrer K, Geley S, Strasser-Wozak EM, et al. CYP11B1 mutations causing nonclassic adrenal hyperplasia due to 11 beta-hydroxylase deficiency. Hum Mol Genet 1997;6:1829–34.

75. Polat S, Kulle A, Karaca Z, et al. Characterisation of three novel CYP11B1 mutations in classic and non-classic 11beta-hydroxylase deficiency. Eur J Endocrinol 2014;170:697–706.

76. Mooij CF, Parajes S, Rose IT, et al. Characterization of the molecular genetic pathology in patients with 11beta-hydroxylase deficiency. Clin Endocrinol 2015;83: 629–35.

77. Biglieri EG, Herron MA, Brust N. 17-hydroxylation deficiency in man. J Clin Invest 1966;45:1946–54.

78. Goldsmith O, Solomon DH, Horton R. Hypogonadism and mineralocorticoid excess. The 17-hydroxylase deficiency syndrome. N Engl J Med 1967;277: 673–7.

79. Geller DH, Auchus RJ, Mendonca BB, et al. The genetic and functional basis of isolated 17,20-lyase deficiency. Nat Genet 1997;17:201–5.

80. Yanase T, Simpson ER, Waterman MR. 17 alpha-hydroxylase/17,20-lyase deficiency: from clinical investigation to molecular definition. Endocr Rev 1991;12: 91–108.

81. Imai T, Yanase T, Waterman MR, et al. Canadian Mennonites and individuals residing in the Friesland region of The Netherlands share the same molecular basis of 17 alpha-hydroxylase deficiency. Hum Genet 1992;89:95–6.

82. Miura K, Yasuda K, Yanase T, et al. Mutation of cytochrome P-45017 alpha gene (CYP17) in a Japanese patient previously reported as having glucocorticoid-responsive hyperaldosteronism: with a review of Japanese patients with mutations of CYP17. J Clin Endocrinol Metab 1996,81.3797–801.

83. Costa-Santos M, Kater CE, Auchus RJ, Brazilian Congenital Adrenal Hyperplasia Multicenter Study Group. Two prevalent CYP17 mutations and genotype-phenotype correlations in 24 Brazilian patients with 17-hydroxylase deficiency. J Clin Endocrinol Metab 2004;89:49–60.

84. Simard J, Ricketts ML, Gingras S, et al. Molecular biology of the 3beta-hydroxysteroid dehydrogenase/delta5-delta4 isomerase gene family. Endocr Rev 2005;26:525–82.

85. Pang SY, Lerner AJ, Stoner E, et al. Late-onset adrenal steroid 3 beta-hydroxysteroid dehydrogenase deficiency. I. A cause of hirsutism in pubertal and postpubertal women. J Clin Endocrinol Metab 1985;60:428–39.

86. Simard J, Rheaume E, Mebarki F, et al. Molecular basis of human 3 beta-hydroxysteroid dehydrogenase deficiency. J Steroid Biochem Mol Biol 1995; 53:127–38.

87. Mermejo LM, Elias LL, Marui S, et al. Refining hormonal diagnosis of type II 3beta-hydroxysteroid dehydrogenase deficiency in patients with premature pubarche and hirsutism based on HSD3B2 genotyping. J Clin Endocrinol Metab 2005;90:1287–93.

88. Lutfallah C, Wang W, Mason JI, et al. Newly proposed hormonal criteria via genotypic proof for type II 3beta-hydroxysteroid dehydrogenase deficiency. J Clin Endocrinol Metab 2002;87:2611–22.

89. Chang YT, Kappy MS, Iwamoto K, et al. Mutations in the type II 3 beta-hydroxysteroid dehydrogenase gene in a patient with classic salt-wasting 3 beta-hydroxysteroid dehydrogenase deficiency congenital adrenal hyperplasia. Pediatr Res 1993;34:698–700.

90. Fluck CE, Tajima T, Pandey AV, et al. Mutant P450 oxidoreductase causes disordered steroidogenesis with and without Antley-Bixler syndrome. Nat Genet 2004;36:228–30.

91. Krone N, Reisch N, Idkowiak J, et al. Genotype-phenotype analysis in congenital adrenal hyperplasia due to P450 oxidoreductase deficiency. J Clin Endocrinol Metab 2012;97:E257–67.

92. Arlt W, Walker EA, Draper N, et al. Congenital adrenal hyperplasia caused by mutant P450 oxidoreductase and human androgen synthesis: analytical study. Lancet 2004;363:2128–35.

93. Huang N, Pandey AV, Agrawal V, et al. Diversity and function of mutations in p450 oxidoreductase in patients with Antley-Bixler syndrome and disordered steroidogenesis. Am J Hum Genet 2005;76:729–49.

94. Fukami M, Horikawa R, Nagai T, et al. Cytochrome P450 oxidoreductase gene mutations and Antley-Bixler syndrome with abnormal genitalia and/or impaired steroidogenesis: molecular and clinical studies in 10 patients. J Clin Endocrinol Metab 2005;90:414–26.

95. Adachi M, Asakura Y, Matsuo M, et al. POR R457H is a global founder mutation causing Antley-Bixler syndrome with autosomal recessive trait. Am J Med Genet A 2006;140:633–5.

96. Lin D, Gitelman SE, Saenger P, et al. Normal genes for the cholesterol side chain cleavage enzyme, P450scc, in congenital lipoid adrenal hyperplasia. J Clin Invest 1991;88:1955–62.

97. Bose HS, Sugawara T, Strauss JF 3rd, et al, International Congenital Lipoid Adrenal Hyperplasia Consortium. The pathophysiology and genetics of congenital lipoid adrenal hyperplasia. N Engl J Med 1996;335:1870–8.

98. Bose HS, Sato S, Aisenberg J, et al. Mutations in the steroidogenic acute regulatory protein (StAR) in six patients with congenital lipoid adrenal hyperplasia. J Clin Endocrinol Metab 2000;85:3636–9.

99. Baker BY, Lin L, Kim CJ, et al. Nonclassic congenital lipoid adrenal hyperplasia: a new disorder of the steroidogenic acute regulatory protein with very late presentation and normal male genitalia. J Clin Endocrinol Metab 2006;91:4781–5.

100. Tajima T, Fujieda K, Kouda N, et al. Heterozygous mutation in the cholesterol side chain cleavage enzyme (p450scc) gene in a patient with 46,XY sex reversal and adrenal insufficiency. J Clin Endocrinol Metab 2001;86:3820–5.

101. Miller WL. Disorders in the initial steps of steroid hormone synthesis. J Steroid Biochem Mol Biol 2017;165(Pt A):18–37.

102. Guran T, Buonocore F, Saka N, et al. Rare causes of primary adrenal insufficiency: genetic and clinical characterization of a large nationwide cohort. J Clin Endocrinol Metab 2016;101:284–92.

103. Therrell BL. Newborn screening for congenital adrenal hyperplasia. Endocrinol Metab Clin North Am 2001;30:15–30.

104. Moran C, Azziz R, Weintrob N, et al. Reproductive outcome of women with 21-hydroxylase-deficient nonclassic adrenal hyperplasia. J Clin Endocrinol Metab 2006;91:3451–6.

105. Levine LS, Pang S. Prenatal diagnosis and treatment of congenital adrenal hyperplasia. J Pediatr Endocrinol 1994;7:193–200.

106. Merce Fernandez-Balsells M, Muthusamy K, Smushkin G, et al. Prenatal dexamethasone use for the prevention of virilization in pregnancies at risk for classical congenital adrenal hyperplasia because of 21-hydroxylase (CYP21A2) deficiency: a systematic review and meta-analyses. Clin Endocrinol 2010;73:436–44.

107. Lo YM, Corbetta N, Chamberlain PF, et al. Presence of fetal DNA in maternal plasma and serum. Lancet 1997;350:485–7.

108. Gotoh H. Gene therapy of a lethal mutation associated with adrenal hyperplasia in mice. Jikken Dobutsu 1993;42:279–81 [in Japanese].

109. Margolis G, Kilham L, Hoenig EM. Experimental adenovirus infection of the mouse adrenal gland. I. Light microscopic observations. Am J Pathol 1974; 75:363–74.
110. Alesci S, Ramsey WJ, Bornstein SR, et al. Adenoviral vectors can impair adrenocortical steroidogenesis: clinical implications for natural infections and gene therapy. Proc Natl Acad Sci U S A 2002;99:7484–9.
111. Stauber E, Card C. Experimental intra-amnionic exposure of bovine fetuses with subgroup 2, type 7 adenovirus. Can J Comp Med 1978;42:466–72.
112. Tajima T, Okada T, Ma XM, et al. Restoration of adrenal steroidogenesis by adenovirus-mediated transfer of human cytochromeP450 21-hydroxylase into the adrenal gland of21-hydroxylase-deficient mice. Gene Ther 1999;6: 1898–903.
113. Ordonez-Sanchez ML, Ramirez-Jimenez S, Lopez-Gutierrez AU, et al. Molecular genetic analysis of patients carrying steroid 21-hydroxylase deficiency in the Mexican population: identification of possible new mutations and high prevalence of apparent germ-line mutations. Hum Genet 1998;102:170–7.

Genetics of Pheochromocytomas and Paragangliomas

An Overview on the Recently Implicated Genes *MERTK, MET, Fibroblast Growth Factor Receptor 1,* and *H3F3A*

Rodrigo Almeida Toledo, PhD[a,b,*]

KEYWORDS

- Pheochromocytomas • Paragangliomas • MERTK • MET • c-MET • H3F3A
- FGFR1 • Exome

KEY POINTS

- Pheochromocytomas and paragangliomas (PPGLs) are among the most hereditable tumors occurring in humans.
- A sole germline mutation in one of the many known susceptibility genes is identified and the cause of approximately 50% of patients with PPGL independently of a clear familial history of PPGLs.
- Two previously unrecognized PPGL syndromes were characterized both clinically and genetically: PPGL-giant cell tumor of the bone caused by the H3 histone family member 3A (*H3F3A*) G34W hotspot mosaic mutation and non-*RET* PPGL-medullary thyroid carcinoma caused by MER proto-oncogene, tyrosine kinase (*MERTK*) germline mutation.

REVIEW OUTLINE

Pheochromocytomas and paragangliomas (PPGLs) are neural crest-derived tumors rising on the adrenal medulla and extra-adrenal gland, respectively. Our knowledge of the molecular pathogenesis of PPGLs has greatly expanded in the recent years because of genomic investigation performed by several local groups and international

Disclosure Statement: The author has nothing to disclose.
[a] Division of Hematology and Medical Oncology, Department of Medicine, Cancer Therapy and Research Center, University of Texas Health Science Center at San Antonio (UTHSCSA), 7703 Floyd Curl Dr, San Antonio, TX 78229, USA; [b] Clinical Research Program, Spanish National Cancer Research Centre, CNIO, Calle de Melchor Fernández Almagro, 3, Madrid 28029, Spain
* Clinical Research Program, Spanish National Cancer Research Centre, CNIO, Calle de Melchor Fernández Almagro, 3, Madrid 28029, Spain.
E-mail address: toledorodrigo79@gmail.com

consortiums. PPGLs are the most hereditable tumors known in humans with more than half of the cases, independent of family history of the disease, caused by a germline pathogenic mutation in one of the various susceptibility genes. In parallel to the analyses of germline susceptibility-associated variants, genomic studies could also focus on the tumor exclusively mutations and managed to decipher for the first time the somatic landscape of PPGLs. Although the mutation rates of PPGLs are one of the smallest among the sequenced tumors, several exciting findings have already been reported and many more are expected in the near future with the completion of other projects.

To date, there are at least 27 genes implicated in the molecular pathogenesis of PPGLs. The complete list and main information on these genes are shown in **Table 1**. Some of these genes are mutated exclusively on the germline and, therefore, are classic susceptibility genes; other genes are found mutated at the germline or somatic levels; in a third group only somatic mutations have been reported so far. Because of space limitation and the fact that genetics and genomics discoveries performed up to 2014 to 2015 were comprehensively reviewed elsewhere,[27,28] the current review focuses on very new findings and discusses the previously unrecognized role of *MERTK*, MET proto-oncogene, receptor tyrosine kinase (*MET*), *fibroblast growth factor (FGF) receptor 1 (FGFR1)*, and *H3F3A* genes in syndromic and nonsyndromic PPGLs. These 4 new genes were selected because, although their association with PPGLs is very recent, mounting evidence was generated that rapidly consolidated the prominence of these genes in the molecular cause of PPGLs.

MERTK PROTO-ONCOGENE MUTATIONS IN MULTIPLE ENDOCRINE NEOPLASIA TYPE 2–LIKE PATIENTS AND PATIENTS WITH PHEOCHROMOCYTOMAS AND PARAGANGLIOMA

Recently, a rare multiple endocrine neoplasia type 2 (MEN2)–like 32-year-old patient diagnosed with medullary thyroid carcinoma (MTC), pheochromocytoma, and recurrent and metastatic paragangliomas carrying no germline mutation on exons 5, 8, 10, 11, and 13 to 16 of the *RET* proto-oncogene was comprehensively investigated. Genomic analysis confirmed the absence of mutation in the hotspot exons and entire coding region and splicing regions of the *RET* gene, and no mutation was observed in the remaining PPGL susceptibility genes or in the *estrogen receptor 2 (ESR2)* gene, in which a frameshift variant has been reported in a young patient with MTC and in relatives with C cell hyperplasia.[29]

Whole-exome sequencing of this MEN2-like patient enables the discovery of the c.2273G>A p.R758H germline mutation on the tyrosine kinase (TK) domain of the *MERTK* receptor gene,[30] previously reported to play an oncogenic role in a variety of human cancers, mostly due to gene amplification.[31] RET and MERTK are both TK receptors that activate MAPK/ERK, PIK3CA, and AKT pathways. They have similarities and important differences (**Fig. 1**). The extracellular portion of RET is formed by 4 cadherin and a cysteine domains, whereas MERTK is formed by 2 immunoglobulin-like and fibronectin type III domains. Intracellular portions of TK receptors are usually more similar; however, some signature domains may be present, and sometimes define, specific TK receptor families. This situation is the case of the TK receptor family of MERTK that, along with *TYRO3* and *AXL*, forms the Tyro-3, Axl, and Mer (TAM) receptor family and is characterized by the unique KWIAIES motif in the TK domain.[31] The KWIAIES domain is also called the TAM-signature domain and defines the TAM TK receptor family.

Following the identification of the *MERTK* mutation in a MEN2-like patient, MERTK and RET protein sequences were carefully compared. Remarkably, it was found that

Table 1
List of genes implicated in pheochromocytomas and paragangliomas

N	Gene	Entrez ID	Locus	Molecular Pathway	Types of Mutations	Frequency of Mutations	References
1	ATRX	546	Xq21.1	Chromatin remodeling	Somatic, inactivating	Uncommon	Castro-Vega et al,[1] 2016; Fishbein et al,[2] 2015
2	BRAF	673	7q34	Pseudohypoxia signaling	Somatic, activating	Rare	Currás-Freixes et al,[3] 2015; Luchetti et al,[4] 2015
3	CDKN2A	Alpha	9p21	Cell cycle regulator	Somatic, inactivating	Rare	Castro-Vega et al,[1] 2016
4	EGLN1/PHD2	54,583	1q42.1	Pseudohypoxia signaling	Germline or somatic, inactivating	Very rare	Ladroue et al,[5] 2008; Yang et al,[6] 2015; TCGA[7]
5	EPAS1/HIF2A	2034	2p21-p16	Pseudohypoxia signaling	Mosaic or somatic, HIF stabilizing	Very common	TCGA[7]; Comino-Mendez et al,[8] 2013; Toledo et al,[9] 2013; Currás-Freixes et al[3]
6	FGFR1	2260	8p11.23-p11.22	MAPK pathway	Somatic, activating	Uncommon	TCGA[7]; Toledo et al,[9] 2013; Welander et al[42]
7	FH	2271	1q42.1	Pseudohypoxia signaling	Germline, inactivating	Rare	Currás-Freixes et al[3]; Castro-Vega et al,[10] 2014; Luchetti et al[11]
8	H3F3A	3020	1q42.12	Chromatin remodeling/MYC pathway	Mosaic, MYCN activator	Rare	Toledo et al,[9] 2013
9	HRAS	3265	11p15.5	MAPK pathway	Somatic, activating	Common	Currás-Freixes et al[3]; Oudijk et al,[12] 2014; Stenman et al,[13] 2016

(continued on next page)

Table 1
(continued)

N	Gene	Entrez ID	Locus	Molecular Pathway	Types of Mutations	Frequency of Mutations	References
10	IDH1	3417	2q33.3	Pseudohypoxia signaling	Somatic, hypoxia independent	Very rare	TCGA[7]; Gaal et al,[14] 2010
11	KIF1B	23,095	1p36.2	Hypoxia-independent pathway	Germline or somatic	Uncommon	Welander et al[42]; Schlisio et al,[15] 2008; Yeh et al,[16] 2008
12	KMT2D	8085	12q13.12	Chromatin remodeling	Germline or somatic	Common	Juhlin et al,[17] 2015
13	MAX	4149	14q23	MYC pathway	Germline or somatic, inactivating	Rare	Burnichon et al,[18] 2012; Cancer Genome Atlas Research Network,[19] 2014
14	MDH2	4191	7cen-q22	Pseudohypoxia signaling	Germline, inactivating	Rare	Cascón et al,[20] 2015
15	MERTK	10,461	2q14.1	MAPK pathway	Germline, activating	Rare	TCGA[7]; Toledo et al,[9] 2013
16	MET	4233	7q31	MAPK pathway	Germline or somatic, activating	Rare germline, common somatic	Toledo[9] ~ 10%, Castro-Vega[1,60] 2.4%, TCGA[7] 0% (somatic)
17	MYCN	4149	14q23	MYC pathway	Somatic, activating	Very rare	Wilzén et al,[21] 2016
18	NF1	4763	17q11.2	MAPK pathway	Germline or somatic, inactivating	Uncommon germline, very common somatic	Burnichon et al,[22] 2012; Welander et al[42]
19	RET	5979	10q11.2	MAPK pathway	Germline or somatic, activating	Common	Curras-Freixes et al[3]; Burnichon et al,[23] 2011
20	SDHA	6389	5p15	Pseudohypoxia signaling	Germline, inactivating	Rare	Burnichon et al,[24] 2009
21	SDHAF2	54,949	11q12.2	Pseudohypoxia signaling	Germline, inactivating	Very rare	Bayley et al,[62] 2010

22	*SDHB*	6390	1p36.13	Pseudohypoxia signaling	Germline, inactivating	Very common	Curras-Freixes et al,[3] Burnichon et al,[18] 2012
23	*SDHC*	6391	1q23.3	Pseudohypoxia signaling	Germline, epimutation, inactivating	Rare	Curras-Freixes et al,[3] Burnichon et al,[22] 2012; Richter et al,[25] 2016
24	*SDHD*	6392	11q23	Pseudohypoxia signaling	Germline, inactivating	Common	Curras-Freixes et al,[3] Burnichon et al,[23] 2011
25	*TMEM127*	55,654	2q11.2	mTOR negative regulator	Germline, inactivating	Rare	Curras-Freixes et al,[3] Yao et al,[26] 2010
26	*TP53*	7157	17p13.1	TP53 multifunction	Somatic, inactivating	Uncommon	Castro-Vega et al,[1] 2016
27	*VHL*	7428	3p25.3	Pseudohypoxia signaling	Germline or somatic, inactivating	Very common	Currás-Freixes et al,[3] 2015; Burnichon et al[23]

Very common	>10%
Common	5%–10%
Uncommon	<5%
Rare	<2%
Very rare	<1%
Unknown	?

Abbreviations: HIF, hypoxia inducible factor; ID, identification; mTOR, mechanistic target of rapamycin.

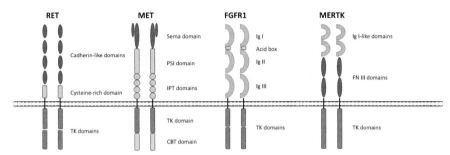

Fig. 1. Protein structures of the RET, MET, MERTK, FGFR1 TK receptors mutated in PPGLs. Ig, immunoglobulin. CBT, docking site; FN, fibronectin domain; IPT, (Ig-like, plexins, transcription factors; PSI, plexins, semaphorins, integrins.

the RET receptor contains a very similar sequence to the KWIAIES motif in its kinase domain with the only difference being the change of an *i*soleucine to a *m*ethionine: KWI *[M]*AIES. Such similarity between the two receptors was apparently previously unrecognized. Other new and interesting findings from the comparison of MERTK and RET protein sequences came from the correlation between the residues where mutations occurred. The amino acid residue found mutated in MERTK, arginine 758, is analogous to the *RET* arginine 912, a residue whereby a germline mutation (R912P) has been reported to cause multiple endocrine neoplasia type 2A (MEN2A) syndrome,[32] suggesting that the specific location of this residue on the TK domain would possibly trigger common molecular targets implicated on both PPGL and MTC. Indeed, other germline and somatic mutations on MERTK R758 were found; this residue seems to be a hotspot mutation, as follows. The MERTK R758C germline mutation was found in one case during the screening of a validation cohort of PPGLs, whereas the R758H mutation found in the germline of the MEN2-like case was also observed in colorectal, esophagus, and prostate tumor projects, as reported on the Catalogue of Somatic Mutations in Cancer (COSMIC, mutation ID COSM1398803) and on The Cancer Genome Atlas (TCGA) projects. A somatic mutation involving a change to a third amino acid (R758S) was also reported by the TCGA.

Functional in vitro studies of MERTK R758H and R758C mutations were performed and showed that, resembling activating *RET* mutations, these mutations lead to activation of downstream MAPK proliferation pathway by the increased of ERK phosphorylation in the presence or absence of the GAS6 ligand.[30] These results suggesting a ligand-independent constitutive activation of the receptor caused by R758H/C mutations contrasted with the lack of effect by the empty vector, wild-type and kinase dead Y754F mutant constructs used as experimental controls.

In addition to mutations occurring on R758 hotspot, several other *MERTK* somatic mutations have been identified in melanomas, lymphomas, and other cancers (TCGA and COSMIC). However, the functional characterization of most of these variants is still lacking and its implication in cancer is uncertain.

MERTK Mutations in Human Disorders

The human *MERTK* gene (NCBI ID: 10,461), also known as c-Mer, is located at the 2q14.1 locus and contains 19 exons that encode a 999 long amino acid TK receptor protein of 160 to 205 KDa, depending on the glycosylation status.[33] The main known function of the TAM receptors is to regulate the innate immune response, especially by modulating activities of macrophages and dendritic cells.[34] Activation of TAM receptors reduces immune system activity, whereas its deficiency leads to autoimmunity disorders. Mutation in *MERTK* (inactivating) was first identified in rats naturally presenting retinal pigment epithelium due to photosensitive disks contained in their outer segments phagocytose deficiency.[35] Later, similar *MERTK* inactivating mutations were observed in patients with recessively transmitted retinitis pigmentosa from multiple consanguineous families, reinforcing its role in apoptotic clearance.[36] Oncogenic effects of MERTK have also been characterized,[31] and ectopic hyperexpression of MERTK in mice leads to lymphoblastic leukemia/lymphoma.[37]

Remarks of MERTK in Pheochromocytomas and Paragangliomas

Germline activating mutation of the *RET* proto-oncogene is found in virtually all patients presenting with the co-occurrence of MTC and PPGLs (often benign pheochromocytomas), classified as MEN2A syndrome. The case in which an R758H-activating germline mutation of *MERTK* was discovered by whole-exome sequencing presented, in addition to MTC and pheochromocytoma, recurrent and metastatic paragangliomas, which have not been reported in the setting of *RET* and MEN2 syndrome. This unique and rare phenotype could be generally termed MEN2-like until further studies clarify the frequency of mutations and possible genotype-phenotype correlations involving *MERTK* on *RET*-negative atypical cases.

FIBROBLAST GROWTH FACTOR RECEPTOR 1 SOMATIC MUTATION IN PHEOCHROMOCYTOMAS AND PARAGANGLIOMAS

Recent genomic studies have shown that *FGFR1* mutations seem to be a rare but recurrent genetic event in PPGLs. Recently, the c.1638C>A p.N546K hotspot oncogenic mutation of the *FGFR1* gene was identified by whole-exome sequencing of the tumor sample of a 28-year-old female patient with a solitary nonmalignant adrenal pheochromocytoma carrying no germline or somatic mutation in PPGL genes, suggesting a sporadic PPGL.[30] Analysis of the patient's blood DNA showed that the mutation was present only in the tumor. Two other female patients diagnosed with solitary, nonmalignant, and apparently sporadic adrenal pheochromocytoma diagnosed at 46 and 64 years of age were also identified by the PPGL TCGA genomic project, whose data are already available publicly, also carrying the *FGFR1* N546K hotspot mutation. A third independent genomic study reported 2 other patients with sporadic PPGL carrying *FGFR1* hotspot somatic mutations; one case carried the *FGFR1* N546K, whereas the other harbored the *FGFR1* K656E.[38] An additional *FGFR1* N546K-mutated PPGL was found within the study's validation cohort including 64 sporadic PPGLs, and to date a total of 6 independent patients have been reported (**Table 2**). Interestingly, all the *FGFR1*-mutated tumors were clinically sporadic; indeed, in 5 of them whereby whole-exome sequencing was performed, no germline mutations were observed in the PPGL genes. In addition, 4 of these cases presented no germline or somatic mutations in the PPGL genes, strengthening the role of *FGFR1* as the driver of these tumors. One case presented *FGFR1* and *myc-associated factor X (MAX)* (also somatic) mutation, indicating that co-occurrence of PPGL somatic driver mutations may also occur.

Importantly, the *FGFR1* mutations identified in PPGLs patients, N546K and K656E, are the two main hotspot mutations of this gene among human cancers as observed in public databases as TCGA and COSMIC (mutation ID COSM19176/ COSM302229). In vitro characterization of these mutants revealed a ligand-independent oncogenic potential through activation of the FGFR1 signaling and constitutive phosphorylation of the MAPK/ERK pathway.[40] Accordingly, to the kinase activation, gene expression analysis clustered *FGFR1*-mutated PPGLs on the cluster

Table 2
Clinical and genetic features of patients with pheochromocytomas and paragangliomas carrying a germline or somatic MET mutation

N	Sample ID	Clinical Features	Age (y)	Sex	Malignancy	Cohort	Nucleotide	Protein	Aminc Acid	Origin	Public Cancer Databases	PPGL Mutation Co-occurrence	Public Control Databases	Reference
2	355	PH	63	M	N	Validation cohort	c.352A>AT	M118L	118	U	Pancreas TCGA	—	Not reported	Toledo & Dahia,[39] 2014
3	370	MTC and PH	35	M	N	Exome investigational	c.607T>A	S203T	203	U	S203Y Colon TCGA; COSM97089	gRET	rs200861145 (AA = 0/ AT = 4/ TT = 6005, 0.0006819)	Toledo & Dahia,[39] 2014
4	105	PH	28	M	N	Exome investigational	c.967A>G	S323G	323	U	Thyroid TCGA[7]	—	rs201467281 (GG = 0/ GA = 5/ AA = 5988, 0.0003491)	Toledo & Dahia,[39] 2014
7	317	PGL	42	F	N	Validation cohort	c.1076G>GA	R359Q	359	U	COSM1286164 mutated neuroblastoma	—	rs201274041 (AA = 0/ AG = 4/ GG = 6103, 0.0002590)	Toledo & Dahia,[39] 2014
12	317	PGL	42	F	N	Validation cohort	c.2962C>T	R988C	988	U	COSM1666978	—	rs3458476 (TT = 0/ TC = 42/ CC = 5938, 0.002853)	Toledo & Dahia,[39] 2014

		Age	Sex		Cohort	cDNA	Protein	Codon	S/U	Annotation		dbSNP (genotype)	Reference
13 318	PGL	49	F	N	Validation cohort	c.2962C>T	R988C	988	U	COSM1666978	—	rs34589476 (TT = 0/ TC = 42/ CC = 5938, 0.002853)	Toledo & Dahia,[39] 2014
14 339	PH	36	M	N	Validation cohort	c.2962C>T	R988C	988	U	COSM1666978	—	rs34589476 (TT = 0/ TC = 42/ CC = 5938, 0.002853)	Toledo & Dahia,[39] 2014
16 174	PH	66	F	N	Validation cohort	c.3029C>CT	T1010I	1010	U	Residue hotspot multiple TCGA projects; COSM29813; COSM707	—	rs56391007 (TT = 0/ TC = 106/ CC = 5852, 0.007928)	Toledo & Dahia,[39] 2014
19 325	PH	49	F	N	Validation cohort	c.3029C>CT	T1010I	1010	U	Residue hotspot multiple TCGA projects; COSM29813; COSM707	—	rs56391007 (TT = 0/ TC = 106/ CC = 5852, 0.007928)	Toledo & Dahia,[39] 2014
1 265	PH	52	M	N	Validation cohort	c.352A>AT	M118L	118	S	Pancreas TCGA	—	Not reported	Toledo & Dahia,[39] 2014
5 203	PH	74	M	N	Exome investigational	c.967A>G	S323G	323	S	Thyroid TCGA[7]	—	rs201467281 (GG = 0/ GA = 5/ AA = 5988, 0.0003491)	Toledo & Dahia,[39] 2014

(continued on next page)

Table 2 (*continued*)

N	Sample ID	Clinical Features	Age (y)	Sex	Malignancy	Cohort	Nucleotide	Protein	Amino Acid	Origin	Public Cancer Databases	PPGL Mutation Co-occurrence	Public Control Databases	Reference
6	162	PH	53	F	N	Validation cohort	c.1063G>A	E355K	355	S	COSM4172536	sNF1	(0.0000258)	Castro-Vega[55]
8	76	PH	42	F	N	Exome investigational	c.1124A>G	N375S	375	S	COSM5020653; COSM5024549	gNF1	Not reported	Castro-Vega[55]
20	119	PH	58	F	N	Validation cohort	c.3029C>T	T1010I	1010	S	Residue hotspot multiple TCGA projects; COSM29813; COSM707	—	rs56391007 (TT = 0/ TC = 106/ CC = 5852, 0.007928)	Castro-Vega[55]
21	125	PH	21	M	N	Validation cohort	c.3029C>T	T1010I	1010	S	Residue hotspot multiple TCGA projects; COSM29813; COSM707	—	rs56391007 (TT = 0/ TC = 106/ CC = 5852, 0.007928)	Castro-Vega[55]
22	130	PH	58	F	N	Validation cohort	c.3028A>G	T1010A	1010	S	Residue hotspot multiple TCGA projects; COSM29813; COSM707	—	(0.00001662)	Castro-Vega[55]
9	493 (II.3)	Familial PH	25	F	N	Exome investigational	c.2416G>A	V806M	806	G	—	—	Not reported	Toledo & Dahia,[39] 2014

10 493 (III.1)	Familial PH	Son of 493 (II.3)	M	N	Family screening	c.2416G>A	V806M	806	G	—	Not reported	Toledo & Dahia,[39] 2014
11 493 (II.3)	Familial PH	Son of 493 (II.3)	M	N	Family screening	c.2416G>A	V806M	806	G	—	Not reported	Toledo & Dahia,[39] 2014
15 1101	PH	51	M	N	Validation cohort	c.3029C>CT	T1010I	1010	G	Residue hotspot multiple TCGA projects; COSM29813; COSM707	rs56391007 (TT = 0/ TC = 106/ CC = 5852, 0.007928)	Toledo & Dahia,[39] 2014
17 11	PH	40	F	N	Validation cohort	c.3029C>CT	T1010I	1010	G	Residue hotspot multiple TCGA projects; COSM29813; COSM707	rs56391007 (TT = 0/ TC = 106/ CC = 5852, 0.007928)	Toledo & Dahia,[39] 2014
18 282	PH	41	M	N	Validation cohort	c.3029C>CT	T1010I	1010	G	Residue hotspot multiple TCGA projects; COSM29813; COSM707	rs56391007 (TT = 0/ TC = 106/ CC = 5852, 0.007928)	Toledo & Dahia,[39] 2014

Abbreviations: F, female; G, germline; ID, identification; M, male; N, no; PGL, paraganglioma; PH, phechromocytoma; S, somatic; U, unknown.

2, also known as the kinase group together with PPGLs carrying mutations in *RET*, *HRAS*, and *NF1*.[38]

FGFR1 mutation frequency in PPGLs varied between 0.5% and 3.8%; however, these numbers are very initial and studies of larger cohorts are needed to better define more accurate mutation rates and whether these is a possible genotype-phenotype correlation. Notably, the *FGFR2* N549K/H/S/D mutation is paralogous to the *FGFR1* N540K and also represents a hotspot mutation in several human cancers (COSMIC and TCGA databases). Activating mutations of *FGFR2* occurs in 12% of endometrial cancers,[41] and *FGFR3* mutations are seen in approximately the same frequency in bladder cancers.[42] Therefore, it will be important to determine whether FGFR1 is the only FGFR receptor somatically mutated in PPGLs or whether other FGFR receptors can also be genetically activated in these tumors. Finally, further studies are warranted to determine whether *FGFR1* rearrangements, as the t(8;13) (p11;q12) translocation involving *ZMYM2*, which is a common cause of myeloproliferative disorders,[43] and gene amplification, commonly seen in lung cancers, can also occur in PPGLs. Other genetic aspects of FGFR-associated disorders in humans are described later as they can offer new insights in the future studies of FGFR1 in PPGLs, particularly the new evidence of mosaic *FGFR1* mutations leading to young sporadic cancer.

Fibroblast Growth Factor Receptor 1 Mutations in Human Disorders

The 18 different FGFs ligands and their correspondent TK receptors 1 to 4 (FGFR1–4) comprise a multifunctional cell signaling transducing network controlling, among other roles, cell growth, migration, and differentiation during embryogenesis. Later in life, FGFs and FGFRs are prominently active on endothelial cells promoting growth of new blood vessel angiogenesis.[44] In accordance with these main roles in embryogenesis and on angiogenesis, one of the hallmarks of cancer, aberrant signaling of FGFR1 to 3 have been well described and are linked to a variety of developmental disorders, as well as in a different context, implicated in tumorigenesis.[44]

FGFR1 mutations are pleiotropic; its effects on different traits depend on the mutation origin, timing of appearance, and its functional consequences. Germline inactivating mutations of *FGFR1* cause isolated hypogonadotropic hypogonadism, Kallmann syndrome, and severe Hartsfield syndrome, whereas heterozygous gain-of-function germline or de novo mutations in *FGFR1*, *FGFR2*, and *FGFR3* genes are the underlying cause of different skeletal syndromes, including Crouzon, Antley-Bixler, Apert, Beare-Stevenson cutis gyrata, Jackson-Weiss, Pfeiffer, Saethre-Chotzen syndromes, as well as several skeletal dysplasias, including achondroplasia, hypochondroplasia, platyspondylic lethal skeletal dysplasia, and thanatophoric dysplasia.[45] Eventually, the same *FGFRx* mutations can be found associated with developmental phenotypes or cancer depending the mutation origin and timing, that is, *FGFR2* S267P de novo mutation found in apparently sporadic cases of Pfeiffer syndrome while its somatic counterpart occurs in gastric cancers. Interestingly, patients carrying mosaic mutations in genes involving RAS-MAPK pathway, like *FGFRs*, are prone to developmental disorders and tumors combined as, for example, patients with encephalocraniocutaneous lipomatosis carrying mosaic *FGFR1* N546K and *FGFR1* K656E mutations.[46]

Remarks of Fibroblast Growth Factor Receptor 1 in Pheochromocytomas and Paragangliomas

Although still early, the new finding of *FGFR1* mutations in PPGLs is reliable and should be immediately incorporated to the constellation of genes involved in these tumors because of several reasons, as follows. *FGFR1* somatic mutations in PPGLs were found by whole-exome sequencing and confirmed by an orthogonal technique[30]; were observed by 3 independent genomic projects that included patients with PPGLs with different ethnic groups, and a total of 6 cases were identified within a little period of time (see **Table 2**); previously identified as the main hotspot mutations of FGFR1 in a broad spectrum of human cancers; previous in vitro characterization have shown oncogenic potential of such mutations; structural analysis has shown a key importance of the N546 residue as involved in the *molecular brake hydrogen-bond network*, one of the typical FGFR mechanistic processes of FGFRs.[47]

In light of these very new data, an extensive effort for analyzing the role and the extension of FGFR1 aberrant activation involvement in large and diversified cohorts of PPGLs is warranted. In order to detect low represented mutations in tumor samples and possible mosaic mutations in blood/saliva samples, it is required that these studies apply high-coverage whole-exome sequencing, deep sequencing, and/or sensitive genotyping methods as digital polymerase chain reaction.

H3F3A POSTZYGOTIC MOSAIC MUTATION CAUSES THE NEW PHEOCHROMOCYTOMAS AND PARAGANGLIOMAS-GCTB SYNDROME

A 31-year-old woman was diagnosed with bilateral pheochromocytomas, later bladder and periaortic paragangliomas, and had a history of recurrent tibial giant cell tumor of the bone (GCT). The independent whole-exome sequencing of the right and left pheochromocytomas and one paraganglioma samples enable the identification of the known cancer mutation *H3F3A* G34W (COSM1732355) in all samples with frequency of the mutant alleles varying from 20% to 46%.[30] Deep sequencing by target next-generation sequencing of these 3 samples originated between 63,000 and 250,000 reads and refined the mutant frequencies to between 43% and 47%. Sequencing of the normal tissue and the GCT reveled 0% and 5% of the mutant allele suggesting a postzygotic and not germline origin of the mutation. The same genotype-phenotype correlation was observed in a second case with PPGL-GCT syndrome (multiple and aggressive paragangliomas, GCTs, and postzygotic *H3F3A* G34W mutation) consolidating the discovery and genetic characterization of this previously unrecognized paraganglioma syndrome.

H3F3A and Mounting Evidence of Involvement of MYC in Pheochromocytomas and Paragangliomas

MYC is one of the most frequently activated oncogene in human cancers, and its role in tumorigenesis is well documented.[48,49] The most common activation event of MYC in cancer is gene amplification followed by gene expression and rarely mutation. Genomic studies have indicated, for the first time, a clear and direct involvement of MYC in PPGLs. Whole-exome sequencing uncovers mutations in the *MAX* gene as a new PPGL susceptibility gene.[50] Germline inactivating *MAX* mutations would lead to increased levels of MYC. In addition, *H3F3A* G34R/L mutations cause intense upregulation of MYCN, which comprises the molecular mechanism thought to drive pediatric glioblastoma.[51] Importantly, the *H3F3A* G34W-mutated PPGLs analyzed by Western blot showed upregulation of MYCN oncoprotein.[30] Lastly, although *MYCN* mutations are not frequent, there is one hotspot mutation, which seems to be activating, that was recurrently found in several human tumors (c.131C>T, P44L, COSM35624). Recent a whole-exome sequencing study revealed the P44L somatic mutation in a malignant PPGL case suggesting a direct involvement of MYCN oncogene in PPGL tumorigenesis.[21]

H3F3A Mutations in Human Disorders

Somatic mutations in the *H3F3A* gene are common in human cancers and occur in a very select manner. For example, *H3F3A* K27M and G34R/V mutations are recurrently found in pediatric gliomas,[52] whereas G34W/L and K36M mutations are found in nearly all (~95%) GTC and chondroblastomas.[53] The presence of H3F3A G34W/L mutations, commonly referred to as oncohystones, is currently being used as a diagnostics tool for GCT.

Nucleosomes are octamer protein structures formed by 2 molecules of core histones H2A, H2B, H3, and H4, and wrapped in the nucleus by approximately 150 base pair of DNA.

The report of the PPGL-GCT syndrome caused by *H3F3A* mosaic mutation represents the first study to identify nonsomatic mutations in this highly essential gene. Germline mutation in *H3F3A* has never been identified and is probably incompatible with life. This idea is in line with no missense polymorphisms of the *H3F3A* gene being reported on the 1000 genomes project.

In addition to the high specificity in terms of residue mutated (K27 or G34) depending on the tumor types, the recurrent co-occurrence of mutation in defined drivers reveals another level of specificity observed in H3F3A cancer mutations. Constellations involving *H3F3A/TP53/ATRX/DAXX* mutations are found very frequently in deadly pediatric brain tumors, such as pediatric glioblastomas (PGBMs) and diffuse intrinsic pontine glioma.[52] The concordance found on PGBMs harboring a somatic *H3F3A* G34R/V mutation with ATR and TP53 mutations was 100%, whereas PGBMs harboring *H3F3A* K27M do not show such association.[52] A recent study showed that *H3F3A* mutations in diffuse intrinsic pontine glioma follows a recurrent spatial and temporal pattern. The study deciphered the clonal evolution of these tumors that start with *H3F3A* mutations as early events followed by mutations on *ACVR1/TP53/PPM1D/PIK3R1*, forming 4 obligatory driver partners (H3K27M/TP53 and/or PPM1D, H3K27M/ACVR1, and H3K27M/PIK3R1).[54] The analysis of the whole-exome sequencing of the 3 *H3F3A*-mutated PPGL tumors did not reveal a clear co-occurrence pattern of driver mutations as reported in very aggressive brain tumors. However, it is possible that mutations in subclones that were low represented in the sequencing analysis could have not been identified.

MET MUTATIONS IN PATIENTS WITH PHEOCHROMOCYTOMAS AND PARAGANGLIOMAS

A missense somatic *MET* mutation previously reported in a variety of human cancers N375S (COSM5020653) was identified by whole-exome sequencing of the tumor sample of a 42-year-old female patient with pheochromocytoma.[55] Target sequencing of a validation cohort reveled somatic missense variants in 4 more PPGLs, including the recurrent I1010L in 3 tumors. A second genomic study confirmed the high frequency of *MET* variants in PPGLs and identified 17 more cases carrying possible pathogenic *MET* missense variants[30]; to date a total of 22 PPGLs cases were reported carrying a MET variant (**Tables 3–7**). Both germline and somatic variants were observed, including the *MET* c.2416G>A V806M variant identified by whole-exome sequencing of a 25-year-old female patient with a history of familial pheochromocytoma.[30] Her father and brother with pheochromocytoma were tested and also carried the V806M variant, whereas the healthy mother was wild type. Somatic mutations of MET are frequently observed in multiple cancers. The functional role of the identified *MET* somatic variants still need to be investigated in the neuro-crest cell context. Remarkably, PPGL cases harboring germline *MET* variants, including the V806M

Table 3
Clinical and genetic features of patients with pheochromocytomas and paragangliomas carrying somatic fibroblast growth factor receptor 1 hotspot mutation

N	Sample ID	Clinical Features	Age (y)	Sex	Malignancy	Cohort	Nucleotide	Protein	Mutation Effect	Origin	Public Cancer Databases	PPGL Mutation Co-occurrence	Public Control Databases	Reference
1	472	Sporadic PH	28	F	N	Exome investigational	c.1638C>A	N546K	Activating mutation	Somatic	COSM302229; COSM19176	No	Not reported	Toledo et al,[30] 2016
2	TCGA-RW-A684-01	Sporadic PH	64	F	N	TCGA genomic investigational	c.1638C>A	N546K	Activating mutation	Somatic	COSM302229; COSM19176	No	Not reported	PPGL TCGA[56]
3	TCGA-QR-A70U-01	Sporadic PH	46	F	N	TCGA genomic investigational	c.1638C>A	N546K	Activating mutation	Somatic	COSM302229; COSM19176	No	Not reported	PPGL TCGA[56]
4	Linköping and Bergen 1	Sporadic PH	NI	NI	NI	Exome investigational	c.1638C>A	N546K	Activating mutation	Somatic	COSM302229; COSM19176	No	Not reported	Welander et al,[38] 2015
5	Linköping and Bergen 2	Sporadic PH	NI	NI	NI	Exome investigational	c.1966A>G	K656E	Activating mutation	Somatic	COSM35673, COSM3734716	No	Not reported	Welander et al,[38] 2015
6	Linköping and Bergen (and France) 3	Sporadic PH	NI	NI	NI	Validation cohort	c.1638C>A	N546K	Activating mutation	NI	COSM302229; COSM19176	NI	Not reported	Welander et al,[38] 2015

Abbreviations: F, female; ID, identification; NI, not informed.

Table 4
Molecular signatures

Molecular Pathway	Gene	Entrez ID	Locus	Types of Mutations	Frequency of Mutations	References
Pseudohypoxia signaling	EGLN1/PHD2	54,583	1q42.1	Germline or somatic, inactivating	Very rare	Ladroue et al,[5] 2008; Yang et al,[6] 2015; TCGA[7]
	EPAS1/HIF2A	2034	2p21-p16	Mosaic or somatic, HIF stabilizing	Very common	TCGA[7]; Comino-Méndez et al,[8] 2013; Toledo et al,[9] 2013; Curras-Freixes[3]
	FH	2271	1q42.1	Germline, inactivating	Rare	Curras-Freixes[3]; Castro-Vega et al,[10] 2014; Luchetti[11]
	IDH1	3417	2q33.3	Somatic, hypoxia independent	Very rare	TCGA[7]; Gaal et al,[14] 2010
	MDH2	4191	7cen-q22	Germline, inactivating	Rare	Cascón et al,[20] 2015
	SDHA	6389	5p15	Germline, inactivating	Rare	Burnichon et al,[24] 2009
	SDHAF2	54,949	11q12.2	Germline, inactivating	Very rare	Bayley et al,[62] 2010
	SDHB	6390	1p36.13	Germline, inactivating	Very common	Curras-Freixes et al[3], Burnichon et al,[18] 2012
	SDHC	6391	1q23.3	Germline, epimutation, inactivating	Rare	Curras-Freixes et al[3], Burnichon et al,[22] 2012; Richter et al,[25] 2016
	SDHD	6392	11q23	Germline, inactivating	Common	Curras-Freixes et al[3], Burnichon et al,[23] 2011
	VHL	7428	3p25.3	Germline or somatic, inactivating	Very common	Curras-Freixes et al,[3] 2015; Burnichon et al[23]
Chromatin remodeling	ATRX	546	Xq21.1	Somatic, inactivating	Uncommon	Castro-Vega et al,[1] 2016; Fishbein et al,[2] 2015
	KMT2D	8085	12q13.12	Germline or somatic	Common	Juhlin et al,[17] 2015
	H3F3A	3020	1q42.12	Mosaic, MYCN activator	Rare	Toledo et al,[9] 2013

Pathway	Gene	ID	Locus	Mutation	Frequency	References
MAPK pathway	FGFR1	2260	8p11.23-p11.22	Somatic, activating	Uncommon	TCGA[7]; Toledo et al,[9] 2013; Welander et al[42]
	HRAS	3265	11p15.5	Somatic, activating	Common	Curras-Freixes et al[3]; Oudijk et al,[12] 2014; Stenman et al,[13] 2016
	MERTK	10,461	2q14.1	Germline, activating	Rare	TCGA[7]; Toledo et al,[9] 2013
	MET	4233	7q31	Germline or somatic, activating	Rare germline, common somatic	Toledo ~10%, Castro-Vega 2.4%, TCGA[7] 0% (somatic)
	NF1	4763	17q11.2	Germline or somatic, inactivating	Uncommon germline, very common somatic	Welander et al[42]; Burnichon et al,[24] 2009
	BRAF	673	7q34	Somatic, activating	Rare	Currás-Freixes et al,[3] 2015; Luchetti et al,[4] 2015
	RET	5979	10q11.2	Germline or somatic, activating	Common	Currás-Freixes et al[3]; Burnichon et al,[18] 2012
MYC pathway	MAX	4149	14q23	Germline or somatic, inactivating	Rare	Burnichon et al,[22] 2012
	MYCN	4149	14q23	Somatic, activating	Very rare	Wilzén et al,[21] 2016
mTOR negative regulator	TMEM127	55,654	2q11.2	Germline, inactivating	Rare	Currás-Freixes et al[3]; Yao et al,[26] 2010
TP53 multifunction	TP53	7157	17p13.1	Somatic, inactivating	Uncommon	Castor-Vega et al,[1] 2016
Cell cycle regulator	CDKN2A	Alpha	9p21	Somatic, inactivating	Rare	Castor-Vega et al,[1] 2016
Hypoxia-independent pathway	KIF1B	23,095	1p36.2	Germline or somatic	Uncommon	Welander et al[42]; Schlisio et al,[15] 2008; Yeh et al,[16] 2008

Abbreviations: ID, identification; mTOR, mechanistic target of rapamycin.

Table 5
Mutation frequency

Frequency of Mutations	Gene	Entrez ID	Locus	Molecular Pathway	Types of Mutations	References
Very common	EPAS1/HIF2A	2034	2p21-p16	Pseudohypoxia signaling	Mosaic or somatic, HIF stabilizing	TCGA[7]; Comino-Mendéz et al,[8] 2013; Toledo et al,[9] 2013; Curras-Freixes et al[3]
	SDHB	6390	1p36.13	Pseudohypoxia signaling	Germline, inactivating	Curras-Freixes et al[3]; Burnichon et al,[23] 2011
	VHL	7428	3p25.3	Pseudohypoxia signaling	Germline or somatic, inactivating	Currás-Freixes et al,[3] 2015; Burnichon et al[23]
Very common somatic, uncommon germline	NF1	4763	17q11.2	MAPK pathway	Germline or somatic, inactivating	Welander et al[42]; Burnichon et al,[24] 2009
Common	HRAS	3265	11p15.5	MAPK pathway	Somatic, activating	Curras-Freixes et al[3]; Oudijk et al,[12] 2014; Stenman et al,[13] 2016
	KMT2D	8085	12q13.12	Chromatin remodeling	Germline or somatic	Juhlin et al,[17] 2015
	RET	5979	10q11.2	MAPK pathway	Germline or somatic, activating	Curras-Freixes et al[3]; Burnichon et al,[18] 2012
	SDHD	6392	11q23	Pseudohypoxia signaling	Germline, inactivating	Curras-Freixes et al[3]; Burnichon et al,[22] 2012
Common somatic, rare germline	MET	4233	7q31	MAPK pathway	Germline or somatic, activating	Toledo ~ 10%, Castro-Vega 2.4%, TCGA[7] 0% (somatic)

	Gene		Locus	Pathway/function	Mutation type	References
Uncommon	ATRX	546	Xq21.1	Chromatin remodeling	Somatic, inactivating	Castro-Vega et al,[1] 2016; Fishbein et al,[2] 2015
	FGFR1	2260	8p11.23-p11.22	MAPK pathway	Somatic, activating	TCGA[7]; Toledo et al,[9] 2013; Welander et al[42]
	KIF1B	23,095	1p36.2	Hypoxia-independent pathway	Germline or somatic	Welander et al[42], Schlisio et al,[15] 2008; Yeh et al,[16] 2008
	TP53	7157	17p13.1	TP53 multifunction	Somatic, inactivating	Castro-Vega,[1] 2016
Rare	BRAF	673	7q34	Pseudohypoxia signaling	Somatic, activating	Currás-Freixes et al,[3] 2015; Luchetti et al,[4] 2015
	CDKN2A	Alpha	9p21	Cell cycle regulator	Somatic, inactivating	Castro-Vega et al,[1] 2016
	FH	2271	1q42.1	Pseudohypoxia signaling	Germline, inactivating	Curras-Freixes et al[3], Castro-Vega et al,[10] 2014; Luchetti[11]
	H3F3A	3020	1q42.12	Chromatin remodeling/ MYC pathway	Mosaic, MYCN activator	Toledo et al,[9] 2013
	MAX	4149	14q23	MYC pathway	Germline or somatic, inactivating	Burnichon et al,[23] 2011
	MDH2	4191	7cen-q22	Pseudohypoxia signaling	Germline, inactivating	Cascon et al,[20] 2015
	MERTK	10,461	2q14.1	MAPK pathway	Germline, activating	TCGA[7]; Toledo et al,[9] 2013
	SDHA	6389	5p15	Pseudohypoxia signaling	Germline, inactivating	Burnichon et al,[24] 2009
	SDHC	6391	1q23.3	Pseudohypoxia signaling	Germline, epimutation, inactivating	Curras-Freixes et al[3], Burnichon et al,[18] 2012; Richter et al,[25] 2016
	TMEM127	55,654	2q11.2	mTOR negative regulator	Germline, inactivating	Curras-Freixes et al[3], Yao et al,[26] 2010

(continued on next page)

Table 5
(continued)

Frequency of Mutations	Gene	Entrez ID	Locus	Molecular Pathway	Types of Mutations	References
Very rare	EGLN1/PHD2	54,583	1q42.1	Pseudohypoxia signaling	Germline or somatic, inactivating	Ladroue et al,[5] 2008; Yang et al,[6] 2015; TCGA[7]
	IDH1	3417	2q33.3	Pseudohypoxia signaling	Somatic, hypoxia independent	TCGA[7]; Yang et al,[14] 2010
	MYCN	4149	14q23	MYC pathway	Somatic, activating	Wilzén et al,[21] 2016
	SDHAF2	54,949	11q12.2	Pseudohypoxia signaling	Germline, inactivating	Bayley et al,[62] 2010
Very common						>10%
Common						5%–10%
Uncommon						<5%
Rare						<2%
Very rare						<1%
Unknown						?

Abbreviations: ID, identification; mTOR, mechanistic target of rapamycin.

Table 6
Origin of mutations

Origin of Mutations	Gene	Entrez ID	Locus	Molecular Pathway	Mutation Effects	Frequency of Mutations	References
Germline	FH	2271	1q42.1	Pseudohypoxia signaling	Inactivating	Rare	Curras-Freixes et al[3]; Castro-Vega et al,[10] 2014; Luchetti[11]
	MDH2	4191	7cen-q22	Pseudohypoxia signaling	Inactivating	Rare	Cascón et al,[20] 2015
	MERTK	10,461	2q14.1	MAPK pathway	Activating	Rare	TCGA,[7]; Toledo et al[9]
	SDHA	6389	5p15	Pseudohypoxia signaling	Inactivating	Rare	Burnichon et al,[22] 2012
	SDHAF2	54,949	11q12.2	Pseudohypoxia signaling	Inactivating	Very rare	Bayley et al,[62] 2010
	SDHB	6390	1p36.13	Pseudohypoxia signaling	Inactivating	Very common	Curras-Freixes et al[3]; Burnichon et al,[23] 2011
	SDHD	6392	11q23	Pseudohypoxia signaling	Inactivating	Common	Curras-Freixes et al[3]; Burnichon et al,[24] 2009
	TMEM127	55,654	2q11.2	mTOR negative regulator	Inactivating	Rare	Curras-Freixes et al[3]; Yao et al,[26] 2010
Germline (including epimutation)	SDHC	6391	1q23.3	Pseudohypoxia signaling	Inactivating	Rare	Curras-Freixes et al[3]; Burnichon et al,[18]

(continued on next page)

Table 6
(continued)

Origin of Mutations	Gene	Entrez ID	Locus	Molecular Pathway	Mutation Effects	Frequency of Mutations	References
Germline or somatic	KMT2D	8085	12q13.12	Chromatin remodeling	Unknown (possibly activating)	Common	Juhlin et al,[17] 2015
	KIF1B	23,095	1p36.2	Hypoxia-independent pathway	Unclear	Uncommon	Welander et al[42]; Schlisio et al,[15] 2008; Yeh et al,[16] 2008
	MAX	4149	14q23	MYC pathway	Inactivating	Rare	Burnichon et al,[22] 2012
	MET	4233	7q31	MAPK pathway	Activating	Rare germline, common somatic	Toledo ~10%, Castro-Vega 2.4%, TCGA[7] 0% (somatic)
	VHL	7428	3p25.3	Pseudohypoxia signaling	Inactivating	Very common	Currás-Freixes et al,[3] 2015; Burnichon et al[23]
	EGLN1/PHD2	54,583	1q42.1	Pseudohypoxia signaling	Inactivating	Very rare	Ladroue et al,[5] 2008; Yang et al,[6] 2015; TCGA[7]
	NF1	4763	17q11.2	MAPK pathway	Inactivating	Uncommon germline, very common somatic	Welander et al[42]; Burnichon et al,[23] 2011
	RET	5979	10q11.2	MAPK pathway	Activating	Common	Currás-Freixes et al[3]; Burnichon et al,[24] 2009

(first row references continued: 2012 Richter et al,[25] 2016)

	Gene	ID	Location	Chromatin remodeling/MYC pathway	MYCN upregulation		Reference
Mosaic	*H3F3A*	3020	1q42.12			Rare	Toledo et al,[9] 2013
Mosaic or somatic	*EPAS1/HIF2A*	2034	2p21-p16	Pseudohypoxia signaling	HIF stabilizing	Very common	TCGA[7]; Comino-Mendéz et al,[8] 2013 Toledo et al,[9] 2013; Curras-Freixes et al[3]
Somatic	*IDH1*	3417	2q33.3	Pseudohypoxia signaling	Hypoxia independent	Very rare	TCGA[7]; Gaal et al,[14] 2010
	ATRX	546	Xq21.1	Chromatin remodeling	Inactivating	Uncommon	Castro-Vega et al,[1] 2016; Fishbein et al,[2] 2015
	BRAF	673	7q34	Pseudohypoxia signaling	Activating	Rare	Currás-Freixes et al,[3] 2015; Luchetti et al,[4] 2015
	CDKN2A	Alpha	9p21	Cell cycle regulator	Inactivating	Rare	Castro-Vega et al,[1] 2016
	FGFR1	2260	8p11.23-p11.22	MAPK pathway	Activating	Uncommon	TCGA[7]; Toledo et al,[9] 2013; Welander et al[42]
	HRAS	3265	11p15.5	MAPK pathway	Activating	Common	Currás-Freixes et al[3]; Oudijk et al,[12] 2014; Stenman et al,[13] 2016
	MYCN	4149	14q23	MYC pathway	Activating	Very rare	Wilzén et al,[21] 2016
	TP53	7157	17p13.1	TP53 multifunction	Inactivating	Uncommon	Castro-Vega et al,[1] 2016

Abbreviations: ID, identification; mTOR, mechanistic target of rapamycin.

Table 7
Mutation effects

Mutation Effects	Gene	Entrez ID	Locus	Molecular Pathway	Origin of Mutations	Frequency of Mutations	References
Activating	BRAF	673	7q34	Pseudohypoxia signaling	Somatic	Rare	Currás-Freixes et al,[3] 2015; Luchetti et al,[4] 2015
	FGFR1	2260	8p11.23-p11.22	MAPK pathway	Somatic	Uncommon	TCGA[7]; Toledo et al,[9] 2013; Welander et al[42]
	HRAS	3265	11p15.5	MAPK pathway	Somatic	Common	Currás-Freixes et al[3]; Oudijk et al,[12] 2014; Stenman et al,[13] 2016
	MERTK	10,461	2q14.1	MAPK pathway	Germline	Rare	TCGA[7]; Toledo et al,[9] 2013
	MET	4233	7q31	MAPK pathway	Germline or somatic	Rare germline, common somatic	Toledo ~10%, Castro-Vega 2.4%, TCGA[7] 0% (somatic)
	MYCN	4149	14q23	MYC pathway	Somatic	Very rare	Wilzén et al,[21] 2016
	RET	5979	10q11.2	MAPK pathway	Germline or somatic	Common	Currás-Freixes et al[3]; Burnichon et al,[18] 2012

	Gene	Number	Locus	Function/Pathway	Type	Frequency	References
Inactivating	ATRX	546	Xq21.1	Chromatin remodeling	Somatic	Uncommon	Castro-Vega et al,[1] 2016; Fishbein et al,[2] 2015
	CDKN2A	Alpha	9p21	Cell cycle regulator	Somatic	Rare	Castro-Vega et al,[1] 2016
	EGLN1/PHD2	54,583	1q42.1	Pseudohypoxia signaling	Germline or somatic	Very rare	Ladroue et al,[5] 2008; Yang et al,[6] 2015; TCGA[7]
	FH	2271	1q42.1	Pseudohypoxia signaling	Germline	Rare	Curras-Freixes et al[3]; Castro-Vega et al,[10] 2014; Luchetti[11]
	MAX	4149	14q23	MYC pathway	Germline or somatic	Rare	Burnichon et al,[22] 2012
	MDH2	4191	7cen-q22	Pseudohypoxia signaling	Germline	Rare	Cascón et al,[20] 2015
	NF1	4763	17q11.2	MAPK pathway	Germline or somatic	Uncommon germline, very common somatic	Welander et al,[42]; Burnichon et al,[23] 2011
	SDHA	6389	5p15	Pseudohypoxia signaling	Germline	Rare	Burnichon et al,[24] 2009
	SDHAF2	54,949	11q12.2	Pseudohypoxia signaling	Germline	Very rare	Bayley et al,[62] 2010
	SDHB	6390	1p36.13	Pseudohypoxia signaling	Germline	Very common	Curras-Freixes et al,[3]; Burnichon et al,[18] 2012
	SDHC	6391	1q23.3	Pseudohypoxia signaling	Germline (including epimutation)	Rare	Curras-Freixes et al,[3]; Burnichon et al,[22] 2012; Richter et al,[25] 2016
	SDHD	6392	11q23	Pseudohypoxia signaling	Germline	Common	Curras-Freixes et al,[3]; Burnichon et al,[23] 2011
	TMEM127	55,654	2q11.2	mTOR negative regulator	Germline	Rare	Curras-Freixes et al,[3]; Yao et al,[26] 2010
	TP53	7157	17p13.1	TP53 multifunction	Somatic	Uncommon	Castro-Vega et al,[1] 2016
	VHL	7428	3p25.3	Pseudohypoxia signaling	Germline or somatic	Very common	Currás-Freixes et al,[3] 2015; Burnichon et al[23]

(continued on next page)

Table 7
(continued)

Mutation Effects	Gene	Entrez ID	Locus	Molecular Pathway	Origin of Mutations	Frequency of Mutations	References
MYCN upregulation	H3F3A	3020	1q42.12	Chromatin remodeling/MYC pathway	Mosaic	Rare	Toledo et al,[9] 2013
Unclear	KIF1B	23,095	1p36.2	Hypoxia-independent pathway	Germline or somatic	Uncommon	Welander et al[42]; Schlisio et al,[15] 2008; Yeh et al,[16] 2008
Unknown (possibly activating)	KMT2D	8085	12q13.12	Chromatin remodeling	Germ ine or somatic	Common	Juhlin et al,[17] 2015
HIF stabilizing	EPAS1/HIF2A	2034	2p21-p16	Pseudohypoxia signaling	Mosaic or somatic	Very common	TCGA[7]; Comino-Mendéz et al,[8] 2013; Toledo et al,[9] 2013; Curras-Freixes et al[3]
Hypoxia independent	IDH1	3417	2q33.3	Pseudohypoxia signaling	Somatic	Very rare	TCGA[7]; Gaal et al,[14] 2010

Abbreviations: ID, identification; mTOR, mechanistic target of rapamycin.

found in the PPGL family, did not present papillary renal carcinoma (PRC). Clinical and functional studies are required to clarify the possible existence of PRC- and PPGL-specific mutations.

THERAPEUTIC OPPORTUNITIES OF TARGETING MET AND *FIBROBLAST GROWTH FACTOR RECEPTOR 1* IN PHEOCHROMOCYTOMAS AND PARAGANGLIOMAS

Because of the activation of TK receptors observed in tumors, a great effort has been done in order to develop small-molecule kinase inhibitors for cancer therapy. The recent observation that MET, FGFR1, and MERTK TK are, in addition to RET, mutated and activated in PPGLs solidify the rationale and opens a new window of opportunity to the study of the efficacy of kinase inhibitors in the treatment of PPGLs, especially advanced and inoperable cases.

The clinical development of inhibitors of MET is more advanced among the new PPGL-mutated kinases. Crizotinib (Xalkori), which targets both MET and anaplastic lymphoma receptor tyrosine kinase (ALK) (ALK) (IC50 [inhibitory concentration] of 11 nM and 24 nM, respectively), is approved by the Food and Drug Administration for metastatic non–small-cell lung cancer (NSCLC) whose tumors are ALK positive. Clinical studies have shown the efficacy of crizotinib in MET-amplified NSCLC; however, the low frequency of such a genetic event in these tumors is a drawback.[57–59] Two independent studies indicated that pathogenic and possibly pathogenic mutations are frequently found in PPGLs.[30,55] More MET-upregulated PPGL tumors can be found once gene amplification, gene fusion, and receptor activation by exon 14 splicing skip are carefully investigated in PPGLs. Clinical trials and clinical research studies are expected in the near future to evaluate the efficacy of crizonitib and cabozantinib, a second clinically developed MET inhibitor already approved for advanced MTC.

FGFR1 inhibitors are also clinically available; however, initial drugs that were developed were not specific and would also inhibit other off-target receptors, even in a more potent manner than they would inhibit the FGFRs. For example, in addition to FGFRs, lucitanib potently inhibits vascular endothelial growth factor receptor (VEGFR) 1 to 3 and colony-stimulating factor 1 receptor (CSF1R) and dovitinib presents even higher nonselective function by inhibiting VEGFR1 to 3, RET, platelet-derived growth factor receptor beta, KIT proto-oncogene receptor tyrosine kinase (KIT), CSF1R, and FLT-3. Lenvatinib, ponatinib, nintedanib, orantinib, and brivanib are other examples of FGFR inhibitors that show important toxicity because of nonselective targeting. Recently, a phase I dose-escalation study was conducted with the JNJ-42756493, an oral pan–FGFR inhibitor, in patients with advanced solid tumors.[60] JNJ-42756493 is being further investigated in patients with solid tumors carrying FGFR1 mutations or gene fusions (clinicaltrials.com = NCT02699606).

MERTK inhibitors are not as developed as inhibitors of MET and FGFR1. MERTK's role as an oncogene has been characterized and its downregulation assessed in vitro and in vivo. It was seen that melanoma cells treated with MERTK-selective inhibitor UNC1062 had many proliferation characteristics decreased as capacity to form colonies and tumors in murine xenograft models.[61]

DIAGNOSTIC EXOME SEQUENCING

Genomic studies have shown high efficiency of whole-exome sequencing to discover mutations on known and new PPGL genes mutated in the germline or in the tumor samples from patients with PPGL.

Many research and clinical laboratories have embraced targeted next-generation sequencing designed to analyze the most commonly mutated or all PPGLs genes as the optimal strategy to the analysis of highly genetic heterogeneous disorders, such as PGGLs. Also, whole-exome sequencing has now become a first-tier tool as a routine diagnostic test for heterogeneous genetic disorders. A consensus guideline by international experts on PPGLs who have implemented target- and/or whole-exome sequencing in their routine genetic analysis and molecular diagnostic of hereditary PPGLs was recently completed.[63]

REFERENCES

1. Castro-Vega LJ, Lepoutre-Lussey C, Gimenez-Roqueplo AP, et al. Rethinking pheochromocytomas and paragangliomas from a genomic perspective. Oncogene 2016;35(9):1080–9.
2. Fishbein L, Khare S, Wubbenhorst B, et al. Whole-exome sequencing identifies somatic ATRX mutations in pheochromocytomas and paragangliomas. Nat Commun 2015;6:6140.
3. Currás-Freixes M, Inglada-Pérez L, Mancikova V, et al. Recommendations for somatic and germline genetic testing of single pheochromocytoma and paraganglioma based on findings from a series of 329 patients. J Med Genet 2015; 52(10):647–56.
4. Luchetti A, Walsh D, Rodger F, et al. Profiling of somatic mutations in phaeochromocytoma and paraganglioma by targeted next generation sequencing analysis. Int J Endocrinol 2015;2015:138573.
5. Ladroue C, Carcenac R, Leporrier M, et al. PHD2 mutation and congenital erythrocytosis with paraganglioma. N Engl J Med 2008;359(25):2685–92.
6. Yang C, Zhuang Z, Fliedner SM, et al. Germ-line PHD1 and PHD2 mutations detected in patients with pheochromocytoma/paraganglioma-polycythemia. J Mol Med (Berl) 2015;93(1):93–104.
7. Cancer Genome Atlas Research Network, Weinstein JN, Collisson EA, et al. The Cancer Genome Atlas Pan-Cancer analysis project. Nat Genet 2013;45(10): 1113–20.
8. Comino-Méndez I, de Cubas AA, Bernal C, et al. Tumoral EPAS1 (HIF2A) mutations explain sporadic pheochromocytoma and paraganglioma in the absence of erythrocytosis. Hum Mol Genet 2013;22(11):2169–76.
9. Toledo RA, Qin Y, Srikantan S, et al. In vivo and in vitro oncogenic effects of HIF2A mutations in pheochromocytomas and paragangliomas. Endocr Relat Cancer 2013;20(3):349–59.
10. Castro-Vega LJ, Buffet A, De Cubas AA, et al. Germline mutations in FH confer predisposition to malignant pheochromocytomas and paragangliomas. Hum Mol Genet 2014;23(9):2440–6.
11. Luchetti A, Walsh D, Rodger F, et al. Profiling of somatic mutations in phaeochromocytoma and paraganglioma by targeted next generation sequencing analysis. Int J Endocrinol 2015;2015:138573.
12. Oudijk L, de Krijger RR, Rapa I, et al. H-RAS mutations are restricted to sporadic pheochromocytomas lacking specific clinical or pathological features: data from a multi-institutional series. J Clin Endocrinol Metab 2014;99(7):E1376–80.
13. Stenman A, Welander J, Gustavsson I, et al. HRAS mutation prevalence and associated expression patterns in pheochromocytoma. Genes Chromosomes Cancer 2016;55(5):452–9.
14. Gaal J, Burnichon N, Korpershoek E, et al. Isocitrate dehydrogenase mutations are rare in pheochromocytomas and paragangliomas. J Clin Endocrinol Metab 2010;95(3):1274–8.

15. Schlisio S, Kenchappa RS, Vredeveld LC, et al. The kinesin KIF1Bbeta acts downstream from EglN3 to induce apoptosis and is a potential 1p36 tumor suppressor. Genes Dev 2008;22(7):884–93.

16. Yeh IT, Lenci RE, Qin Y, et al. A germline mutation of the KIF1B beta gene on 1p36 in a family with neural and nonneural tumors. Hum Genet 2008;124(3):279–85.

17. Juhlin CC, Stenman A, Haglund F, et al. Whole-exome sequencing defines the mutational landscape of pheochromocytoma and identifies KMT2D as a recurrently mutated gene. Genes Chromosomes Cancer 2015;54(9):542–54.

18. Burnichon N, Cascón A, Schiavi F, et al. MAX mutations cause hereditary and sporadic pheochromocytoma and paraganglioma. Clin Cancer Res 2012; 18(10):2828–37.

19. Cancer Genome Atlas Research Network. Comprehensive molecular characterization of urothelial bladder carcinoma. Nature 2014;507(7492):315–22.

20. Cascón A, Comino-Méndez I, Currás-Freixes M, et al. Whole-exome sequencing identifies MDH2 as a new familial paraganglioma gene. J Natl Cancer Inst 2015; 107(5) [pii:djv053].

21. Wilzén A, Rehammar A, Muth A, et al. Malignant pheochromocytomas/paragangliomas harbor mutations in transport and cell adhesion genes. Int J Cancer 2016;138(9):2201–11.

22. Burnichon N, Buffet A, Parfait B, et al. Somatic NF1 inactivation is a frequent event in sporadic pheochromocytoma. Hum Mol Genet 2012;21(26):5397–405.

23. Burnichon N, Vescovo L, Amar L, et al. Integrative genomic analysis reveals somatic mutations in pheochromocytoma and paraganglioma. Hum Mol Genet 2011;20(20):3974–85.

24. Burnichon N, Rohmer V, Amar L, et al, PGL.NET Network. The succinate dehydrogenase genetic testing in a large prospective series of patients with paragangliomas. J Clin Endocrinol Metab 2009;94(8):2817–27.

25. Richter S, Klink B, Nacke B, et al. Epigenetic mutation of the succinate dehydrogenase C promoter in a patient with two paragangliomas. J Clin Endocrinol Metab 2016;101(2):359–63.

26. Yao L, Schiavi F, Cascon A, et al. Spectrum and prevalence of FP/TMEM127 gene mutations in pheochromocytomas and paragangliomas. JAMA 2010;304(23): 2611–9.

27. Dahia PL. Pheochromocytoma and paraganglioma pathogenesis: learning from genetic heterogeneity. Nat Rev Cancer 2014;14(2):108–19.

28. Favier J, Amar L, Gimenez-Roqueplo AP. Paraganglioma and phaeochromocytoma: from genetics to personalized medicine. Nat Rev Endocrinol 2015;11(2): 101–11.

29. Smith J, Read ML, Hoffman J, et al. Germline ESR2 mutation predisposes to medullary thyroid carcinoma and causes up-regulation of RET expression. Hum Mol Genet 2016;25(9):1836–45.

30. Toledo RA, Qin Y, Cheng ZM, et al. Recurrent mutations of chromatin-remodeling genes and kinase receptors in pheochromocytomas and paragangliomas. Clin Cancer Res 2016;22(9):2301–10.

31. Graham DK, Dawson TL, Mullaney DL, et al. Cloning and mRNA expression analysis of a novel human protooncogene, c-mer. Cell Growth Differ 1994;5(6): 647–57.

32. Jimenez C, Dang GT, Schultz PN, et al. A novel point mutation of the RET protooncogene involving the second intracellular tyrosine kinase domain in a family with medullary thyroid carcinoma. J Clin Endocrinol Metab 2004;89(7):3521–6.

33. Sather S, Kenyon KD, Lefkowitz JB, et al. A soluble form of the Mer receptor tyrosine kinase inhibits macrophage clearance of apoptotic cells and platelet aggregation. Blood 2007;109(3):1026–33.

34. Rothlin CV, Ghosh S, Zuniga EI, et al. TAM receptors are pleiotropic inhibitors of the innate immune response. Cell. 2007;131(6):1124–36.

35. Bok D, Hall MO. The role of the pigment epithelium in the etiology of inherited retinal dystrophy in the rat. J Cell Biol. 1971;49(3):664–82.

36. Gal A, Li Y, Thompson DA, et al. Mutations in MERTK, the human orthologue of the RCS rat retinal dystrophy gene, cause retinitis pigmentosa. Nat Genet 2000;26(3):270–1.

37. Keating AK, Salzberg DB, Sather S, et al. Lymphoblastic leukemia/lymphoma in mice overexpressing the Mer (MerTK) receptor tyrosine kinase. Oncogene 2006; 25(45):6092–100.

38. Welander J, Söderkvist P, Gimm O. Genetic alterations in pheochromocytoma and paraganglioma [thesis]. Linköping (Sweden): Linköping University Electronic Press; 2015. p. 64.

39. Toledo RA, Dahia PL. Next-generation sequencing for the genetic screening of phaeochromcytomas and paragangliomas: riding the new wave, but with caution. Clin Endocrinol (oxf) 2014;80(1):23–4.

40. Jones DT, Hutter B, Jäger N, et al, International Cancer Genome Consortium Ped-Brain Tumor Project. Recurrent somatic alterations of FGFR1 and NTRK2 in pilocytic astrocytoma. Nat Genet 2013;45(8):927–32.

41. Dutt A, Salvesen HB, Chen TH, et al. Drug-sensitive FGFR2 mutations in endometrial carcinoma. Proc Natl Acad Sci U S A 2008;105(25):8713–7.

42. Welander J, Andreasson A, Juhlin CC, et al. Rare germline mutations identified by targeted next-generation sequencing of susceptibility genes in pheochromocytoma and paraganglioma. J Clin Endocrinol Metab 2014;99(7):E1352–60.

43. Ren M, Cowell JK. Constitutive Notch pathway activation in murine ZMYM2-FGFR1-induced T-cell lymphomas associated with atypical myeloproliferative disease. Blood 2011;117(25):6837–47.

44. Katoh M. FGFR inhibitors: effects on cancer cells, tumor microenvironment and whole-body homeostasis (review). Int J Mol Med 2016;38(1):3–15.

45. Passos-Bueno MR, Wilcox WR, Jabs EW, et al. Clinical spectrum of fibroblast growth factor receptor mutations. Hum Mutat 1999;14(2):115–25.

46. Bennett JT, Tan TY, Alcantara D, et al. Mosaic activating mutations in FGFR1 cause encephalocraniocutaneous lipomatosis. Am J Hum Genet 2016;98(3): 579–87.

47. Klein T, Vajpai N, Phillips JJ, et al. Structural and dynamic insights into the energetics of activation loop rearrangement in FGFR1 kinase. Nat Commun 2015;6: 7877.

48. Adams JM, Harris AW, Pinkert CA, et al. The c-myc oncogene driven by immunoglobulin enhancers induces lymphoid malignancy in transgenic mice. Nature 1985;318(6046):533–8.

49. Bamford S, Dawson E, Forbes S, et al. The COSMIC (Catalogue of Somatic Mutations in Cancer) database and website. Br J Cancer 2004;91(2):355–8.

50. Comino-Méndez I, Gracia-Aznárez FJ, Schiavi F, et al. Exome sequencing identifies MAX mutations as a cause of hereditary pheochromocytoma. Nat Genet 2011;43(7):663–7.

51. Bjerke L, Mackay A, Nandhabalan M, et al. Histone H3.3. mutations drive pediatric glioblastoma through upregulation of MYCN. Cancer Discov 2013;3(5):512–9.

52. Schwartzentruber J, Korshunov A, Liu XY, et al. Driver mutations in histone H3.3 and chromatin remodelling genes in paediatric glioblastoma. Nature 2012; 482(7384):226–31.
53. Behjati S, Tarpey PS, Presneau N, et al. Distinct H3F3A and H3F3B driver mutations define chondroblastoma and giant cell tumor of bone. Nat Genet 2013; 45(12):1479–82.
54. Nikbakht H, Panditharatna E, Mikael LG, et al. Spatial and temporal homogeneity of driver mutations in diffuse intrinsic pontine glioma. Nat Commun 2016;7:11185.
55. Castro-Vega LJ, Letouzé E, Burnichon N, et al. Multi-omics analysis defines core genomic alterations in pheochromocytomas and paragangliomas. Nat Commun 2015;6:6044.
56. Fishbein L, Leshchiner I, Walter V, et al. Comprehensive Molecular Characterization of Pheochromocytoma and Paraganglioma. Cancer Cell 2017;31(2):181–93.
57. Landi L, Cappuzzo F. Targeting MET in NSCLC: looking for a needle in a haystack. Transl Lung Cancer Res 2014;3(6):389–91.
58. Lemke G, Rothlin CV. Immunobiology of the TAM receptors. Nat Rev Immunol 2008;8(5):327–36.
59. Lu Q, Lemke G. Homeostatic regulation of the immune system by receptor tyrosine kinases of the Tyro 3 family. Science 2001;293(5528):306–11.
60. Tabernero J, Bahleda R, Dienstmann R, et al. Phase I dose-escalation study of JNJ-42756493, an oral pan-fibroblast growth factor receptor inhibitor, in patients with advanced solid tumors. J Clin Oncol 2015;33(30):3401–8.
61. Schlegel J, Sambade MJ, Sather S, et al. MERTK receptor tyrosine kinase is a therapeutic target in melanoma. J Clin Invest 2013;123(5):2257–67.
62. Bayley JP, Kunst HP, Cascon A, et al. SDHAF2 mutations in familial and sporadic paraganglioma and phaeochromocytoma. Lancet Oncol 2010;11(4):366–72.
63. NGS in PPGL (NGSnPPGL) Study Group, Toledo RA, Burnichon N, et al. Consensus Statement on next-generation-sequencing-based diagnostic testing of hereditary phaeochromocytomas and paragangliomas. Nat Rev Endocrinol 2016. [Epub ahead of print].

Genetics of Multiple Endocrine Neoplasia Type 1/Multiple Endocrine Neoplasia Type 2 Syndromes

CrossMark

Samuel M. Hyde, MS, CGC[a,b], Gilbert J. Cote, PhD[c],
Elizabeth G. Grubbs, MD, MS[a,*]

KEYWORDS

- Multiple endocrine neoplasia type 1 • Multiple endocrine neoplasia type 2
- Hereditary • Genetic testing • Genetic counseling

KEY POINTS

- Genetic testing is an important part of diagnosing, managing, and treating multiple endocrine neoplasia type 1 (MEN1) and multiple endocrine neoplasia type 2 (MEN2) syndromes.
- Approaches to genetic testing for MEN1 and MEN2 have changed, as has understanding of these conditions.
- In some cases, genetic testing for MEN1 and MEN2 can provide uninformative or unclear results that do not necessarily clarify a suspected diagnosis.
- Genetic test results should be carefully interpreted in the context of a patient's personal and/or family history.

INTRODUCTION

The breadth and depth of knowledge about MEN1 and MEN2 are impressive; years of study by many dedicated researchers have allowed characterizing and refining estimates of disease penetrance, expressivity, optimal management, and the spectrum of disease-causing genotypes. This work has permitted risk stratification for medullary thyroid carcinoma (MTC) based on *RET* genotype in MEN2,[1] which has led to genotype-phenotype correlations that are at the crux of management

Disclosure Statement: The authors have nothing to disclose.
[a] Department of Surgical Oncology, University of Texas MD Anderson Cancer Center, 1400 Pressler Street, Houston, TX 77030, USA; [b] Department of Clinical Cancer Genetics, University of Texas MD Anderson Cancer Center, 1400 Pressler Street, Houston, TX 77030, USA; [c] Department of Endocrine Neoplasia and Hormonal Disorders, University of Texas MD Anderson Cancer Center, 1400 Pressler Street, Houston, TX 77030, USA
* Corresponding author.
E-mail address: eggrubbs@mdanderson.org

Endocrinol Metab Clin N Am 46 (2017) 491–502
http://dx.doi.org/10.1016/j.ecl.2017.01.011
0889-8529/17/© 2017 Elsevier Inc. All rights reserved.
endo.theclinics.com

recommendations for patients; in cases of MEN1, a better understanding of the age-related penetrance and expression of disease manifestations has helped guide clinicians in determining to whom and when to offer germline *MEN1* testing.[2] For both MEN1 and MEN2 patients and their family members, undergoing genetic testing has expanded understanding of the respective mutation spectrums, while parallel advances in genetic testing technology have also increased the possibility of inconclusive genetic test results (ie, variants of uncertain clinical significance [VUS]). These realities, in the context of certain clinical and/or family histories, can give rise to scenarios that challenge the way of approaching the management of these diseases and the counseling provided to patients and their family members. Examples of such scenarios are discussed to illustrate the evolving understanding of these hereditary conditions.

A HISTORICAL PERSPECTIVE

The recognition of MEN1 and MEN2 as discernable endocrine tumor predisposition syndromes came during the greater first half of the twentieth century. In 1903, Jacob Erdheim,[3] a German pathologist, first described on autopsy an acromegalic man with a pituitary tumor and parathyroid adenomatosis, a constellation of findings that, along with pancreatic islet tumors, was also identified in several related individuals by Paul Wermer,[4] who first suggested that this represented an autosomal dominant, hereditary trait; this syndrome was first named Wermer syndrome but is now known as MEN1. John Sipple[5] was the first, in 1961, to publish on the association of MTC and pheochromocytoma as a second, distinct multiple endocrine neoplasia syndrome; it was only 5 years later that Williams and Pollock published their account of related patients with MTC, gastrointestinal tract ganglioneuromatosis, and mucosal neuromas.[6] Respectively, these syndromes are MEN2A and MEN2B, which were both eventually found to be caused by mutations in the *RET* proto-oncogene.[7,8] Around this same time, mutations in *MEN1* were identified in families affected by MEN1.[9] In the decades that followed these discoveries, the clinical manifestations (both endocrine and nonendocrine) and their molecular etiologies have been well studied and reviewed in the literature, permitting a remarkable understanding of disease penetrance, expressivity, genotype-phenotype correlations, and tumorigenesis.[10–12]

EVOLUTION OF GENETICS TESTING FOR MEN1 AND MEN2

Clinically available genetic testing for MEN1 and MEN2 is now widely available and is an important component of diagnosing affected patients and their family members. Although the diagnoses of MEN1 and MEN2 were, for many years, based on personal and/or family history of endocrine neoplasias, genetic testing to confirm or exclude the presence of a disease-causing mutation can allow for earlier identification of affected family members and can, in some cases, be used to guide management. The American Thyroid Association now recommends that every individual diagnosed with MTC be offered germline *RET* testing to assess for an underlying MEN2-associated gene mutation,[13] and, although there is no similar recommendation for patients suspected to have MEN1, guidelines exist for when genetic testing should be offered based on personal and/or family history of MEN1-associated manifestations.[2,14,15] Consideration of clinical diagnostic criteria for these conditions, however, is still important, particularly in cases of MEN1, where genetic testing sometimes fails to identify a disease-causing mutation in affected individuals and families.[15,16] In these cases, screening recommendations may still be formulated for at-risk family members even in the absence of an identifiable, pathogenic *MEN1* mutation.

For both MEN1 and MEN2, germline genetic testing has changed over the years. As genetic testing technology has allowed for more comprehensive analysis of *MEN1* and *RET*, the number of recognized variants in these genes that both contribute and do not contribute to the diseases has increased dramatically. Repositories that collect these data from genetic testing laboratories and the literature are publically available and can prove helpful in better understanding certain genetic test results.[17,18] The spectrum of MEN2-associated *RET* mutation includes only sequence variants, making deletion/duplication analysis unnecessary. The clinical significance of a *RET* mutation depends on where in the final protein structure the altered codon is located; a majority of pathogenic *RET* mutations are located within a subset of coding exons (**Fig. 1**). Such mutation hotspots do not exist within *MEN1*, where pathogenic mutations have been identified throughout the coding region as well as within the intronic and promoter regions (see **Fig. 1**). A majority of MEN1-associated *MEN1* mutations are sequence variants, and, of these, frameshift mutations are the most common; however, gross deletions of the gene or of parts of the gene have been identified in affected individuals,[15] making deletion/duplication analysis of *MEN1* an important part of clinical genetic testing.

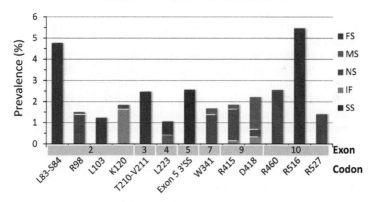

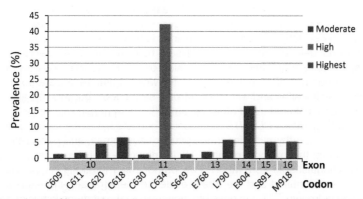

Fig. 1. Prevalence of hot-spot germline mutations in MEN1 (top) and MEN2 (bottom), greater than 1% frequency required for inclusion. FS, frame shift; IF, inframe indel; MS, missense; NS, nonsense; SS, splice site. (*Data from* Refs.[30,34,35,37,38])

RET testing for MEN2 initially began with select sequence analysis of the most commonly mutated codons, including 634, 883, 918, and the cysteine residues of exon 10 (eg, 609, 618, and 620). Later, *RET* sequence analysis was expanded to include the entirety of the coding exons in which these residues are located and where the vast majority of MEN2-associated mutations occur, which include exons 10, 11, and 13 to 16. With the widespread use of next-generation sequencing technology to perform genetic testing, certain laboratories offer comprehensive sequence analysis of all 20 coding *RET* exons; however, some debate exists over when to proceed with comprehensive analysis. Between 1996 and 2014, the relative distribution of MEN2-associated *RET* mutations across these exons shifted dramatically (reviewed by Grubbs and Gagel[19]) and with it the understanding of hereditary MTC/MEN2A has matured significantly. For example, a classification of mutations into groups based on disease aggressiveness and age of onset of disease was initiated in 1996 and has evolved over the past 2 decades; the current 2015 American Thyroid Association guidelines recommend a new grouping of moderate-risk, high-risk, and highest-risk mutations (see **Fig. 1**) with associated suggested treatment. Additionally a recent change in nomenclature now recognizes that familial MTC should not be considered a form of hereditary MTC distinct from MEN2A[13] as it previously was. More widespread *RET* testing has also allowed for the characterization and, in some cases, recharacterization of certain *RET* variants, examples of which include the now recognized as benign Y791F variant.[20–24] Still, there remain many missense *RET* variants for which data are either completely lacking or inconclusive with regard to their contribution to hereditary MTC.

Genetic testing for MEN1 has been less dynamic over the years, but in parallel the understanding of *MEN1* genotypes pales in comparison to that of *RET*. There currently exist no clinically relevant genotype-phenotype correlations for MEN1; however, studies have found that mutations targeting the JunD interacting domain of *MEN1* are associated with an increased risk of disease-associated death,[25] and that some alterations may only predispose to familial isolated primary hyperparathyroidism and not pituitary or pancreatic neuroendocrine tumors.[26,27] In the absence of genotype-phenotype data, there has been an emphasis on understanding intrafamilial disease correlations and a better understanding of MEN1-related causes of death.[28,29] Germline *MEN1* testing began with sequence analysis of the coding exons 2 to 10 and later included sequence analysis of the intervening intronic sequences and that of the noncoding exon 1. The most recent update to *MEN1* genetic testing was the addition of deletion/duplication analysis to assess for exon-level alterations not capable of detection via traditional Sanger sequencing or of next-generation sequencing; most laboratories that provide testing offer both comprehensive sequencing and deletion/duplication analyses; however, in some cases the latter must be specifically requested. The expansion of *MEN1* testing, like with *RET*, has increased the number of germline variants for which conclusive data do not exist, particularly at splice sites and within the intronic sequences, but this has also helped solidify the pathogenic nature of other variants.[30]

Most recently, germline *CDKN1B* mutations in humans have been associated with a predisposition to parathyroid adenomas, pituitary adenomas, and pancreatic neuroendocrine tumors; this phenocopy of MEN1 is known as MEN4 and, thus far, seems clinically indistinguishable from MEN1. Few pathogenic mutations in *CDKN1B*, however, have been identified and the true prevalence, penetrance, and expressivity of MEN4 remain unknown.[31,32] It is possible, however, that mutations in this gene could account for some proportion of individuals meeting clinical diagnostic criteria for MEN1 who do not have an identifiable *MEN1* pathogenic mutation.

INTERPRETING GENETIC TEST RESULTS

Any genetic test can yield positive (ie, pathogenic), negative, and/or inconclusive results, and clinicians who order genetic testing should be prepared to receive these 3 results; they should also adequately prepare patients for these possible scenarios. For a positive genetic test result, how management and screening will change for a patient and what recommendations will be made for family members should be considered. With negative test results, it is important to remember that no genetic test is 100% sensitive and that negative results can be uninformative; a negative genetic test results does not always rule out the possibility of a hereditary predisposition in the family, and thoughtful consideration should be given to what questions have not been answered with a negative test result. Lastly, for VUSs, it is important to remember that non-negative genetic test results do not mean that an explanation has been identified; these results are inherently uninformative, and, although in some situations steps can be taken to further understand these variants in the context of a personal or family history, this is not always the case. A plan for follow-up with the patient and recommendations for family members in these cases is typically based on family history, not the presence or absence of an uncertain variant. The potential germline results that may be encountered when evaluating for MEN1 and MEN2 are discussed and scenarios from the authors' clinical experiences are provided.

THE POSITIVE TEST RESULT

When a positive test result returns for a *RET* or *MEN1* mutation in the proband, the clinician must guide the further treatment of the individual patient as well as address the genetic testing needs of the patient's family members, most often in collaboration with a genetic counselor. At-risk family members deciding whether or not to undergo predictive genetic testing should have the opportunity to discuss the medical and psychological consequences of genetic testing, and particularly careful counseling should be provided to families in which there are at-risk minors. As the first member of a family diagnosed with the germline mutation, the proband has a diagnosis of 1 or more of the diseases associated with the syndrome, and further treatment will involve surveillance for the known disease and screening for additional syndromic-associated diseases. An asymptomatic mutation carrier, especially if diagnosed at a younger age, may not have any diseases associated with the syndrome, and screening for specific related disorders should be performed.

A patient with a *MEN1* germline mutation requires screening for primary hyperparathyroidism, pituitary adenomas, and pancreatic neuroendocrine tumors. The authors also recommend screening for bronchial and thymic carcinoids. Although these lesions are less common manifestations of MEN1, their high malignant potential warrants consideration of their presence. The age at which to begin preventative screening for the MEN1-associated diseases depends on the particular disorder; however, the clinician should always be aware of signs and symptoms that could suggest an earlier presentation than anticipated. **Table 1** shows the authors' recommended biochemical and radiographic screening measures. The authors prefer the use of MRI to CT for screening purposes to reduce patient exposure to radiation over the lengthy follow-up period of this syndrome. The clinician should be aware that the biochemical tests for the pancreatic neuroendocrine tumors, in particular chromogranin A, pancreatic polypeptide, and glucagon, have not been shown optimally sensitive for disease detection[33] and should be used in combination with imaging and clinical evaluation. Additionally, although adrenal lesions can be associated with MEN1, the

Table 1
Screening measures in multiple endocrine neoplasia type 1 and multiple endocrine neoplasia type 2–associated diseases

| | | Screening Measures | |
		Biochemical	Radiographic
MEN1-associated diseases	Primary hyperparathyroidism	Annual serum calcium, albumin, intact parathyroid hormone, 25-hydroxy vitamin D, 24-h urine calcium (less frequent)	Intermittent bone mineral density, frequency based on findings
	Pituitary adenoma	Annual serum prolactin, IGF-1	Triennial MRI of sella
	Pancreatic neuroendocrine tumor	Annual gastrin[a], CgA, PP, proinsulin, insulin, fasting glucose, proinsulin	Triennial MRI of abdomen
	Bronchial or thymic carcinoid		Triennial MRI of chest
MEN2-associated diseases	MTC	Calcitonin, CEA	Comprehensive neck ultrasound
	Pheochromocytoma	Plasma metanephrines	
	Primary hyperparathyroidism	Annual serum calcium, albumin, intact parathyroid hormone, 25-hydroxyvitamin D, 24-h urine calcium (less frequent)	Intermittent bone mineral density, frequency based on findings

Abbreviations: CEA, carcinoembryonic antigen; CgA, chromogranin A; IGF, insulinlike growth factor; PP, pancreatic polypeptide.
[a] With withdrawal of proton pump inhibitors for greater than 7 days.

authors do not recommend any routine biochemical screening for functionality. The clinician should evaluate, however, the adrenal glands on the triennial MRI of the abdomen and lesions that arise should be evaluated both biochemically and radiographically. The age for initiation of screening for MEN1-related diseases should be made on an individual basis with the treating clinician; usually, evaluation for primary hyperparathyroidism begins in childhood whereas the remainder of the diseases are evaluated starting in adolescence.

Clinical scenario

Two brothers, ages 18 and 21 years old, presented to the endocrine clinic for evaluation and screening recommendations regarding their diagnosis of MEN1. The brothers were identified to have MEN1 after undergoing predictive MEN1 genetic testing when their father was diagnosed with MEN1 in his 40s. Both were recommended to have initial screening for primary hyperparathyroidism, pituitary adenoma, pancreatic neuroendocrine tumor, and bronchial/thymic carcinoid. The patients' father has 4 children in total: the 2 brothers described, another 8-year-old son, and a 13-year-old daughter. The family chose to have all children tested at the same time, and the youngest son also tested positive for the familial mutation; the daughter tested negative. The 8-year-old son underwent initial screening for primary hyperparathyroidism with a serum calcium and parathyroid hormone measurement.

Identification of a germline *RET* mutation in a patient requires screening for MTC, primary hyperparathyroidism, and pheochromocytoma in MEN2A and MTC and for pheochromocytoma in MEN2B. Screening measures are outlined in **Table 1** and are usually recommended to be initiated at detection of the mutation. Discussion of the treatment of the diseases associated with MEN1 and MEN2 is beyond the scope of this article; however, references from the American Thyroid Association and Thakker and colleagues are provided.[2,13]

Clinical scenario

A 77-year-old woman was diagnosed with apparently sporadic medullary thyroid cancer at age 75 and underwent *RET* testing. She was subsequently diagnosed with MEN2A secondary to a p.V804M pathogenic *RET* mutation. The patient presented to the authors' institution for further evaluation and recommendations regarding long-term follow-up for MEN2A. The authors advised initial screening for primary hyperparathyroidism and pheochromocytoma and continued annual observation. She has a 57-year-old son who underwent predictive *RET* testing and tested positive for the V804M mutation, as did his 17-year-old son; screening in these individuals for the 3 syndrome-associated diseases was recommended. The proband has a living 86-year-old brother who was not interested in pursuing genetic testing. His next living descendant is a grandson in his 30s who was highly recommended to pursue predictive testing to inform his and his son's risk for MTC, pheochromocytoma, and primary hyperparathyroidism.

THE NEGATIVE TEST RESULT

An asymptomatic patient being evaluated because of an affected family member should undergo testing for the specific *MEN1* or *RET* mutation that their relative harbors. If this testing reveals no mutation, the family member can be assured that no further follow-up is necessary either for them or for their direct descendants. Given the concern for potential confusion if multiple samples are drawn under the same surname at the same time, the authors recommend consideration of testing asymptomatic family members at different settings. This practice helps avoid the opportunity for sample identification uncertainty.

A patient with 1 or more of the diseases associated with MEN1 who has a negative germline test must be considered differently. This scenario may occur in approximately 5% to 10% of patients with the syndrome.[34] Estimates of false-negative *MEN1* genetic testing in the literature vary widely, because this is dependent on how patients were ascertained for genetic testing (presence of 1 tumor at a young age, presence of multiple tumors, positive family history, and so forth). If they have a clinical diagnosis of MEN1, meaning they possess 2 or more MEN1-associated tumors, or they have a familial diagnosis, signifying they have a MEN1-associated tumor and a first-degree relative with a diagnosis of MEN1, they are screened in the same manner as if they have a positive germline test for the syndrome. This individual and clinician should consider the potential benefit of repeat germline *MEN1* testing as indicated and depending on the comprehensiveness of initial germline testing; it is important to be aware of and understand the technical limitations of genetic testing, including as it pertains to *MEN1*, whether or not deletion/duplication analysis was performed, and coverage of the promoter and intronic sequences. The realistic potential causes of having a clinical diagnosis of MEN1 and no correlating *MEN1* mutation detected on germline testing include (1) patients harboring *MEN1* mutations that were not included in the regions targeted by sequencing, such as in the promoter or within the introns[34]; (2) patients with genetic alterations, such as large deletions or gene rearrangements not detected by sequencing; (3) patients who are sporadic phenocopies, especially in the case of a single affected individual or (4) patients harboring germline mutations in other genes.[32] MEN4, described previously, is one such example of the latter and testing for this syndrome should be considered if *MEN1* testing is negative in this population.

Certainly, the lack of a positive test in the clinical setting of MEN1 is unsettling for the patient and clinician, in part because the extent to which following potentially affected family members is challenging. Because no relative can be excluded by a genetic test, the notion of performing the extensive screening, outlined in **Table 1**, for all potentially affected family members can be daunting, both logistically and psychologically for the individual relative. In this setting, the authors recommend a baseline and intermittent biochemical screening for primary hyperparathyroidism given the frequency of this disease and relative ease of screening. Screening for pituitary, pancreatic neuroendocrine tumors and thoracic-based carcinoids should be carried out with thought to the age and potential signs and symptoms of the individual. Importantly, communication about the potential of developing MEN1-related disease should occur with the possibly affected family members so they may share with their health care providers. The authors offer own recent experience.

Clinical scenario

A 44-year-old man with history of a pituitary adenoma and primary hyperparathyroidism diagnosed at ages 43 and 44, respectively, presented to the authors' institution for further evaluation. There was no family history of MEN1 tumors, but the patient met clinical diagnostic criteria for MEN1; he underwent comprehensive *MEN1* testing, which was negative. The patient then underwent comprehensive *CDKN1B* testing for MEN4, which was also negative. The patient's case was presented at a multidisciplinary endocrine conference to determine how to optimally perform follow-up and to discuss recommendations for his children. Decision was made for annual MEN1 pancreatic screening for the patient along with his parathyroid and pituitary follow-up. For his children, the conclusion was to check calcium levels every few years and to possibly expand screening if any child was ever diagnosed with PHPT.

RET testing is performed in apparently sporadic patients usually because of a diagnosis of MTC and should include exons 8, 10 to 11, and 13 to 15. Usually this initial testing is all that is required and, if negative, the patient and family require no further screening. If there is an increased concern for a hereditary form of MTC, however, including a family history of MEN2-related diseases, young age of diagnosis, or pathology characteristics, such as extensive C-cell hyperplasia and multifocality, whole-gene sequencing should be considered to capture the rarer *RET* alterations. If patients have a clinical diagnosis of MEN2, meaning 2 or more syndrome-associated diseases or a family history of MTC, and no *RET* mutation is detected, they should be screened as outlined in **Table 1**. Fortunately this is a rare event.[35] It is reasonable for at-risk family members of such patients to undergo baseline and occasional biochemical screening for MTC given the relative noninvasive nature of this approach.

THE INCONCLUSIVE RESULT, OR VARIANT OF UNCERTAIN SIGNIFICANCE

Receiving VUSs is challenging because, by definition, the associated disease risk is ambiguous. The clinician must balance the potential creation of baseless anxiety by providing non-negative test results with failing to provide potentially important information to patients and their families.[36] In cases of an individual diagnosed with 1 or more of the syndrome-associated diseases and a VUS, the authors counsel the patient carefully as to the indeterminate and uninformative nature of the results and recommend continued intermittent screening for the syndrome-related diseases. Such follow-up is not trivial; the time and expense involved in observing for these diseases is not insignificant and should be patterned on the concern level for the individual patient and the particular VUS. The patient should also understand that as additional data are accumulated, the VUS could be reclassified as benign or pathogenic and that continued follow-up with a health care provider on this subject should be performed; the reclassification of a VUS as benign or pathogenic would also have implications on the family members of the proband, particularly in the case of a pathogenic reclassification in which case at-risk family members would then be recommended to pursue testing for the familial mutation.

Even more challenging for clinicians is how to handle testing and screening of an affected individual's family members, which is typically not recommended when a VUS is identified. In this setting, a detailed family history is essential; additional relatives with syndrome-associated diseases heightens the concern of pathogenicity of the genetic alteration, and targeted testing for the VUS in those family members may be informative. Testing family members for MEN2-associated VUSs should be considered only after careful consideration of a proband's personal and family history, the data available on that particular VUS in the literature, and genetic counseling. In cases of certain MEN2-associated VUSs in which familial screening is chosen, consideration should be given to affected family members undergoing initial evaluation for associated diseases given that screening is straightforward and noninvasive. Because of the gain associated with early detection of C-cell hyperplasia, a personalized approach to follow-up screening that factors both disease presentation in the family and patient preference is recommended. A similar approach may be taken in MEN1-related VUSs with the understanding that screening for all associated tumors is more arduous; a personalized approach based on the phenotypic presentation within the kindred is essential. Given the challenges associated with VUSs in MEN1 and MEN2, the authors offer vignettes of experiences in the recent past.

Clinical scenario

A 29-year-old man was diagnosed with single-gland primary hyperparathyroidism after approximately a decade of hypercalcemia and several years of annual nephrolithiasis. He was also noted to have bilateral upper and lower extremity lipomas. His family history was significant for kidney stones in his father and multiple maternal aunts/uncles. He was identified to have a *MEN1* VUS, and parental studies were recommended to determine if this VUS was inherited or occurred de novo; the potential pathogenicity of the variant would be supported if a de novo occurrence was found. Since then, the patient's mother has tested negative for this specific VUS and paternal studies are pending. The patient was counseled carefully that at this point; based on the available data, it is unclear whether or not he is at increased risk for additional MEN1 manifestations; further characterization of this VUS could help guide future screening recommendations. For the time being, given his young age at presentation, he will continue to be intermittently screened for the presence of MEN1-associated diseases.

Clinical scenario

A 37-year-old woman presented to the authors' institution for MEN1 screening given her 53-year-old mother's history of multiple endocrine tumors, single-gland primary hyperparathyroidism diagnosed at 40 years, and bilateral, nonfunctioning adrenal adenomas, who was identified to have a *MEN1* VUS. The patient had baseline MEN1 laboratory studies, which were all within normal limits, and was counseled that the authors would not recommend targeted genetic testing for the VUS at this time, because it would likely not provide useful information about her risk to develop manifestations of MEN1. The patient was educated as to the manifestations of MEN1 and strongly encouraged to recontact the authors if she were to ever develop any of these symptoms or diseases, in which case targeted testing for the familial VUS could be informative.

Clinical scenario

A 55-year-old woman with a history of apparently sporadic medullary thyroid cancer initially diagnosed at age 27 presented to the authors' institution for transition of long-term follow-up. She underwent *RET* testing in 2010 (sequencing of exons 10, 11, and 13–16 only) at an outside facility and was identified as having a *RET* VUS. The patient was counseled that it is reasonable to test her adult children for this particular VUS to determine who should be followed with biochemical screening for MTC (annual calcitonin), but it was stressed that prophylactic thyroidectomy in the absence of evidence of malignancy would not be recommended based on the presence of the VUS alone. The patient was also counseled about the differences between select exon *RET* testing and comprehensive analysis of exons 1 to 20. In this setting, the authors pursued this approach, especially given her young age of initial diagnosis, to confirm that there is no clearly pathogenic *RET* mutation for which her children would preferentially be tested.

The challenges posed by detecting VUS in MEN1 and MEN2 demand the continued search to determine genotype-phenotype relationships, a task that is often difficult in these rare syndromes. In these settings, it is essential to use registries to accumulate data on germline alterations along with the associated clinical presentations and relevant family data to firmly establish genotype-phenotype correlations and pathogenic characterization of these mutations. Expert guidelines and the creation of treatment recommendations to provide assistance for clinicians encountering such mutations would be beneficial.

SUMMARY

Genetic test results, even for familiar conditions like MEN1 and MEN2, can sometimes be ambiguous and uninformative even after interpreted in the context of a patient's clinical and/or family history. These results do not always provide data that help guide recommendations regarding counseling, management, and/or screening and surveillance, and careful consideration is necessary. Moving forward, it is important to consider what types of endeavors may help clinicians, and the profession as a whole, address these scenarios. This could include (1) garnering collective input from experts in the field of endocrinology, genetics, and genetic counseling in the form of guidelines, best practices, and/or decisional algorithms; (2) increasing access to genetic counseling services through potentially novel service-delivery models; (3) improving data collection through the use of registries, family history questionnaires, and interinstitutional collaborations; and (4) encouraging conversation between clinicians and their institutions regarding strategies used when faced with these types of scenarios.

REFERENCES

1. Eng C, Clayton D, Schuffenecker I, et al. The relationship between specific RET proto-oncogene mutations and disease phenotype in multiple endocrine neoplasia type 2. International RET mutation consortium analysis. JAMA 1996; 276(19):1575–9.
2. Thakker RV, Newey PJ, Walls GV, et al. Clinical practice guidelines for multiple endocrine neoplasia type 1 (MEN1). J Clin Endocrinol Metab 2012;97(9): 2990–3011.
3. Erdheim J. Zur normalen und pathologischen Histologie der Glandula thyreoidea, parathyreoidea und Hypophysis. Beitr Path Anat 1903;33:58.
4. Wermer P. Genetic aspects of adenomatosis of endocrine glands. Am J Med 1954;16(3):363–71.

5. Sipple J. The association of pheochromocytoma with carcinoma of the thyroid gland. Am J Med 1961;31:163–6.
6. Williams DC, Pollock DF. Multiple mucosal neuromata with endocrine tumours: a syndrome allied to von Recklinghausen's disease. J Pathol Bact 1966;91:71–80.
7. Hofstra RM, Landsvater RM, Ceccherini I, et al. A mutation in the RET proto-oncogene associated with multiple endocrine neoplasia type 2B and sporadic medullary thyroid carcinoma. Nature 1994;367(6461):375–6.
8. Mulligan LM, Kwok JB, Healey CS, et al. Germ-line mutations of the RET proto-oncogene in multiple endocrine neoplasia type 2A. Nature 1993;363(6428): 458–60.
9. Chandrasekharappa SC, Guru SC, Manickam P, et al. Positional cloning of the gene for multiple endocrine neoplasia-type 1. Science 1997;276(5311):404–7.
10. Marx SJ. Molecular genetics of multiple endocrine neoplasia types 1 and 2. Nat Rev Cancer 2005;5(5):367–75.
11. Marquard J, Eng C. Multiple endocrine neoplasia type 2. In: Pagon RA, Adam MP, Ardinger HH, et al, editors. GeneReviews(R) [Internet]. Seattle (WA): 1993. Available at: https://www.ncbi.nlm.nih.gov/books/NBK1257/.
12. Giusti F, Marini F, Brandi ML. Multiple endocrine neoplasia type 1. In: Pagon RA, Adam MP, Ardinger HH, et al, editors. GeneReviews(R) [Internet]. Seattle (WA): 1993. Available at: https://www.ncbi.nlm,nih.gov/books/NBK1538.
13. Wells SA Jr, Asa SL, Dralle H, et al. Revised American Thyroid Association guidelines for the management of medullary thyroid carcinoma. Thyroid 2015;25(6): 567–610.
14. Falchetti A. Genetic screening for multiple endocrine neoplasia syndrome type 1 (MEN-1): when and how. F1000 Med Rep 2010;2:14.
15. Tham E, Grandell U, Lindgren E, et al. Clinical testing for mutations in the MEN1 gene in Sweden: a report on 200 unrelated cases. J Clin Endocrinol Metab 2007; 92(9):3389–95.
16. Ellard S, Hattersley AT, Brewer CM, et al. Detection of an MEN1 gene mutation depends on clinical features and supports current referral criteria for diagnostic molecular genetic testing. Clin Endocrinol 2005;62(2):169–75.
17. Landrum MJ, Lee JM, Benson M, et al. ClinVar: public archive of interpretations of clinically relevant variants. Nucleic Acids Res 2016;44(D1):D862–8.
18. Margraf RL, Crockett DK, Krautscheid PM, et al. Multiple endocrine neoplasia type 2 RET protooncogene database: repository of MEN2-associated RET sequence variation and reference for genotype/phenotype correlations. Hum Mutat 2009;30(4):548–56.
19. Grubbs EG, Gagel RF. My, how things have changed in multiple endocrine neoplasia type 2A! J Clin Endocrinol Metab 2015;100(7):2532–5.
20. Toledo RA, Hatakana R, Lourenco DM Jr, et al. Comprehensive assessment of the disputed RET Y791F variant shows no association with medullary thyroid carcinoma susceptibility. Endoc Related Cancer 2015;22(1):65–76.
21. Machens A, Frank-Raue K, Lorenz K, et al. Clinical relevance of RET variants G691S, L769L, S836S and S904S to sporadic medullary thyroid cancer. Clin Endocrinol 2012;76(5):691–7.
22. Siqueira DR, Romitti M, da Rocha AP, et al. The RET polymorphic allele S836S is associated with early metastatic disease in patients with hereditary or sporadic medullary thyroid carcinoma. Endocrine-related cancer 2010;17(4):953–63.
23. Colombo-Benkmann M, Li Z, Riemann B, et al. Characterization of the RET protooncogene transmembrane domain mutation S649L associated with nonaggressive medullary thyroid carcinoma. Eur J Endocrinol 2008;158(6):811–6.

24. Muzza M, Cordella D, Bombled J, et al. Four novel RET germline variants in exons 8 and 11 display an oncogenic potential in vitro. Eur J Endocrinol 2010;162(4): 771–7.
25. Thevenon J, Bourredjem A, Faivre L, et al. Higher risk of death among MEN1 patients with mutations in the JunD interacting domain: a Groupe d'etude des Tumeurs Endocrines (GTE) cohort study. Hum Mol Genet 2013;22(10):1940–8.
26. Hannan FM, Nesbit MA, Christie PT, et al. Familial isolated primary hyperparathyroidism caused by mutations of the MEN1 gene. Nat Clin Pract Endocrinol Metab 2008;4(1):53–8.
27. Warner J, Epstein M, Sweet A, et al. Genetic testing in familial isolated hyperparathyroidism: unexpected results and their implications. J Med Genet 2004;41(3): 155–60.
28. Thevenon J, Bourredjem A, Faivre L, et al. Unraveling the intrafamilial correlations and heritability of tumor types in MEN1: a Groupe d'etude des Tumeurs Endocrines study. Eur J Endocrinol 2015;173(6):819–26.
29. Goudet P, Murat A, Binquet C, et al. Risk factors and causes of death in MEN1 disease. A GTE (Groupe d'Etude des Tumeurs Endocrines) cohort study among 758 patients. World J Surg 2010;34(2):249–55.
30. Concolino P, Costella A, Capoluongo E. Multiple endocrine neoplasia type 1 (MEN1): An update of 208 new germline variants reported in the last nine years. Cancer Genet 2016;209(1–2):36–41.
31. Pellegata NS, Quintanilla-Martinez L, Siggelkow H, et al. Germ-line mutations in p27Kip1 cause a multiple endocrine neoplasia syndrome in rats and humans. Proc Natl Acad Sci U S A 2006;103(42):15558–63.
32. Thakker RV. Multiple endocrine neoplasia type 1 (MEN1) and type 4 (MEN4). Mol Cell Endocrinol 2014;386(1–2):2–15.
33. Qiu W, Christakis I, Silva A, et al. Utility of chromogranin A, pancreatic polypeptide, glucagon and gastrin in the diagnosis and follow-up of pancreatic neuroendocrine tumours in multiple endocrine neoplasia type 1 patients. Clin Endocrinol 2016;85(3):400–7.
34. Lemos MC, Thakker RV. Multiple endocrine neoplasia type 1 (MEN1): analysis of 1336 mutations reported in the first decade following identification of the gene. Hum Mutat 2008;29(1):22–32.
35. Romei C, Mariotti S, Fugazzola L, et al. Multiple endocrine neoplasia type 2 syndromes (MEN 2): results from the ItaMEN network analysis on the prevalence of different genotypes and phenotypes. Eur J Endocrinol 2010;163(2):301–8.
36. Cheon JY, Mozersky J, Cook-Deegan R. Variants of uncertain significance in BRCA: a harbinger of ethical and policy issues to come? Genome Med 2014; 6(12):121.
37. Raue F, Frank-Raue K. Genotype-phenotype correlation in multiple endocrine neoplasia type 2. Clinics 2012;67(Suppl 1):69–75.
38. Machens A, Niccoli-Sire P, Hoegel J, et al. Early malignant progression of hereditary medullary thyroid cancer. N Engl J Med 2003;349(16):1517–25.

Clinical Implications for Germline *PTEN* Spectrum Disorders

Joanne Ngeow, MBBS, MRCP, MPH[a,b], Kaitlin Sesock, MSc[b,c,d],
Charis Eng, MD, PhD[b,c,d,e,f,*]

KEYWORDS

- *PTEN* • *PTEN* hamartoma tumor syndrome • Cowden syndrome

KEY POINTS

- Cowden syndrome is a multiple hamartoma syndrome with a high risk for benign and malignant tumors of the thyroid, breast, kidney, and endometrium.
- Affected individuals usually have macrocephaly at birth, and skin features such as trichilemmomas and papillomatous papules present by the late 20s.
- The lifetime risk of developing breast cancer is 85%; the lifetime risk of thyroid cancer is approximately 35%; the lifetime risk of endometrial cancer may approach 28% and renal cancer 34%.
- The diagnosis of *PTEN* hamartoma tumor syndrome is established in a proband by identification of a heterozygous germline *PTEN* pathogenic variant on molecular genetic testing.
- When a proband is identified, genetic testing of asymptomatic at-risk relatives can identify those who have the family-specific pathogenic variant for high-risk cancer surveillance.

INTRODUCTION

PTEN-related disorders represent a group of autosomal-dominant heritable conditions associated with germline mutations in the tumor suppressor gene, *PTEN*, including Cowden syndrome (CS), Bannayan-Riley-Ruvalcaba syndrome, and Proteus-like

---

The authors have nothing to disclose.
[a] Cancer Genetics Service, Division of Medical Oncology, National Cancer Centre, 11 Hospital Drive, Singapore 169610, Singapore; [b] Genomic Medicine Institute, Cleveland Clinic, 9500 Euclid Avenue, NE-50, Cleveland, OH 44195, USA; [c] Lerner Research Institute, Cleveland Clinic, 9500 Euclid Avenue, NE-50, Cleveland, OH 44195, USA; [d] Taussig Cancer Institute, Cleveland Clinic, 9500 Euclid Avenue, NE-50, Cleveland, OH 44195, USA; [e] Department of Genetics and Genome Sciences, Case Western Reserve University School of Medicine, 10900 Euclid Avenue, Cleveland, OH 44106, USA; [f] Germline High Risk Focus Group, CASE Comprehensive Cancer Center, Case Western Reserve University, 10900 Euclid Avenue, Cleveland, OH 44106, USA
* Corresponding author. Cleveland Clinic Genomic Medicine Institute, 9500 Euclid Avenue, NE-50, Cleveland, OH 44195.
E-mail address: engc@ccf.org

Endocrinol Metab Clin N Am 46 (2017) 503–517
http://dx.doi.org/10.1016/j.ecl.2017.01.013
0889-8529/17/© 2017 Elsevier Inc. All rights reserved.

syndrome.[1,2] The first report of CS, the most well-documented clinical condition within this spectrum, was made in 1962 by Dr Macey Dennis and Dr Kenneth M. Lloyd describing a woman, Rachel Cowden, who presented with multiple anomalies including cystic breast disease, multinodular goiter, and oral papillomatosis.[3,4] Rachel Cowden died of metastatic breast cancer in her 30s.[3] The phenotypic spectrum of CS has expanded since its initial description as we longitudinally follow patients and their families. Increasingly, we are recognizing other manifestations associated with CS, such as autism spectrum disorders and other cancer types.[4–6]

The diagnostic criteria for CS were described initially by the International Cowden Consortium in 1995, and these criteria continue to evolve as researchers further delineate the clinical spectrum of CS (**Box 1**).[7] Several mucocutaneous findings are considered to be pathognomonic for CS, including trichilemmomas and other facial papules, acral keratoses, and oral papillomas.[2,4] Individuals with a diagnosis of CS were

---

Box 1
National Comprehensive Cancer Network 2013 Cowden syndrome criteria

Major criteria

Breast cancer

Endometrial cancer (epithelial)

Thyroid cancer (follicular)

Gastrointestinal hamartomas (including ganglioneuromas but excluding hyperplastic polyps; >3)

Lhermitte-Duclos disease (adult)

Macrocephaly (>97th percentile: 58 cm for adult women, 60 cm for adult men)

Macular pigmentation of the glans penis

Multiple mucocutaneous lesions (any of the following):
  Multiple trihilemmomas (>3, ≥1 proven by biopsy)
  Acral keratoses (>3 palmoplantar keratotic pits and/or acral hyperkeratotic papules)
  Mucocutaneous neuromas (>3)
  Oral papillomas (particularly on tongue and gingival), multiple (>3) *or* biopsy proven *or* dermatologist diagnosed

Minor criteria

Autism spectrum disorder

Colon cancer

Esophageal glycogenic acanthosis (>3)

Lipomas (>3)

Intellectual disability (ie, intelligence quotient <75)

Renal cell carcinoma

Testicular lipomatosis

Thyroid cancer (papillary or follicular variant of papillary)

Thyroid structural lesions (eg, adenoma, multinodular goiter)

Vascular anomalies (including multiple intracranial developmental venous anomalies)

Data from Daly MB, Pilarski R, Axilbund JE, et al. Genetic/familial high-risk assessment: breast and ovarian, version 2.2015. J Natl Compr Canc Netw 2016;14(2):153–62.

traditionally thought to be at increased risk of developing benign and malignant tumors of the thyroid and breast.[5,6] Benign findings include lipomas, colonic polyps, and thyroiditis, which are commonly seen in the general population.[6,8] Other associated features such as Lhermitte-Duclos disease are less common, but are important for clinicians to know as possible "red flags" signaling a CS diagnosis. The overlap between the common benign features of CS and the presence of these features in the general population has caused difficulty in elucidating the true prevalence of CS.[2,9] Previous reports approximate an incidence of 1 in 200,000 for CS, although this is likely to be an underestimate.[2,9] In conjunction with the identification of germline *PTEN* mutations in individuals with CS,[4,10] more recent research has recognized additional cancer risks, including endometrial, colorectal, and renal carcinomas, and melanoma as well as an association between germline *PTEN* mutations and neurodevelopmental disorders such as autism spectrum disorder.[11–13]

Bannayan-Riley-Ruvalcaba syndrome, also known as Bannayan-Zonana or Riley-Smith syndrome, was first described as a disorder of pediatric onset associated with macrocephaly, lipomas, thyroiditis, hamartomatous gastrointestinal polyps, penile freckling, and vascular malformations.[4,14–17] Previous literature reported that about 60% of individuals with a diagnosis of Bannayan-Riley-Ruvalcaba syndrome carry a germline *PTEN* mutation.[4,15–17] Bannayan-Riley-Ruvalcaba syndrome has been shown to be allelic to CS by the identification of identical *PTEN* mutations in families segregating both clinical disorders.[2,15–18] Proteus and Proteus-like syndromes are associated with the overgrowth of various tissues, and individuals with both conditions have been found to carry a detectable germline *PTEN* mutation, thus expanding the clinical spectrum of *PTEN*-related disorders.[2,4,15–18]

Owing to the phenotypic variability of the heritable conditions associated with germline *PTEN* mutations, the term *PTEN* hamartoma tumor syndrome (PHTS) is used to describe all individuals, irrespective of the clinical diagnosis or syndrome, with an identified germline *PTEN* mutation.[2] Early literature estimated that about 80% of individuals with a diagnosis of CS had a germline *PTEN* mutation.[10] A study by Tan and colleagues[19] looked at a diverse cohort of individuals with CS accrued from the community and found that germline *PTEN* mutations are present in about 25% of affected individuals. It is important for clinicians to be aware of the wide spectrum of clinical features of PHTS to help differentiate a diagnosis of PHTS from other hereditary cancer syndromes.[20,21]

MOLECULAR GENETICS

The spectrum of germline mutations seen in PHTS extends throughout the coding sequence of *PTEN*. Located on human chromosome subband 10q23.3, the 9-exon *PTEN* gene encodes a 403-amino acid phosphatase with 4 major domains.[12,22,23] *PTEN* is a tumor suppressor gene that participates in the PI3K/AKT/mTOR pathway and is increasingly shown to be involved in many different cellular pathways (**Fig. 1**). The main canonical function of *PTEN* is to antagonize AKT by dephosphorylating phosphatidylinositol 3,4,5-triphosphate (PIP3) to phosphatidylinositol 3,4,5-diphosphate (PIP2).[24–27] Germline mutations in *PTEN* cause an upregulation of the AKT pathway leading to decreased apoptosis and increased cell growth.[24,28,29] Within the N-terminal tail are several key motifs, including the phosphatidyl-inositol-bisphosphate (PIP_2) binding motif and both nuclear and cytoplasmic localization sequences. The protein phosphatase domain contains the catalytic core of the protein, stretching from amino acid 123 to 130. A C2 domain facilitates membrane binding, and the PDZ-binding motif within the C-terminal tail allows protein–protein

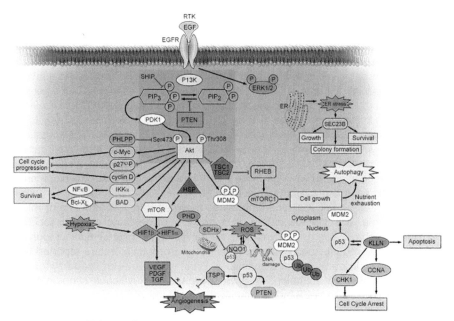

Fig. 1. *PTEN* cellular pathway involvement. Diagram depicts the canonical and non-canonical signaling involving Cowden syndrome (CS)/CS-like–related predisposition genes (*PTEN, AKT, PIK3CA, SDHx, KLLN,* and *SEC23B*). (*Adapted from* Figs. of Refs.[24–29])

interaction.[12,22–24] About one-half of the mutations in *PTEN* occur within the phosphatase domain, which is where the enzymatic activity of *PTEN* occurs. A catalytic core domain lies within the phosphatase domain, and many mutations are found within this area core motif, which disrupt its important enzymatic function.[12,22–24]

Pathogenic variants have been described in all 9 exons of *PTEN*, with various types of mutations identified, including missense, nonsense, splice site variants, intragenic deletions/insertions, and large deletions (**Fig. 2**).[23,30,31] Virtually all germline *PTEN* missense mutations within the coding region are pathogenic.[19,23] Common nonsense/frameshift mutations have been well-described in exons 5, 6, 7, and 8 of *PTEN* as well as specific truncation mutations in exons 5, 7, and 8, which are overrepresented in the *PTEN* mutation spectra[13,24] (see **Fig. 2**). The exon 5 hotspot includes the catalytic core of *PTEN*, and mutations within this 7-amino acid stretch affect probands with a wide variety of clinical presentations. Large deletions and duplications affecting *PTEN* are less common in PHTS than single base pair alterations, although they can be found over the entire coding sequence (see **Fig. 2**). Unfortunately, even the largest cohorts of patients with PHTS are insufficient to identify clear genotype–phenotype associations.

Over the last decade, it became obvious that there are individuals with classic CS without germline *PTEN* mutations. Recent research efforts have resulted in several other germline susceptibility genes for such individuals. Approximately 10% of individuals with classic CS or CS-like phenotypes carry germline heterozygous variants in the genes encoding 3 of the 4 subunits of succinate dehydrogenase or mitochondrial complex II.[32] Single-exon *KLLN*, on 10q23, encodes KILLIN, and shares a bidirectional promoter with *PTEN*. Up to 30% of individuals with CS/CS-like phenotypes, without germline *PTEN* or *SDHx* mutations, were recently found to have germline *KLLN*

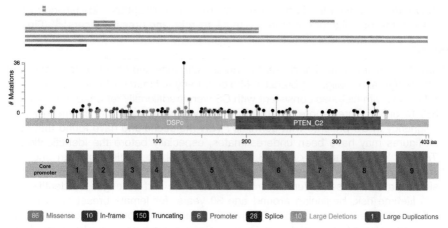

| 86 | Missense | 10 | In-frame | 150 | Truncating | 6 | Promoter | 28 | Splice | 10 | Large Deletions | 1 | Large Duplications |

Fig. 2. *PTEN* germline mutational spectra in 291 probands. The domain structure of phosphatase and tensin homologue (PTEN). PTEN is a 403-amino acid protein that is composed of functional domains: a dual-specificity phosphatase, catalytic domain (DSPc), a C2 domain, a carboxy-terminal tail, and a PDZ-binding domain. PDZ domains are significant regions for protein-protein interactions that play a vital role in cellular signal transduction. The *N*-terminal domain contains the phosphatase domain (the enzymatic activity of PTEN) and it is, therefore, not surprising that the majority of PTEN mutations occur within this domain. The top solid bars represent large deletions and large duplications within the *PTEN* gene. Frequency of point mutations reported in probands is shown which correlates with the vertical height of the line (*middle*). Mutations have been identified in the promoter and all 9 exons of *PTEN* (*bottom*). A key at the bottom of the figure denotes the total number of unique alterations within each category of mutation identified in 291 probands. Missense mutations = green; in-frame mutations = brown; truncating mutations = black; promoter alterations = red; splice alterations = purple; large deletions = orange; large duplications = pink. (*From* Tan MH, Mester J, Peterson C, et al. A clinical scoring system for selection of patients for PTEN mutation testing is proposed on the basis of a prospective study of 3042 probands. Am J Hum Genet 2011;88(1):42–56; with permission.)

promoter hypermethylation.[33] Another 9% of unrelated CS individuals without germline *PTEN* mutations were found to have germline *PIK3CA* mutations and 2% harbored germline *AKT1* mutations.[34] Functionally, we saw a significant increase of phosphorylated-AKT1 levels in these patients' lymphoblastoid cell lines supporting their potential role as novel CS susceptibility genes.[34] More recently, germline heterozygous gain-of-function mutations in *SEC23B* have been identified in approximately 5% of CS patients and enriched in apparently sporadic thyroid cancer patients.[35] Gain-of-function germline mutations in *EGFR* have been seen in a unique CS family presenting with Lhermitte-Duclos disease.[36]

CANCER CLINICAL FEATURES

Before the association of germline *PTEN* mutations with CS, it was recognized that individuals with CS were at an increased risk of developing thyroid and breast cancers.[6] Additional research performed over recent years has expanded the spectra of cancers associated with germline *PTEN* mutations to include cancers of the endometrium, kidney, and colon, and melanoma as well as benign findings such as GI polyposis.[2,6,8,13] To date, 3 studies have reexamined the lifetime risks for malignancy and germline

PTEN mutations, with the largest study by Tan and colleagues[13] identifying significantly increased risks for endometrial, renal, thyroid, and breast cancers[1,37] (**Fig. 3**).

Breast

Many CS patients may first present to breast surgeons and oncologists because of both benign and malignant breast pathology. Early estimates of breast cancer risk for females with histories consistent with CS were traditionally reported to be around 25% to 50%.[6] Three more recent studies have reexamined the lifetime risks for malignancy in CS patients with germline *PTEN* mutations and have found that early risk figures may have been underestimates, especially before the identification of *PTEN*.[1,4,13,37] The largest of the 3 most recent cohort studies, by Tan and colleagues,[13] identified increased risks for several types of cancer, with the highest risk estimate increase for female breast cancer. Tan and colleagues[13] identified an 85% lifetime risk, beginning around age 30 years, for female breast cancer, with 50% penetrance by age 50 years. This risk figure is comparable to that quoted for patients with Hereditary Breast and Ovarian Cancer syndrome.[4] A similar study by

Lifetime Risks of Cancer for Patients with PHTS

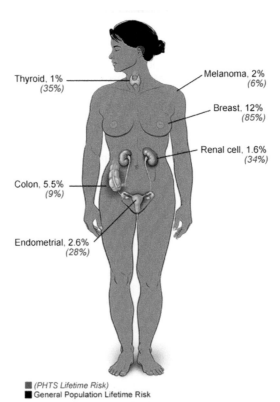

Thyroid, 1%
(35%)

Melanoma, 2%
(6%)

Breast, 12%
(85%)

Renal cell, 1.6%
(34%)

Colon, 5.5%
(9%)

Endometrial, 2.6%
(28%)

■ (PHTS Lifetime Risk)
■ General Population Lifetime Risk

Fig. 3. Lifetime cancer risks for individuals with germline *PTEN* mutations. Lifetime cancer risks for *PTEN* hamartoma tumor syndrome are shown in black; organ-specific lifetime risk for cancer in the general population is shown in brackets in gray. (*From* Tan MH, Mester JL, Ngeow J, et al. Lifetime cancer risks in individuals with germline PTEN mutations. Clin Cancer Res 2012;18(2):400–7; with permission.)

Bubien and colleagues[1] found a cumulative 77% risk for female breast cancer at age 70 years for women with *PTEN* mutations. In addition, Nieuwenhuis and colleagues[37] identified a 67% risk for females with germline *PTEN* mutations developing breast cancer by age 60 years.

Several studies have also considered *PTEN* mutation status related to primary and second primary breast cancer diagnoses, and found that women with *PTEN* mutations are at increased risk for both.[4,38] These studies also identified that women with *PTEN* mutations who have had a diagnosis of breast cancer have a 29% risk of developing a secondary breast cancer within 10 years.[4,38] Women may choose to pursue prophylactic mastectomy for these reasons, particularly if the patients have associated benign breast lesions, making breast cancer surveillance difficult. Breast cancer has been described in males with *PTEN* mutations, but an overall increased risk for male breast cancer was not established in a recent study of more than 3000 patients, although the adults in the cohort were mostly female patients.[19,39]

Thyroid

The only population-based clinical epidemiologic study, performed before the discovery of *PTEN*, suggested that two-thirds of CS patients have benign thyroid disease, and 10% have malignant thyroid neoplasias.[6] However, a systematic study of thyroid neoplasms from a prospectively accrued series of individuals with CS and CS-like features have revised the lifetime thyroid cancer risk for individuals with germline *PTEN* mutations upwards to be around 34%, with the earliest age at diagnosis of 7 years.[1,13,37] Thyroid pathology in PHTS typically affects follicular cells,[40,41] with follicular thyroid carcinoma (FTC) considered a major diagnostic criterion and an important feature in PHTS. Benign thyroid lesions, such as thyroid nodules, multinodular goiter, and Hashimoto's thyroiditis, are also common in individuals with germline *PTEN* mutations.[4] An individual's risk of developing epithelial thyroid cancer was increased by 70-fold when compared with the general population.[19] FTC was overrepresented in a cohort of germline *PTEN* mutation positive individuals, the ratio of FTC to the more common papillary thyroid cancer was 1 in 2 among PHTS patients as compared with approximately 1 in 14 in the general population.[42] Several reports of thyroid cancer in children with germline *PTEN* mutations[43] have been described, emphasizing the need to begin thyroid screening annually at the time of PHTS diagnosis.[4,44]

The prevalence of germline *PTEN* mutations in unselected differentiated thyroid cancer is low (<1%).[45,46] A pediatric onset of thyroid cancer, male gender, history of thyroid nodules and/or thyroiditis, and FTC histology were factors that were found to be predictive of PHTS in a cohort of patients with CS and CS-like disease and with thyroid cancer.[42] These "red flags" and/or a family history of cancers, and physical signs such as macrocephaly and mucocutaneous features should alert the clinician to the possibility of CS.

Gastrointestinal Tract

Whether GI neoplasias, especially malignancies, are true component phenotypes of CS was not certain owing to the lack of systematic studies. In the largest study to date, Heald and colleagues[8] demonstrated almost all (>90%) *PTEN* mutation carriers who had a colonoscopy performed as part of clinical care, had colorectal polyps typically with a mix of histologic subtypes. Patients who developed colorectal carcinomas also tended to have multiple, and mixed, polyps. A small increase in the lifetime risk for colorectal cancer has been associated with PHTS (9%).[13] These findings led to a change in clinical practice; colorectal surveillance should now be offered to any

PTEN mutation carrier, especially those with multiple lower GI polyps. In *PTEN* mutation carriers, upper GI polyps do occur with some frequency, and, for a subset of patients, they do experience symptoms. Notably, a significant proportion (approximately 20%) of those with upper GI examinations had glycogenic acanthosis.[8,47,48]

Endometrial

Individuals with germline *PTEN* mutations have a 28% lifetime risk of developing endometrial cancer.[13] A recent study showed that age less than 50 years at presentation of endometrial carcinoma, macrocephaly, and/or prevalent or synchronous renal cell carcinoma in these women could predict for germline *PTEN* mutation.[42] The mean age of endometrial cancer diagnosis in those with *PTEN* mutations was 44 years, with three-quarters diagnosed at less than 50 years of age. This observation may guide the age range for consideration of surveillance or prophylactic surgery. Individuals with germline *PTEN* mutations are also additionally at increased risk of developing benign findings of the endometrium, such as uterine fibroids.[13]

Renal

Patients with PHTS have a 34% lifetime risk of developing renal cell carcinoma (RCC).[13] The reported histology of each mutation positive patient's RCC was variable. However, on central pathology re-review of 8 patients, 6 examined lesions were determined to be of papillary subhistology, with the other 2 patients' tumors consistent with the initial report of chromophobe RCC. Immunohistochemistry demonstrated complete loss of PTEN protein in all *PTEN* mutation positive patients' papillary RCCs and patchy positivity in 1 chromophome RCC. Physicians caring for PHTS patients should have a low threshold for investigating possible RCC in patients with relevant complaints. Renal ultrasound examination is not sensitive for detecting papillary RCC, especially if small, and so PHTS patients should have alternate renal imaging (computed tomography san or MRI).[49] Recent research has also identified a small increase in the estimated lifetime risk for melanoma (6%) for individuals with germline *PTEN* mutations.[4,13]

NONCANCER CLINICAL FEATURES
Neurologic

The first case study of a child with a *PTEN* mutation and autism described a boy who inherited a nonsense mutation from his mother, who herself was diagnosed with CS but did not have social or intellectual disabilities.[12] After this report, which recommended *PTEN* mutation scanning in cases of macrocephaly with pervasive developmental delay, came the first estimate of mutation frequency in a prospective series of patients with macrocephaly and autism. In 2005, Butler and colleagues[11] reported 3 *PTEN* mutations in a series of 18 children with macrocephaly and autism spectrum disorder. This benchmark prevalence of 17% remains near the weighted average reported across nearly 10 subsequent studies.[50] Together, these results provide a strong case for the association of germline *PTEN* mutation in children with autism spectrum disorder and macrocephaly. These data form the basis for the recommendation of genetic testing in this subset of autism spectrum disorder patients. The degree of macrocephaly observed in patients with autism spectrum disorder and *PTEN* mutations is often more severe than that seen in those with wild-type *PTEN*. A 2011 study examined OFCs in a cohort of 181 *PTEN* mutation carriers, finding their average head size to be +3.5 standard deviations (SDs) from average in adults and +5 SDs in the pediatric subset.[21] Recently, a series of case reports demonstrated epileptic seizures in *PTEN* mutation-positive patients, often linked to underlying cortical dysplasia.[51] Further studies are needed to fully understand the full neurologic sequelae of *PTEN* mutation carriers including cognitive profile.

Metabolic, Immunologic, and Others

Pal and colleagues[52] studied the impact of *PTEN* haploinsufficiency in a cohort of patients and identified that it is a monogenic cause of profound constitutive insulin sensitization. Fasting insulin levels were significantly lower in the *PTEN* mutation carriers than in controls; because the liver is the principal insulin-responsive tissue, the fasting insulin level predominantly reflects insulin resistance in the liver. The authors observed a significant association between *PTEN* haploinsufficiency and increased insulin sensitivity of muscle tissue and that PTEN deficiency enhances insulin signaling in both muscle and liver tissue in humans, possibly by way of its action on the PI3K–AKT pathway. The *PTEN* mutation carriers were obese as compared with population-based controls. This increased body mass in the patients was owing to augmented adiposity without corresponding changes in fat distribution. The authors demonstrated an apparently divergent effect of *PTEN* mutations: increased risks of obesity and cancer but a decreased risk of type 2 diabetes owing to enhanced insulin sensitivity. These data support a large body of studies linking PTEN with the insulin receptor substrate 1/2 (IRS1/2) pathways.[43,53]

Clinicians have observed that PHTS patients commonly suffer from a range of immune-related disorders such as thyroiditis[42] and eosinophilic esophagitis.[54] Indeed, a recent study showed that autoimmunity and peripheral lymphoid hyperplasia was found in 43% of 79 PHTS patients. In a recent study, we reported that immune dysregulation in PHTS patients included lymphopenia, $CD4^+$ T-cell reduction and changes in T- and B-cell subsets.[36]

IDENTIFYING PATIENTS FOR GENETICS RISK ASSESSMENT

CS can be differentiated from other hereditary cancer syndromes including hereditary breast ovarian cancer syndrome, Lynch syndrome, and other hamartomatous polyposis syndromes based on personal as well as family history but, given the protean nature of CS and lack of general awareness among clinicians, this differentiation can be challenging.[20] Additionally, because of the high frequency of de novo *PTEN* germline mutations,[55] a family history of associated cancers may not be apparent. Furthermore, many of the benign features of CS are common in the general population making the diagnosis of CS a challenge for most clinicians. An occipitofrontal head circumference in adults of greater than 2 SDs is seen in the majority of adult PHTS patients; this is one useful clinical feature that can help to flag which cancer patients are at risk of PHTS. Any cancer patient with a large occipitofrontal head circumference should be assessed for personal/family history of other CS-related features (eg thyroiditis, polyps, developmental delay/autism and other malignancies) and be referred for genetic risk assessment.[20,21,56]

To aid in the clinical diagnosis, a clinical predictor (Cleveland Clinic *PTEN* Risk Calculator) was developed based on clinical features derived from a prospective study of more than 3000 patients suspected of having CS.[19] The questionnaire-based clinical decision tool is available online (http://www.lerner.ccf.org/gmi/ccscore/) to assist clinicians at the point of patient care. Based on a patient's presentation, a score (CC score) will be derived that corresponds with an estimated risk for germline *PTEN* mutation to guide clinicians for referral to genetics professionals. A CC score at a threshold of 15 (CC15) corresponds with a 10% a priori risk of a germline *PTEN* mutation detection, which is the lowest among different strategies tested. At a cost-effectiveness threshold of $100,000 per quality-adjusted life-year, CC15 is the optimal strategy for female patients older than 50 years, and CC10 is the optimal strategy for female patients younger than 50 years of age and male patients of all ages.[57] Thus, patients with a CC score of greater than 10 should be considered for genetic risk assessment referral. Additionally, the American College of Medical Genetics published a practical guide for which patients should be referred for genetic assessment for CS. They recommend referral for anyone meeting any 3 criteria from the major or minor diagnostic criteria (see **Box 1**). Referral should be considered for any individual with a personal history of or first-degree relative with (1) Lhermitte–Duclos disease diagnosed after age 18 or (2) any 3 criteria from the major or minor diagnostic criteria list in the same person.[58]

For pediatric cases, we recommend that the presence of macrocephaly (occipito-frontal head circumference > 2 SD over the population mean, or 97.5th percentile) was a necessary criterion for diagnosis, based on 100% prevalence at the point of diagnosis.[19] Neurologic (autism and developmental delay) and dermatologic (lipomas, oral papillomas) features represented extremely common secondary features; either or both systems were involved in 100% of patients with germline *PTEN* mutation. However, given that dermatologic features may often be overlooked, less prevalent features in patients at first presentation in the pediatric setting are likely to be at least as important, such as vascular (such as arteriovenous) malformations, gastrointestinal polyps, thyroid goiter, and early onset cancers (thyroid and germ cell), and warrant consideration for *PTEN* testing (**Table 1**).

SURVEILLANCE AND MANAGEMENT OF COWDEN SYNDROME

The mucocutaneous manifestations of CS are rarely life threatening. If asymptomatic, observation alone is prudent. When symptomatic, topical agents (eg, 5-fluorouracil), curettage, cryosurgery, or laser ablation may provide only temporary relief.[59] Treatment for the benign and malignant manifestations of PHTS is similar to their sporadic counterparts. Some women at increased risk for breast cancer consider prophylactic mastectomy, especially if complicated by existing benign breast disease and/or if repeated breast biopsies have been necessary. The recommendation of prophylactic mastectomy is a generalization for women at increased risk for breast cancer from a variety of causes, not just from PHTS and is best managed by breast surgeons with a specialty interest in high-risk breast cancer patients.

Table 1
Pediatric criteria for consideration of *PTEN* hamartoma tumor syndrome

Required Criteria	Secondary Criteria
Macrocephaly (≥2 SD)	At least 1 of the following should be present: • Autism or developmental delay • Dermatologic features (lipomas, oral papillomas, trichilemmomas, penile freckling) • Vascular features (arteriovenous malformations or hemangiomas) • Gastrointestinal polyps • Pediatric-onset thyroid cancer or germ cell tumors

Data from Tan MH, Mester J, Peterson C, et al. A clinical scoring system for selection of patients for PTEN mutation testing is proposed on the basis of a prospective study of 3042 probands. Am J Hum Genet 2011;88(1):42–56.

The most serious consequences of PHTS relate to the increased risk of cancers, including breast, thyroid, endometrial, and, to a lesser extent, renal cancers. In this regard, the most important aspect of management of any individual with a *PTEN* mutation is increased cancer surveillance to detect any tumors at the earliest, most treatable stages. Current surveillance and management guidelines for adults can be found in **Table 2**. Management of the malignant and benign manifestations of PHTS varies depending on the age of the individual.[13] For adults, current recommendations include annual a comprehensive physical examination and dermatologic examination beginning at the age of 18 years.[13] Screening for additional cancer types may begin at the ages listed in **Table 1**, or 5 to 10 years before the youngest diagnosis of that particular type of cancer in the family if this is earlier.[4,13] For children, it is currently recommended to perform an annual dermatologic examination and annual thyroid ultrasound examination at the age of PHTS diagnosis.[13] Earlier screening may be advisable because thyroiditis and nodules are seen by the time patients reach adolescence, and cancer diagnosis occurs on average 14 years earlier than expected. Furthermore, the thyroid cancer risks observed may justify prophylactic total thyroidectomy in select PHTS patients undergoing surgery for benign thyroid disease.[44]

FUTURE CONSIDERATIONS AND SUMMARY

Patients with PHTS may present to a variety of different subspecialties with benign and malignant clinical features. They have increased lifetime risks of breast, endometrial, thyroid, renal, and colon cancers as well as neurodevelopmental disorders such autism spectrum disorder. Patients and affected family members can be offered

Table 2
Cancer risks and screening recommendations for *PTEN* hamartoma tumor syndrome

Cancer	General Population Risk (%)	Lifetime Risk with *PTEN* Hamartoma Tumor Syndrome (%)	Age at Presentation	Screening Recommendations
Breast	12	~85	40s	Starting at age 30 Annual mammogram Consider MRI for patients with dense breasts
Thyroid	1	35	30s–40s	Baseline ultrasound examination at diagnosis Annual ultrasound and clinical examination
Endometrial	2.6	28	40s–50s	Starting at age 30 Annual endometrial biopsy or transvaginal ultrasound examination
Renal cell	1.6	34	50s	Starting at age 40 Renal imaging every 2 y
Colon	5	9	40s	Starting at age 40 Colonoscopy every 2 y
Melanoma	2	6	40s	Annual dermatologic examination

Data from Tan MH, Mester JL, Ngeow J, et al. Lifetime cancer risks in individuals with germline PTEN mutations. Clin Cancer Res 2012;18(2):400–7.

gene-directed surveillance and management. Patients who are unaffected can be spared unnecessary investigations. With longitudinal follow-up, we are likely to identify other noncancer manifestations associated with PHTS such as metabolic, immunologic, and neurologic features.

ACKNOWLEDGMENTS

We would like to thank Ms Lamis Yehia and the Centre for Medical Art and Photography, Cleveland Clinic for their kind assistance for the artwork presented.

REFERENCES

1. Bubien V, Bonnet F, Brouste V, et al. High cumulative risks of cancer in patients with PTEN hamartoma tumour syndrome. J Med Genet 2013;50(4):255–63.
2. Eng C. PTEN hamartoma tumor syndrome (PHTS). In: Pagon RA, Adam MP, Ardinger HH, editors. GeneReviews(R). Seattle (WA): University of Washington, Seattle; 1993.
3. Lloyd KM 2nd, Dennis M. Cowden's disease. A possible new symptom complex with multiple system involvement. Ann Intern Med 1963;58:136–42.
4. Mester J, Eng C. Cowden syndrome: recognizing and managing a not-so-rare hereditary cancer syndrome. J Surg Oncol 2015;111(1):125–30.
5. Brownstein MH, Wolf M, Bikowski JB. Cowden's disease: a cutaneous marker of breast cancer. Cancer 1978;41(6):2393–8.
6. Starink TM, van der Veen JP, Arwert F, et al. The Cowden syndrome: a clinical and genetic study in 21 patients. Clin Genet 1986;29(3):222–33.
7. Pilarski R, Eng C. Will the real Cowden syndrome please stand up (again)? Expanding mutational and clinical spectra of the PTEN hamartoma tumour syndrome. J Med Genet 2004;41(5):323–6.
8. Heald B, Mester J, Rybicki L, et al. Frequent gastrointestinal polyps and colorectal adenocarcinomas in a prospective series of PTEN mutation carriers. Gastroenterology 2010;139(6):1927–33.
9. Nelen MR, Padberg GW, Peeters EA, et al. Localization of the gene for Cowden disease to chromosome 10q22-23. Nat Genet 1996;13(1):114–6.
10. Liaw D, Marsh DJ, Li J, et al. Germline mutations of the PTEN gene in Cowden disease, an inherited breast and thyroid cancer syndrome. Nat Genet 1997; 16(1):64–7.
11. Butler MG, Dasouki MJ, Zhou XP, et al. Subset of individuals with autism spectrum disorders and extreme macrocephaly associated with germline PTEN tumour suppressor gene mutations. J Med Genet 2005;42(4):318–21.
12. Goffin A, Hoefsloot LH, Bosgoed E, et al. PTEN mutation in a family with Cowden syndrome and autism. Am J Med Genet 2001;105(6):521–4.
13. Tan MH, Mester JL, Ngeow J, et al. Lifetime cancer risks in individuals with germline PTEN mutations. Clin Cancer Res 2012;18(2):400–7.
14. Gorlin RJ, Cohen MM Jr, Condon LM, et al. Bannayan-Riley-Ruvalcaba syndrome. Am J Med Genet 1992;44(3):307–14.
15. Marsh DJ, Coulon V, Lunetta KL, et al. Mutation spectrum and genotype-phenotype analyses in Cowden disease and Bannayan-Zonana syndrome, two hamartoma syndromes with germline PTEN mutation. Hum Mol Genet 1998; 7(3):507–15.
16. Marsh DJ, Dahia PL, Zheng Z, et al. Germline mutations in PTEN are present in Bannayan-Zonana syndrome. Nat Genet 1997;16(4):333–4.

17. Marsh DJ, Kum JB, Lunetta KL, et al. PTEN mutation spectrum and genotype-phenotype correlations in Bannayan-Riley-Ruvalcaba syndrome suggest a single entity with Cowden syndrome. Hum Mol Genet 1999;8(8):1461–72.

18. Zhou XP, Marsh DJ, Hampel H, et al. Germline and germline mosaic PTEN mutations associated with a Proteus-like syndrome of hemihypertrophy, lower limb asymmetry, arteriovenous malformations and lipomatosis. Hum Mol Genet 2000;9(5):765–8.

19. Tan MH, Mester J, Peterson C, et al. A clinical scoring system for selection of patients for PTEN mutation testing is proposed on the basis of a prospective study of 3042 probands. Am J Hum Genet 2011;88(1):42–56.

20. Mester JL, Moore RA, Eng C. PTEN germline mutations in patients initially tested for other hereditary cancer syndromes: would use of risk assessment tools reduce genetic testing? Oncologist 2013;18(10):1083–90.

21. Mester JL, Tilot AK, Rybicki LA, et al. Analysis of prevalence and degree of macrocephaly in patients with germline PTEN mutations and of brain weight in Pten knock-in murine model. Eur J Hum Genet 2011;19(7):763–8.

22. Fanning AS, Anderson JM. PDZ domains: fundamental building blocks in the organization of protein complexes at the plasma membrane. J Clin Invest 1999; 103(6):767–72.

23. Zbuk KM, Eng C. Cancer phenomics: RET and PTEN as illustrative models. Nat Rev Cancer 2007;7(1):35–45.

24. Mester J, Eng C. When overgrowth bumps into cancer: the PTEN-opathies. Am J Med Genet C Semin Med Genet 2013;163C(2):114–21.

25. Neshat MS, Mellinghoff IK, Tran C, et al. Enhanced sensitivity of PTEN-deficient tumors to inhibition of FRAP/mTOR. Proc Natl Acad Sci U S A 2001;98(18): 10314–9.

26. Podsypanina K, Lee RT, Politis C, et al. An inhibitor of mTOR reduces neoplasia and normalizes p70/S6 kinase activity in Pten+/- mice. Proc Natl Acad Sci U S A 2001;98(18):10320–5.

27. Sekulic A, Hudson CC, Homme JL, et al. A direct linkage between the phosphoinositide 3-kinase-AKT signaling pathway and the mammalian target of rapamycin in mitogen-stimulated and transformed cells. Cancer Res 2000;60(13):3504–13.

28. Furnari FB, Lin H, Huang HS, et al. Growth suppression of glioma cells by PTEN requires a functional phosphatase catalytic domain. Proc Natl Acad Sci U S A 1997;94(23):12479–84.

29. Weng LP, Smith WM, Dahia PL, et al. PTEN suppresses breast cancer cell growth by phosphatase activity-dependent G1 arrest followed by cell death. Cancer Res 1999;59(22):5808–14.

30. Pezzolesi MG, Zbuk KM, Waite KA, et al. Comparative genomic and functional analyses reveal a novel cis-acting PTEN regulatory element as a highly conserved functional E-box motif deleted in Cowden syndrome. Hum Mol Genet 2007;16(9):1058–71.

31. Teresi RE, Zbuk KM, Pezzolesi MG, et al. Cowden syndrome-affected patients with PTEN promoter mutations demonstrate abnormal protein translation. Am J Hum Genet 2007;81(4):756–67.

32. Ni Y, Zbuk KM, Sadler T, et al. Germline mutations and variants in the succinate dehydrogenase genes in Cowden and Cowden-like syndromes. Am J Hum Genet 2008;83(2):261–8.

33. Bennett KL, Mester J, Eng C. Germline epigenetic regulation of KILLIN in Cowden and Cowden-like syndrome. JAMA 2010;304(24):2724–31.

34. Orloff MS, He X, Peterson C, et al. Germline PIK3CA and AKT1 mutations in Cowden and Cowden-like syndromes. Am J Hum Genet 2013;92(1):76–80.
35. Yehia L, Niazi F, Ni Y, et al. Germline heterozygous variants in SEC23B are associated with Cowden syndrome and enriched in apparently sporadic thyroid cancer. Am J Hum Genet 2015;97(5):661–76.
36. Colby S, Yehia L, Niazi F, et al. Exome sequencing reveals germline gain-of-function EGFR mutation in an adult with Lhermitte-Duclos disease. Cold Spring Harb Mol Case Stud 2016;2(6):a001230.
37. Nieuwenhuis MH, Kets CM, Murphy-Ryan M, et al. Cancer risk and genotype-phenotype correlations in PTEN hamartoma tumor syndrome. Fam Cancer 2014;13(1):57–63.
38. Ngeow J, Stanuch K, Mester JL, et al. Second malignant neoplasms in patients with Cowden syndrome with underlying germline PTEN mutations. J Clin Oncol 2014;32(17):1818–24.
39. Fackenthal JD, Marsh DJ, Richardson AL, et al. Male breast cancer in Cowden syndrome patients with germline PTEN mutations. J Med Genet 2001;38(3):159–64.
40. Harach HR, Soubeyran I, Brown A, et al. Thyroid pathologic findings in patients with Cowden disease. Ann Diagn Pathol 1999;3(6):331–40.
41. Parisi MA, Dinulos MB, Leppig KA, et al. The spectrum and evolution of phenotypic findings in PTEN mutation positive cases of Bannayan-Riley-Ruvalcaba syndrome. J Med Genet 2001;38(1):52–8.
42. Ngeow J, Mester J, Rybicki LA, et al. Incidence and clinical characteristics of thyroid cancer in prospective series of individuals with Cowden and Cowden-like syndrome characterized by germline PTEN, SDH, or KLLN alterations. J Clin Endocrinol Metab 2011;96(12):E2063–71.
43. Ozes ON, Akca H, Mayo LD, et al. A phosphatidylinositol 3-kinase/Akt/mTOR pathway mediates and PTEN antagonizes tumor necrosis factor inhibition of insulin signaling through insulin receptor substrate-1. Proc Natl Acad Sci U S A 2001;98(8):4640–5.
44. Milas M, Mester J, Metzger R, et al. Should patients with Cowden syndrome undergo prophylactic thyroidectomy? Surgery 2012;152(6):1201–10.
45. Nagy R, Ganapathi S, Comeras I, et al. Frequency of germline PTEN mutations in differentiated thyroid cancer. Thyroid 2011;21(5):505–10.
46. Dahia PL, Marsh DJ, Zheng Z, et al. Somatic deletions and mutations in the Cowden disease gene, PTEN, in sporadic thyroid tumors. Cancer Res 1997;57(21):4710–3.
47. Nishizawa A, Satoh T, Watanabe R, et al. Cowden syndrome: a novel mutation and overlooked glycogenic acanthosis in gingiva. Br J Dermatol 2009;160(5):1116–8.
48. McGarrity TJ, Wagner Baker MJ, Ruggiero FM, et al. GI polyposis and glycogenic acanthosis of the esophagus associated with PTEN mutation positive Cowden syndrome in the absence of cutaneous manifestations. Am J Gastroenterol 2003;98(6):1429–34.
49. Mester JL, Zhou M, Prescott N, et al. Papillary renal cell carcinoma is associated with PTEN hamartoma tumor syndrome. Urology 2012;79(5):1187.e1-7.
50. Tilot AK, Frazier TW 2nd, Eng C. Balancing proliferation and connectivity in PTEN-associated autism spectrum disorder. Neurotherapeutics 2015;12(3):609–19.
51. Conti S, Condo M, Posar A, et al. Phosphatase and tensin homolog (PTEN) gene mutations and autism: literature review and a case report of a patient with Cowden syndrome, autistic disorder, and epilepsy. J Child Neurol 2012;27(3):392–7.

52. Pal A, Barber TM, Van de Bunt M, et al. PTEN mutations as a cause of constitutive insulin sensitivity and obesity. N Engl J Med 2012;367(11):1002–11.
53. Simpson L, Li J, Liaw D, et al. PTEN expression causes feedback upregulation of insulin receptor substrate 2. Mol Cell Biol 2001;21(12):3947–58.
54. Henderson CJ, Ngeow J, Collins MH, et al. Increased prevalence of eosinophilic gastrointestinal disorders in pediatric PTEN hamartoma tumor syndromes. J Pediatr Gastroenterol Nutr 2014;58(5):553–60.
55. Mester J, Eng C. Estimate of de novo mutation frequency in probands with PTEN hamartoma tumor syndrome. Genet Med 2012;14(9):819–22.
56. Shiovitz S, Everett J, Huang SC, et al. Head circumference in the clinical detection of PTEN hamartoma tumor syndrome in a clinic population at high-risk of breast cancer. Breast Cancer Res Treat 2010;124(2):459–65.
57. Ngeow J, Liu C, Zhou K, et al. Detecting germline PTEN mutations among at-risk patients with cancer: an age- and sex-specific cost-effectiveness analysis. J Clin Oncol 2015;33(23):2537–44.
58. Hampel H, Bennett RL, Buchanan A, et al. A practice guideline from the American College of Medical Genetics and Genomics and the National Society of Genetic Counselors: referral indications for cancer predisposition assessment. Genet Med 2015;17(1):70–87.
59. Hildenbrand C, Burgdorf WH, Lautenschlager S. Cowden syndrome-diagnostic skin signs. Dermatology 2001;202(4):362–6.

Genetics of Disorders of Sex Development

The DSD-TRN Experience

Emmanuèle C. Délot, PhD[a],*,
Jeanette C. Papp, PhD[b], the DSD-TRN Genetics Workgroup,
David E. Sandberg, PhD[c], Eric Vilain, MD, PhD[d]

KEYWORDS

- Disorders of sex development • Genotype • Phenotype • Genomic sequencing

KEY POINTS

- Although many next-generation sequencing platforms are being developed around the world, implementation is facing multiple hurdles from clinicians' habits, institutional constraints, and insurance coverage.
- A strong hurdle to the full adherence of clinical teams to the Disorders of Sex Development-Translational Research Network (DSD-TRN) guidelines for standardization of reporting and practice is the current lack of integration of the standardized clinical forms into the various electronic medical records at different sites.
- Time allocated to research (eg, registry data entry) is also severely limited at most sites for lack of funding supporting this new effort of development and implementation of best practices.
- In spite of these hurdles, genetic information for half the enrolled patients is already available in the DSD-TRN registry, and early results demonstrate the value of such an infrastructure.

Samples of a physical examination form, an intake form, a cumulative genetics form, and monthly clinic reports are available on http://www.endo.theclinics.com.

The authors have nothing to disclose.
[a] Departments of Human Genetics and Pediatrics, David Geffen School of Medicine, University of California, Los Angeles, Room 5301A, 695 Charles East Young Drive South, Los Angeles, CA 90095, USA; [b] Department of Human Genetics, David Geffen School of Medicine, University of California, Los Angeles, Room 5506, 695 Charles East Young Drive South, Los Angeles, CA 90095, USA; [c] Division of Pediatric Psychology, Department of Pediatrics & Communicable Diseases and the Child Health Evaluation and Research Center, University of Michigan Medical School, 1500 East Medical Center Drive, Ann Arbor, MI 48109, USA; [d] Departments of Human Genetics, Urology, and Pediatrics, David Geffen School of Medicine, University of California, Los Angeles, Room 4554B, 695 Charles East Young Drive South, Los Angeles, CA 90095, USA
* Corresponding author.
E-mail address: edelot@ucla.edu

Endocrinol Metab Clin N Am 46 (2017) 519–537
http://dx.doi.org/10.1016/j.ecl.2017.01.015
0889-8529/17/© 2017 Elsevier Inc. All rights reserved.

The Disorders of Sex Development (DSD) Consensus Conference, held in Chicago in 2005, identified several domains of care where improvement was needed.[1] In particular, it called for the establishment of an infrastructure for collaborative interdisciplinary clinical practice and research, with the goal of integrating scientific understanding of DSD with real-time standardization and improvement in clinical practice. The DSD-Translational Research Network (DSD-TRN) was created in response, the first such North American infrastructure, a network of 4 (now expanded to 10) research and clinical sites and a central registry, with the collaboration of Accord Alliance, a nonprofit convener of diverse DSD stakeholders. To address the variability within and across medical, surgical, and behavioral health aspects of care, the DSD-TRN is dedicated to the standardization of diagnostic and treatment protocols in order to enhance clinical and scientific discovery, as well as quality of life outcomes for patients and their families. A critical aspect of this standardization of practice is a commitment to an early and comprehensive diagnostic process (including genetic), associated with extensive standardized phenotyping and psychosocial screening and support of patients and families. A recent review of the state of clinical, biochemical, genetic, and psychosocial evaluations of the newborn or adolescent with DSD, 10 years after the consensus statement, continued to highlight the need for a thorough diagnostic process that sets in motion informed discussions with parents (and newly diagnosed adolescent patients) regarding treatment options.[2] Developmental pathways of sex determination and differentiation impacted in isolated and syndromic DSD conditions were recently reviewed.[3–5] This article will briefly review the main categories of genetic causes of DSD and the diagnostic revolution promised by the advent of new genomic technology, and will present the DSD-TRN guidelines for genetic diagnosis, features of the registry for future research, and a peek into some early registry data.

DISORDERS OF SEX DEVELOPMENT PHENOTYPIC AND GENOTYPIC SPECTRUM

The term DSD encompasses a wide phenotypic spectrum, and, while DSDs associated with uncertain gender assignment are relatively rare, the prevalence of DSDs as a whole might have been underestimated. Depending on what conditions are included, combined incidences from 1 case per 200 patients to 1% to 2% are routinely quoted, with great differences between conditions.[2] Hypospadias (atypical location of the urethral meatus) is reported to have increased to approximately 1 case per 125 newborn boys, and cryptorchidism (failure of testicular descent) is seen in as many as 3% of full-term newborn boys.[6] Evidence is emerging that these conditions may represent part of a phenotypic spectrum, sharing a genetic etiology with more complex forms of DSDs.[7]

DSDs have been historically classified according to overlapping categories:

Sex chromosome complement—46,XX, 46,XY, other, mosaic
Gonadal structure—testicular DSD, ovotesticular DSD, gonadal dysgenesis
Gonadal functional status—gonadal dysgenesis, disorders of androgen biosynthesis

When presenting as developmental disorders, DSDs may be isolated, or part of a syndrome, typically of unknown etiology:

- Isolated hypospadias (46,XY)
- Cloacal exstrophy/OEIS spectrum (46,XX or 46,XY)
- Müllerian structures, developmental anomalies (MRKH, vaginal atresia, Müllerian agenesis; 46,XX)

In addition, DSDs can be found as part of complex multiorgan developmental syndromes.[5]

Known genetic causes of DSDs range from chromosomal aneuploidies, such as Turner syndrome or Klinefelter syndrome, to small copy number variants (CNVs) of open reading frames or promoter regions, to discrete variants in single genes. Major single gene etiologies of isolated or syndromic DSD are listed in **Table 1**. Broad categories include

Sex chromosome complement variants—Turner syndrome (45, X, typically mosaic), Klinefelter syndrome (47,XXY, possibly mosaic), variants of higher chromosomal count,[8] mosaic 45,X/46,XY mixed gonadal dysgenesis, and 46,XX/46,XY ovotesticular DSD

46,XX disorders of ovarian development—These include 46,XX testicular and ovotesticular DSDs, as well as 46,XX gonadal dysgenesis. Known etiologies for isolated testicular and ovotesticular DSDs overlap and include (typically de novo) SRY translocation (~ 85% of 46,XX testicular and ~ 10% of ovotesticular DSDs, respectively), and SOX9 or SOX3 gene CNVs. Variants in RSPO1 cause a rare form of syndromic 46,XX testicular DSD.[9] 46,XX gonadal dysgenesis leads to premature ovarian failure (POF) caused by failure of ovarian development or resistance to gonadotropins. Rare mutations in the FSH receptor (FSHR, autosomal recessive), BMP15 (X-linked), NR5A1 (autosomal dominant), and STAG3 explain a few of the cases.[10–12]

46,XY disorders of testicular development (including complete and partial gonadal dysgenesis, Swyer syndrome). The main cause is mutations or deletions of SRY. Rarer causes are variants in DHH, NR5A1 (SF1), MAP3K1, CBX2, duplication of NROB1 (DAX1) or WNT4, and 9p24.3 (including DMRT1) deletion.[13] Patterns of inheritance include sex limited autosomal recessive and dominant, X-linked and Y-linked. It is therefore critical to assess genetic etiology for genetic counseling of these conditions.

46,XX and 46,XY disorders of steroid hormone biosynthesis—Congenital adrenal hyperplasia[14] results from mutations in the biosynthetic pathways of adrenal hormones, including the androgen biosynthesis pathway. Frequency is the same in males and females; however, the resulting DSD is different. The most frequent form (>90%) is associated with recessive mutations in the CYP21A2 gene. The main DSD concern is that of virilization of women, but effect is poorly described in 46,XY individuals.

- Much rarer causes include: STAR and 3-βHSD deficiencies (which result in androgen deficiency and male hypovirilization), and 11-hydroxylase (CYP11B1) deficiency (causing excess androgen and virilization of affected women).
- POR deficiency causes a distinct form of autosomal recessive CAH that can result in DSD in both 46,XX and 46,XY individuals, including infertility, PCOS, primary amenorrhea, with Antley Bixler syndrome at the most severe end of the phenotypic spectrum.[15]
- Aromatase deficiency (CYP19A1 gene, recessive inheritance) causes elevated levels of androgens in utero and deficit of estrogen later, and may present as virilized genitalia in a 46,XX newborn or primary amenorrhea in adolescence.
- Androgen biosynthesis defects, such as 5ARD or 17βHSD3 deficiency (both autosomal recessive), result in DSD in 46,XY individuals.[16,17]

46,XY disorders of hormonal action include

- Androgen insensitivity syndrome (AIS)—Variants in the X-linked androgen receptor (AR) cause complete or partial AIS, frequent forms of 46,XY DSD.

Table 1
Primary gene list used at the UCLA Clinical Genome Center to call DSD variants

Gene	Alternative Names	Coverage (February 2012-February 2015) (%)	Coverage since March 2015 (%)	Reported Associated Phenotype
Sex Determination (gonadal dysgenesis, testicular and ovotesticular DSD)				
BMP15		—	100	46,XX premature ovarian failure
CBX2	CDCA6	99	100	46,XY sex reversal
DHH	HHG	85	100	46,XY partial or complete gonadal dysgenesis
DMRT1	DMT1	93	100	46,XY gonadal dysgenesis
DMRT2		76	100	46,XY gonadal dysgenesis
FSHR	ODG1/LGR1	—	100	46,XX premature ovarian failure
GATA4		64	(82)	46,XY ambiguous genitalia
HHAT		94	99	46,XY gonadal dysgenesis
MAP3K1	MEKK	89	98	46,XY sex reversal
NR0B1	DAX1/AHCH	98	100	46,XY sex reversal
NR5A1	SF1	97	100	46,XY sex reversal; 46,XX premature ovarian failure
RSPO1	RSPONDIN	100		46,XX sex reversal and palmoplantar hyperkeratosis
SOX3	PHP	78	100	46,XX sex reversal
SOX9	SRA1	100		46,XX sex reversal and campomelic dysplasia
SRY	TDF	100		46,XX (ovo)testicular DSD and 46,XY gonadal dysgenesis
STAG3	STROMALIN-3	—	(93)	46,XX premature ovarian failure
WNT4	SERKAL	92	100	46,XY DSD 46,XY complete gonadal dysgenesis
WT1	AWT1/WAGR	77	100	Wilms tumor-aniridia-genital anomalies-retardation syndrome
WWOX	SDR41C1/WOX1/FOR	95	100	46,XY gonadal dysgenesis
ZFPM2	FOG2	99	100	46,XY gonadal dysgenesis

Sex differentiation (eg, steroid synthesis/receptors)

Gene	Alias			Phenotype
AKR1C2	BABP/DD/DD2/HAKRD/MCDR2	(91)	—	46,XY DSD
AKR1C4	3-a-HSD, C11/CDR/DD4/HAKRA	100		46,XY DSD
AMH	MIS	59	98	Persistent Müllerian duct syndrome (PMDS)
AMHR2	MISR2	100		PMDS
AR	AIS	95	99	Androgen insensitivity syndrome (CAIS/PAIS)
ARX	CT121/EIEE1/ISSX	50	(89)	X-linked lissencephaly with ambiguous genitalia (XLAG)
ATRX	RAD54	100		Alpha-thalassemia X-linked intellectual disability syndrome
CYP11A1	P450SCC	100		CAH, 11-hydroxylase deficiency
CYP17A1		100		CAH, 17-hydroxylase deficiency
CYP19A1		100		46,XX virilization
CYP21A2	CA21H/CAH1/CPS1	79	(90)	CAH, 21-hydroxylase deficiency
DHCR7		—	100	Smith Lemli Opitz syndrome
FGFR2		100		Apert syndrome
FOXL2	BPES	79	97	Blepharophimosis, ptosis, and epicanthus inversus
HSD17B3	SDR12C2	100		17β-hydroxysteroid dehydrogenase III deficiency (46,XY DSD)
HSD3B2	SDR11E2	100		CAH, 3β-hydroxysteroid dehydrogenase deficiency (46,XY DSD)
KDM5D	JARID1D/HYA	—	(60)	Y chromosome infertility
LHCGR	LCGR/LGR2/LHR/ULG5	92	100	Leydig cell hypoplasia
MAMLD1	CG1/F18/CXORF6	69	100	Hypospadias (46,XY)
POR		100		Cytochrome P450 oxidoreductase deficiency
SRD5A2		100		Steroid 5-alpha-reductase deficiency
STAR	StAR/STARD1	100		CAH, cholesterol desmolase deficiency
VAMP7	SYBL1/TI-VAMP	50	100	46,XY undervirilization

(continued on next page)

Table 1
(continued)

Gene	Alternative Names	Coverage (February 2012-February 2015) (%)	Coverage since March 2015 (%)	Reported Associated Phenotype
Central causes of hypogonadism				
ARL6	BBS3	100		Bardet Biedl syndrome
BBS1	BBS2L2	99	100	Bardet Biedl syndrome
BBS2	RP74	100		Bardet Biedl syndrome
BBS4		99	100	Bardet Biedl syndrome
BBS5		100		Bardet Biedl syndrome
BBS7	BBS2L1/FLJ10715	100		Bardet Biedl syndrome
BBS9	B1/PTHB1	100		Bardet Biedl syndrome
BBS10	FLJ23560	100		Bardet Biedl syndrome
BBS12	FLJ35630/FLJ41559	100		Bardet Biedl syndrome
CHD7	FLJ20357/FLJ20361/KIAA1416	100		Kallman syndrome; normosmic IGD; CHARGE syndrome
FGF8	AIGF	79	97	IGD with anosmia (Kallman syndrome) and normosmic IGD
FGFR1	BFGFR/CD331/CEK/FLG	98	100	Kallman syndrome, normosmic IGD, and Pfeiffer syndrome
FRAS1		—	100	Fraser syndrome
FREM2	ECM3homolog	—	100	Fraser syndrome
GNRH1	GNRH/GRH/LHRH	100		Isolated abnormality in GnRH secretion or response
GNRHR	LHRHR	100		Isolated abnormality in GnRH secretion or response
GRIP1		—	100	Fraser syndrome
HESX1	ANF/RPX	100		Combined pituitary hormone deficiency

HFE	HLA-H	100	Hemochromatosis
KAL1	anosmin-1/KALIG-1	95	IGD with anosmia (Kallman syndrome)
KISS1R	AXOR12/HOT7T175	54	Isolated abnormality in GnRH secretion or response
LEP		100	Morbid obesity
LEPR	CD295/OBR	95	Morbid obesity
LHX3	LIM3	87	Combined pituitary hormone deficiency
MKKS	BBS6	100	Bardet Biedl syndrome/McKusick-Kaufman syndrome
PCSK1	PC1/PC3/SPC3	98	Morbid obesity
PROK2	BV8/KAL4/MIT1/PK2	76	IGD with anosmia (Kallman syndrome) and normosmic IGD
PROKR2	GPR73b/GPRg2/PKR2	100	IGD with anosmia (Kallman syndrome) and normosmic IGD
PROP1		100	Combined pituitary hormone deficiency
PTPN11	NS1	99	Noonan syndrome 1
SOS1	GINGF	100	Noonan syndrome 4
TAC3	NKB/ZNEUROK1	100	Isolated abnormality in GnRH secretion or response
TACR3	neurokinin beta receptor/NK3R	100	Isolated abnormality in GnRH secretion or response
TRIM32	BBS11	100	Bardet Biedl syndrome
TTC8	BBS8	100	Bardet Biedl syndrome/retinitis pigmentosa, autosomal recessive

Improved coverage with the v.3 capture protocol is shown in the fourth column. Genes with 100% coverage are indicated in bold. Genes with coverage above 97% are indicated in bold. Genes with lower coverage are indicated within parenthesis. Genes not showing a coverage value in the third column were added to the list after February 2015. Coverage was not indicated in the fourth column when capture was unchanged from the previous iteration.
Abbreviations: CAH, congenital adrenal hyperplasia; IGD, isolated GnRH deficiency.

- Persistent Müllerian duct syndrome is caused by mutations in the genes coding for the anti-Müllerian hormone or its receptors. Inheritance is autosomal recessive, but the phenotype is expressed only in 46,XY individuals.[18]
- LH receptor—Inactivating mutations cause Leydig cell agenesis/hypoplasia, an extremely rare autosomal (sex-limited) recessive form of DSD. Conversely, constitutively active variants cause an autosomal-dominant familial form of precocious puberty in boys.[19]

IMPROVE AND ACCELERATE THE PATH TO AN ACCURATE DIAGNOSIS FOR DISORDERS OF SEX DEVELOPMENT

In spite of this long list of known genetic etiologies, currently known genes explain about only half of the cases. Many patients with DSD have historically experienced long diagnostic odysseys, in part because of uncoordinated diagnostic approaches, and many more never receive a definitive diagnosis. This, of course, is a common concern for patients with rare disorders.[20] About 10 years ago, a European survey of 6000 patients with rare, but well-known genetic entities (not including DSDs) showed that time between first symptoms and definitive diagnostic extended from 5 to 30 years for 1 in 4 patients. Of those who received an early diagnosis, this diagnosis proved to be wrong in 40% of the cases, leading to inappropriate treatments.[21]

In DSD care, an accurate diagnosis is critical to predicting the occurrence of life-threatening crises (such as in salt-wasting forms of CAH), response to hormone replacement therapy (eg, androgen in/sensitivity), eventual gender, fertility, recurrence risk, and cancer risk. In addition, the well-documented empowerment of patients with rare chronic disorders after a diagnosis is reached allows them to plan for health-related and psychological effects of their condition for an optimal quality of life.[3,22]

Many DSDs are caused by enzymatic defects in synthesis of steroid hormones. Testing for those is rapid and relatively inexpensive, and may be critical, as in CAH. However, because of phenotypic overlap between the various forms of DSDs, endocrine testing alone frequently yields an ambiguous diagnosis.[23,24] A genetic diagnosis is indispensable in these cases, as well as for the enzymes for which no diagnostic endocrine test exists, for variants affecting proteins other than enzymes, as well as to counsel families for further pregnancies and prenatal diagnosis. Also because of phenotypic overlap, serial single candidate gene testing, which has been the traditional approach for DSD genetic testing, is highly inefficient and can become prohibitively expensive.[25,26] Over the past decade, chromosomal microarrays have proven indispensable tools for diagnosis of DSD caused by CNVs, and should be prioritized in cases of syndromic DSD.[5,27–30] Genome-wide maps of CNVs of known pathogenicity as well as of uncertain clinical significance will continue to support clinical diagnosis and drive research for new etiologies.[31] The advent of next-generation sequencing in the realm of clinical diagnosis in the past 4 to 5 years is now allowing providers to rethink the diagnostic process.

GENOMIC SEQUENCING AS A PRIMARY DIAGNOSTIC TOOL FOR DISORDERS OF SEX DEVELOPMENT

The University of California Los Angeles (UCLA) Clinical Genomic Center has been at the forefront of this effort, being one of the original two academic centers to offer clinical exome testing in the United States, starting at the beginning of 2012, and has reported high diagnostic success for rare disorders.[32] This diagnostic rate, around a third for trio cases, has proven remarkably similar across platforms, types of disorders, or countries.[33–38] In spite of high costs and poor insurance coverage, exome sequencing is cost-effective in specific clinical scenarios, such as when multiple genetic etiologies result in overlapping phenotypes,[36,39] as is the case in DSDs. The early results of large-scale studies of clinical utility and cost-effectiveness of genomic sequencing such as the MedSeq Project are encouraging.[40] Finally, turn-around time has rapidly gone down—now routinely 4 weeks at the UCLA center, including sequencing and interpretation, and down to 1 week for exceptional urgent cases—making the use of next-generation sequencing as a first-tier diagnostic test a realistic possibility in DSD care.

As a consequence, DSD-TRN best practice guidelines recommend early, comprehensive genetic testing as a means to improve the path to an accurate diagnosis and optimized management for DSD patients.[25] An early success of the DSD-TRN using exome sequencing resulted from a collaboration of 3 DSD-TRN teams, UCLA, Seattle Children's Hospital, and University of Michigan.[41] For all of these patients, many of whom had previously undergone extensive, unsuccessful genetic and endocrine testing, exome sequencing streamlined the diagnostic process. It yielded a diagnosis in cases where endocrine testing had been ambiguous, in genes for which clinical testing as single-gene testing was not available in the United States, and, in several cases, it critically modified clinical management, compared with the working diagnosis the patient had previously been carrying, or even oriented gender identity.[25]

DISORDERS OF SEX DEVELOPMENT TRANSLATIONAL RESEARCH NETWORK RECOMMENDATIONS FOR DISORDERS OF SEX DEVELOPMENT GENOMIC TESTING

The primary gene list used at the UCLA Clinical Genomic Center currently has 78 genes (see **Table 1**), allowing testing at the same time for many DSD genes that may not be available for individual clinical testing. The adoption in March 2015 of an enhanced capture protocol (http://pathology.ucla.edu/cgc-resources) has greatly increased the coverage for all DSD genes. This resolved a few limitations of the test, such as the poor coverage of *AMH* (under 60%) or *SOX3* (78%) in the previous capture process. Sixty-five of the 78 genes are now covered at 100% (vs only half with the previous protocol), and another 7 genes are covered at 97% or above.

In addition, there is a secondary gene list, including genes that cause urogenital conditions in animal models or are involved in molecular pathways with genes known to cause DSD in people. Variants in such preclinical genes are reported with the hope of providing the clinical team with avenues to orient further exploration (endocrine, imaging) of the patient's phenotype toward a definitive diagnosis.

Samples should be submitted as trios of patient plus biological parents, as this enhances diagnostic yield by at least 50%.[32,34]

In addition to the UCLA Clinical Genomic Center, DSD-TRN network sites have used other sequencing resources for a variety of reasons, such as the State of New York's mandate that priority be given to in-state companies, development of in-house facilities, or the ease of pricing out-of-pocket expenses for patients offered by companies such as GeneDx. However, a unique strength of the UCLA facility is the weekly Genomic Data Board, a group of approximately 20 clinical and molecular geneticists, laboratory directors, genetic counselors, bench researchers, and referring clinicians who participate in the interpretation of exome results. Bioinformatic work is performed in advance of each meeting, and a data file organized through in-house-developed tools,[32] reports patient information, clinical keywords, regions of homozygosity, variants, and information on variants such as minor allele frequency (an indicator of pathogenic likelihood), protein damage prediction, and tissue expression patterns. The multidisciplinary expertise of the team, including multiple DSD specialists, as well as having all the sequences interpreted by the same team, is expected to enhance variant calling accuracy and reliability.

Regardless of origin of the sequence, for patients who agree to participate in the DSD-TRN database, an annotated set of variants for each exome will be made accessible to network investigators through secure electronic access to the registry. Future research using these data will allow comparison of variant calling across platforms, research into new etiologies, and call reassessment as new genetic causative genes are discovered.

STANDARDIZED DEEP PHENOTYPING IN DISORDERS OF SEX DEVELOPMENT TRANSLATIONAL RESEARCH NETWORK PRACTICE

Accurately predicting natural history and consequences of intervention is predicated on understanding risk (ie, accurate phenotype/genotype correlation). It is also critical to the ability to interpret the variants identified by exome sequencing. In parallel with extensive genotyping, the DSD-TRN therefore undertook an effort to collect comprehensive, standardized phenotyping data, with the goals of informing clinical care and uncovering fine, cryptic phenotype/genotype correlations not currently apparent.

The aim is to describe precisely, reliably, and quantitatively, the traits involved in the phenotype of sex development, including genito-urinary anatomy, comprehensive endocrine profile, mental health, social environment, family and pregnancy history, environmental exposures, and genetic profile. To collect this information, the network developed standardized clinical forms for all specialties involved in the interdisciplinary care of families living with DSD. Almost 2000 discrete data points per patient are collected:

- Endocrine profile—A main form plus 3 forms for the most common stimulation tests used to diagnose DSDs (hCG, ACTH, GnRH) document the patient's history of endocrine testing. For each analyte, a standard set of features is collected: laboratory where testing was performed, normal range of value for this laboratory for this patient's age/sex if available, measured value of the analyte, and a call (normal, abnormal, cannot judge). Most importantly, this is completed by an "opinion of the endocrinologist" comment, to ensure accuracy of complex interpretation for patients whose sex may be incongruent with their chromosomes, who may present atypical anatomy and function, or who may be under hormone replacement therapy.
- Urogenital Anatomy Forms Urogenital Anatomy Forms to be completed at each patient encounter and for each imaging, to document anatomy longitudinally across development, endocrine interventions, and/or surgeries.
- A schedule of psychosocial questionnaires document risk and resilience factors in the family, the patient's psychosocial and educational adaptation, self- and body-image, and gender development over time.
- A physical examination form, filled at each encounter, tracks the evolution of all systems, including genital anatomy (Supplementary Fig. 1).

STANDARDIZATION OF DIAGNOSTIC PROCESS AND GENETIC PRACTICE REPORTING

The genetic diagnostic process by clinical teams and for individual patients is captured by multiple different documents.

Documentation of Family History

Obtaining extensive family background information is a hallmark of DSD-TRN practice, toward an optimal diagnostic process. This information is collected mostly in the intake form, and includes extensive data about parental health and reproductive history, pregnancy exposures, prenatal testing, birth circumstances, and congenital defects (Supplementary Fig. 2).

Documentation of Genetic Testing and Diagnosis

A cumulative genetics form collects results of all genetic tests performed on patients and family members over time (Supplementary Fig. 3). Results reporting for all tests (karyotype, chromosomal microarray, SRY status, variants from exome sequencing, or single gene testing) is standardized to ensure data accuracy and comparison across providers. Negative results are also recorded, to document the diagnostic process. Year of testing is recorded to help interpretation of result if techniques have evolved and to quantify time to diagnosis. The front page of the form highlights genetic diagnosis as well as interpretation by the geneticist. For patients participating in the registry, annotated sequencing variants are uploaded to the registry to support further research into etiology and fine genotype/phenotype correlations.

A definitive genetic diagnosis is considered reached when the phenotype of the patient can be explained by any of the following:

- Aneuploid or mosaic complement of sex chromosomes
- CNV that has previously been described in DSDs
- Likely pathogenic or pathogenic variant identified in known DSD gene

A normal karyotype discordant with genital phenotype (eg, 46,XY karyotype in a phenotypic female) is not considered a diagnosis.

Documentation of Genetic Practice

The physical examination form contains a series of questions documenting what genetic counseling was provided to patients at each encounter. This is eventually to be completed by a mirror form filled by patients after the encounter, to document the family's understanding and support practice improvement. Pursuit of a genetic diagnosis is documented in the teams' monthly clinic reports, where each team details what genetic tests have been ordered and whether a genetic diagnosis has been pursued/achieved for each patient in clinic (Supplementary Fig. 4).

In parallel, the physical examination form tracks the evolution of the working diagnosis until a definitive genetic diagnosis has been achieved. For example, a working diagnostic could evolve from ambiguous genitalia at the first encounter with a newborn, to 46,XX DSD with ambiguous genitalia once a karyotype has been performed, then 46,XX ovotesticular DSD once pathology of the gonad has been ascertained and, perhaps, finally 46,XX ovotesticular DSD with *SOX9* duplication when a definitive genetic diagnosis has been achieved. Analysis of working diagnosis registry data should allow one to determine evolution of time to diagnosis over time, as well as condition-to-condition and site-to-site variability. In association with psychosocial data, it should allow assessment of the influence of an accurate diagnosis on clinical management and quality-of-life outcomes for various DSD conditions.

Collectively, clinical specialty forms serve multiple purposes:
- Supporting the clinical team's adherence to network best practice guidelines by providing the list of data points that needs to be documented for each patient
- Ensuring phenotypic description and genetic variant reporting is standardized

- Clarifying electronic medical records, by grouping in a single set of standard documents all historical and longitudinal patient information
- Supporting interdisciplinary team function and decision-making by showcasing interpretation of results by each specialist for the information of other providers
- For patients who agree to participate in the study, the forms serve as registry data-collecting tools

PRELIMINARY DISORDERS OF SEX DEVELOPMENT TRANSLATIONAL RESEARCH NETWORK REGISTRY FINDINGS
Diagnostic Effort by the Disorders of Sex Development Translational Research Network Team Increased the Percentage of Patients with a Firm Diagnosis from 24% to 46%

A survey of the database in August 2016 showed that a genetics form was entered into the registry for 144 out of the 303 probands enrolled (a form was also entered for 7 affected siblings) (**Table 2**). Data entry varied greatly between sites, from just under 6% (2 sites) to 100% of completion (3 sites). Out of the 144 probands, 35 had a

Table 2
Diagnostic effort by the DSD-TRN team increased the percentage of patients with a firm diagnosis from 24% to 46%

A			
(Total = 144 Forms)	Yes	No	Not Answered
Patient had diagnosis prior to 1st visit	35	101	8
Patient currently has diagnosis	65	71	8
Patient has diagnosis (manual assessment)	66	77	1 uncertain diagnosis

B									
Site	1	2	3	4	5	6	7	8	9
Dx	15	11	10	13	5	0	0	0	9
no Dx	8	21	5	12	14	1	10	4	5
% Dx	66%	37%	67%	52%	26%	0%	0%	0%	64%
# Reported	23	30	15	25	19	1	10	4	14
# Enrolled	54	31	15	39	19	17	43	72	14
% Reported	43%	97%	100%	64%	100%	6%	23%	6%	100%
% with Dx	28%	36%	67%	33%	26%	0%	0%	0%	64%

Forms entered for siblings and 2 forms mistakenly entered in duplicate were discarded prior to analysis to ensure search in unique proband data. First, an automated query for "patient has diagnosis" (true/false) and "patient had diagnosis prior to first visit to DSD-TRN team" (true/false) was run. Follow-up manual curating made use of the built-in redundancy features of the forms, designed for such data quality control. It included searching for (1) positive answers to "gene with diagnostic variant", confirmed with entry of actual variant; (2) "CNV found" with a pathogenic or likely pathogenic call in the CMA results; (3) abnormal/mosaic karyotype, with actual data entry of mosaic percentages or sex chromosome complement. Eight forms out of 144 had no response in the "patient has/had diagnosis" fields. Answers were found using other variables for 7 of the 8 forms. Another 6 forms had erroneous reporting; 3 forms were reported as not having a diagnosis when manual validation did find one, and 3 forms were reported as having a diagnosis when in fact a normal karyotype was reported, without specific gene variants. This constitutes an approximate 10% error in data entry or recording. Teams are subsequently notified of these errors for rectification as part of the practice improvement process.

In B, the ratio (%Dx) of number of patients with (Dx) or without (no Dx) a firm genetic diagnosis is reported per clinical site. The total number of genetic forms in the registry (# reported = Dx + noDx) compared with the total number of patients enrolled in the study (# Enrolled) gives an estimate of data entry completion (% reported) and of percentage of patients with a diagnosis available in the registry (% with Dx = Dx/Total enrolled) at a specific site.

diagnosis prior to their first visit to the interdisciplinary DSD-TRN team. Clinical care by the DSD-TRN team resulted in establishing a firm diagnosis in 30% of the remaining patients (30 of 101 patients), for a total of 66 of 144 (46%) patients currently with a firm diagnosis. Diagnostic success too was variable from site to site, with 3 sites reporting zero diagnosis and 4 sites more than 50% of patients with a firm genetic diagnosis.

The accuracy of this percentage must be viewed cautiously, as no genetic data are available in the registry for half of the enrolled probands. When the number of diagnoses reported achieved was compared with total number of enrolled patients, the ratios fell around a quarter to a third of patients with a firm genetic diagnosis, more in line with typical diagnostic success for DSD. One suspects there might be a bias in favor of prioritizing form completion and registry data entry for patients in whom a genetic diagnosis has been pursued, if not achieved, and that teams may more rarely create mostly blank registry forms for patients when no genetic testing has been pursued. Two sites, where reporting had been completed, maintained an exceptional diagnostic rate of 64% and 67% in their patients.

The Conditions of 6% of Probands Reported in the Disorders of Sex Development Translational Research Network Registry are Familial

Over 40% of probands had a reported call for "Is proband condition familial?" (17 yes, 44 no de novo) **(Table 3)**. However, data QC through search of other variables showed that testing of other family members had been pursued in a limited number of cases. A *SOX9* duplication and a nondiagnostic rearrangement involving 2 autosomes were confirmed to be *de novo* by karyotype of the parents. Two chromosomal microarrays, identifying diagnoses of Klinefelter and deletion of the entire *AR* gene, were performed in trios confirming the *de novo* status. In 2 patients, the parental origin of compound heterozygous variants was identified by trio exome, but the condition was not familial. In contrast, 9 cases were proven familial (8 reported, 1 not reported) through the existence of affected family members (2 Swyer syndromes without genetic diagnosis, 2 *MAP3K1*, 1 *CYP21A2* CAH, and 4 AIS with *AR* variants).

Table 3				
The conditions of 6% of probands reported in the DSD-TRN registry are familial				
	Familial	**De novo**	**Unknown**	**Not Answered**
"Familial" reported	17	44	66	17
Accurate "familial/de novo/inherited" call	Yes: 8 Unk.: 9	Yes: 6 Unk.:38	Unk.:66	Yes: 1 Unk.: 16
Actual familial cases	9	6	129	—

Reported numbers for each answer options to the question "Is condition familial?" ("yes, familial", "no, de novo", "unknown") are shown in the "familial reported" row. Manual curating of the responses by cross-examining other data points is shown in the "accurate call" row, as Yes (accurate reporting) or Unk. (should have been reported as Unknown). Other variables examined to determine the accuracy of the call included karyotype mother/father/siblings, CMA and exome variants parent of origin, existing genetics form for an affected sibling, and phenotype/genotype shared by family member. Actual calls as they would be expected to be reported are shown in the "actual familial cases" row.

Frequency of Specific Genetic Diagnoses in the Disorders of Sex Development Translational Research Network Registry

Karyotype was reported in almost all (92%) patients **(Table 4)**. Of those reported, approximately 15% had sex chromosome complement anomalies, 16 of 18 in mosaic

Table 4
Frequency of genetic diagnoses in the disorders of sex development translational research network registry

Karyotype		Genetic Diagnosis	
Sex Chromosome aneuploidy	19	Mosaic 45,X/46,XY	13 (10 idicY)
		46,XX Xq del	2
		Klinefelter 47,XXY	3 (2 mosaic)
		49,XXXXY	1
46,XX	46	CAH *CYP21A2*	14
		SRY+	3
		SOX9 Dup (mosaic)	1
		Kabuki syndrome	1
		No diagnosis	27
46,XY	64	PAIS/CAIS (*AR*)	15
		SRD5A2	4
		17βHSD	4
		MAP3K1	2
		WAGR (11p del)	1
		Smith Lemli Opitz	1
		No diagnosis	37
Not reported	15	*SRD5A2*	1
		Unknown	14

form. Normal 46,XX and 46,XY karyotypes were found in 36% and 50%, respectively. Of the 15 with no reported karyotypes, most were conditions where genetic diagnosis is rarely attained or may be viewed as unnecessary by some: 6 CAH, 2 cloaca, 4 MRKH, 1 SRD5A2 deficiency, and 2 without a clear working diagnosis.

Mosaic Turner syndrome accounted for the vast majority of sex chromosome complement anomalies. A majority of those had a marker Y chromosome (isodicentric Y). Such marker chromosomes, which are rare in the general population, are found with elevated frequency in people with infertility (45 times more frequent) or developmental delay (60 times).[42] Their frequency in Turner syndrome, as well as the wide associated phenotypic range, became rapidly apparent during the clinical case videoconferences held by the DSD-TRN.[43]

CAH was the predominant diagnosis, with 14 cases of genetically documented *CYP21A2* deficiency in 46,XX individuals and 4 cases of *17βHSD* deficiency in 46,XY individuals. No other etiologies of CAH were reported. Search on the working diagnosis of the physical examination form identified one more *17βHSD* deficiency, one *CYP11A2* deficiency, and another 19 potential CAH cases for which no genetics form has been filed or genetic testing was not pursued.

In 46,XY individuals, the most frequent diagnosis was likely pathogenic or pathogenic variants in the *AR* receptor, leading to complete or partial AIS. No mutations or deletions of SRY were reported. The next most common diagnosis was 5α-reductase deficiency, with 5 cases.

Efficacy and Completion of the Diagnostic Process

Chromosomal microarrays
CMA was performed in 43 (30%) of patients for whom a genetics form was entered in the registry, whether they had syndromic or isolated DSDs (**Table 5**). Six diagnoses were made: 2 loss and 1 gain of portion of Y chromosome, 1 Klinefelter syndrome, 1 deletion of entire *AR* gene, and 1 WAGR syndrome. In addition, CNVs of unknown

Table 5			
The diagnostic process is not exhausted in 97% of undiagnosed cases			

A			
	CMA Performed	**CMA Not Performed**	**Not Reported**
Have Dx	20	35	9
Don't have Dx	23	37	20

B				
Method	**Karotype/FISH**	**Single gene**	**CMA**	**Exome**
Diagnosis achieved	19	36	6	4
Test performed	129	47	43	9

The number of patients for whom a chromosomal microarray (CMA) was performed is indicated in A. Numbers were similar among patients who have a firm genetic diagnostic and among those who do not. B shows the method by which diagnosis was eventually achieved in comparison with the number of patients for whom the test was performed.

clinical significance were identified in another 5 patients, 4 of whom had a firm diagnosis obtained by another method. These may represent avenues of research to identify modifier genes.

Chromosomal microarrays have clear demonstrated diagnostic value, especially in syndromic cases and for isolated DSDs due to typically submicroscopic CNVs (eg, SOX3, SOX9, NR0B1, WNT4).[7,27] In the DSD-TRN registry, CMA identified absence or excess of whole chromosomes, as the diagnosis of Klinefelter, or of an entire gene (AR).

Single gene testing
Thirty-five patients had molecular diagnoses after single-gene testing. This included 14 cases of CYP21A2-deficiency CAH, which were likely tested to confirm a suspected endocrine diagnosis. Serial single-gene testing was reported in 47 patients. In 12 patients, it yielded no diagnosis, with an average of 1.6 genes tested per patient. In 8 patients with a diagnosis and multiple testing, 2.7 genes were tested on average. Genes tested that turned out to be wrong guesses were: AR (11), 5ARD2 (6), SRY (3), WT1 (3), LHCGR (2), HSD17B3 (2), and 1 each for AKR1C4, AMH, AMHR2, CYP11B1, DHH, FGFR1, KAL1, MAMLD1, MAPK8, NR0B1, PTEN, SOX9, WNT4, and ZFPM2. Thus, while AR and 5ARD2 were the most frequently diagnostic genes in 46,XY individuals (15 and 5, respectively), they were wrongly suspected equally frequently (11 and 6).

Exome sequencing
Although few exomes have yet been reported in the registry, diagnosis success was high, with a definitive diagnosis identified in 44%. As previously reported, trio exome was more efficient than singleton exome; 3 of 5 trio exomes versus only 1 of 4 singleton exomes reached a diagnosis.

Completion of genetic diagnostic process
Among the 77 patients for whom no diagnosis has been reached, 2 patients have exhausted the genetic diagnostic options currently available on a clinical basis (karyotype, FISH, CMA, trio exome). Three have undergone singleton exome (and CMA) and might benefit from reassessment of their variants using parental controls, given the higher diagnostic rate of trio exome. Another 14 patients had CMA but no exome performed, and 58 patients had neither CMA nor exome. Therefore, available genetic diagnostic options have not been exhausted in the vast majority (97%) of patients who remain without a diagnosis.

SUMMARY

Although documented evidence is scarce, a review of longitudinal quality-of-life outcomes for patients with DSD in varied settings indicates better outcomes when care is provided by a multidisciplinary team at a tertiary center.[44] This model was advocated by the Chicago Consensus[1] and is being put into place in many centers.[45] The DSD-TRN is the first network to harness the work of such teams through a common registry, expertise-sharing via clinical case videoconferences, and adherence to common best-practice recommendations. The network has undertaken a massive effort of both the standardization and the documentation of the diagnostic process. The authors and others have provided evidence for the prioritization of genetic testing, including new genomic technologies, to streamline the diagnostic process in DSD care.[23,25,33,41,46,47] With time to results of exome sequencing now in the same range as some hormonal tests, and price similar to an MRI, use of genomic technologies as a first-tier diagnostic tool should become the norm in the near future.

Even though there are still a significant number of unsolved cases even after exome sequencing, strategies to improve the interpretation and diagnostic yield have emerged. One is the reanalysis of the exome data, at least 1 year after the original analysis. As more cases become analyzed in the literature, several variants have become significant, with an increased diagnostic yield of about 10%.[48,49] Whole-genome sequencing may identify variants in known DSD genes in regions not captured by exome sequencing (promoter or deep intronic). Another promising approach to improve the diagnostic interpretation is the analysis of the transcriptome (eg, by RNA sequencing) and the combination of RNA and DNA variant exploration.[50,51]

Although many next-generation sequencing platforms are indeed being developed around the world, implementation is facing multiple hurdles, from clinicians' habits, to institutional constraints, to insurance coverage. In addition, a strong hurdle to the full adherence of clinical teams to the DSD-TRN guidelines for standardization of reporting and practice is the current lack of integration of the standardized clinical forms into the various electronic medical records at the different sites. Time allocated to research (such as registry data entry) is also severely limited at most sites for lack of funding supporting this new effort of development and implementation of best practices. In spite of these hurdles, genetic information for half the enrolled patients is already available in the DSD-TRN registry, and early results demonstrate the value of such an infrastructure. The long-term value of an accurate diagnosis goes beyond the molecular diagnostic yield, as it supports reproductive decision making for families, identification of at-risk family members, quality of life, and general empowerment of patients. Although those outcomes (including psychosocial) may vary, they can and must be measured, in DSD practice as in the case of any other chronic condition.[52] This effort should allow production of evidence for the efficacy of various methods toward an accurate diagnosis and, most importantly, the effects of a reliable diagnosis on evolving health-related quality-of-life outcomes for patients and families living with DSDs.

ACKNOWLEDGMENTS

The Genetics Workgroup that created the standardized forms included Emmanuèle C. Délot, Michelle Fox, Wayne Grody, Hane Lee, Jeanette C. Papp, Eric Vilain (UCLA), Catherine Keegan (University of Michigan), Linda Ramsdell (Seattle Children's Hospital), and Janet Green (Accord Alliance). The group now also includes Hayk Barseghyan, Naghmeh Dorrani (UCLA), Lauren Mohnach (University of Michigan), Margaret A. Pearson (Phoenix Children's Hospital), Jullianne Diaz, Eyby Leon (National

Children's Hospital), Robert J. Hopkin, Jodie Johnson, Howard Saal, (Cincinnati Children's Hospital), Ina Amarillo (Washington University, St Louis), Margaret Adam (Seattle Children's Hospital).

SUPPLEMENTARY DATA

Supplementary figures related to this article can be found at http://dx.doi.org/10.1016/j.ecl.2017.01.015.

REFERENCES

1. Lee PA, Houk CP, Ahmed SF, et al. Consensus statement on management of intersex disorders. Pediatrics 2006;118(2):e488.
2. Lee PA, Nordenström A, Houk CP, et al. Global disorders of sex development update since 2006: perceptions, approach and care. Horm Res Paediatr 2016; 85(3):158–80.
3. Arboleda VA, Sandberg DE, Vilain E. DSDs: genetics, underlying pathologies and psychosexual differentiation. Nature reviews. Endocrinology 2014;10(10):603–15.
4. Auchus RJ, Miller WL. Defects in androgen biosynthesis causing 46,XY disorders of sexual development. Semin Reprod Med 2012;30(5):417–26.
5. Hutson JM, Grover SR, O'Connell M, et al. Malformation syndromes associated with disorders of sex development. Nat Rev Endocrinol 2014;10(8):476–87.
6. Pohl HG, Joyce GF, Wise M, et al. Cryptorchidism and hypospadias. J Urol 2007; 177(5):1646–51.
7. Baetens D, Mladenov W, Delle Chiaie B, et al. Extensive clinical, hormonal and genetic screening in a large consecutive series of 46,XY neonates and infants with atypical sexual development. Orphanet J Rare Dis 2014;9(1):1–13.
8. Tartaglia N, Ayari N, Howell S, et al. 48,XXYY, 48,XXXY and 49,XXXXY syndromes: not just variants of Klinefelter syndrome. Acta Paediatr 2011;100(6):851–60.
9. Délot E, Vilain E. Nonsyndromic 46,XX testicular disorders of sex development. In: Pagon RA, Adam MP, Ardinger HH, et al, editors. GeneReviews® [Internet]. Seattle (WA): University of Washington, Seattle; 2003. p. 1993–2016. Available at: http://www.ncbi.nlm.nih.gov/books/NBK1416/.
10. Bramble MS, Goldstein EH, Lipson A, et al. A novel follicle-stimulating hormone receptor mutation causing primary ovarian failure: a fertility application of whole exome sequencing. Hum Reprod 2016;31(4):905–14.
11. Caburet S, Arboleda VA, Llano E, et al. Mutant cohesin in premature ovarian failure. N Engl J Med 2014;370(10):943–9.
12. Hiort O, Wieacker P. 46,XX gonadal dysgenesis. 2011. Available at: http://www.orpha.net/consor/cgi-bin/OC_Exp.php?Expert=243. Accessed February 22, 2017.
13. Mohnach L, Fechner P, Keegan C. Nonsyndromic disorders of testicular development. In: Pagon RA, Adam MP, Ardinger HH, et al, editors. GeneReviews® [Internet]. Seattle (WA): University of Washington, Seattle; 2008. p. 1993–2016. Available at: http://www.ncbi.nlm.nih.gov/books/NBK1547/.
14. Nimkarn S, Gangishetti PK, Yau M, et al. 21-hydroxylase-deficient congenital adrenal hyperplasia. In: Pagon RA, Adam MP, Ardinger HH, et al, editors. GeneReviews ® [Internet]. Seattle (WA): University of Washington, Seattle; 2002. p. 1993–2016. Available at: http://www.ncbi.nlm.nih.gov/books/NBK1171/.
15. Cragun D, Hopkin R. Cytochrome P450 oxidoreductase deficiency. In: Pagon RA, Adam MP, Ardinger HH, et al, editors. GeneReviews® [Internet]. Seattle (WA): University of Washington, Seattle; 2005. p. 1993–2016. Available at: http://www.ncbi.nlm.nih.gov/books/NBK1419/.

16. Mendonca BB, Gomes NL, Costa EM, et al. 46,XY disorder of sex development (DSD) due to 17beta-hydroxysteroid dehydrogenase type 3 deficiency. J Steroid Biochem Mol Biol 2017;165(Pt A):79–85.

17. Okeigwe I, Kuohung W. 5-Alpha reductase deficiency: a 40-year retrospective review. Curr Opin Endocrinol Diabetes Obes 2014;21(6):483–7.

18. Josso N, Belville C, di Clemente N, et al. AMH and AMH receptor defects in persistent Mullerian duct syndrome. Hum Reprod Update 2005;11(4):351–6.

19. Themmen APN, Verhoef-Post M. LH receptor defects. Semin Reprod Med 2002; 20(3):199–204.

20. Shashi V, McConkie-Rosell A, Rosell B, et al. The utility of the traditional medical genetics diagnostic evaluation in the context of next-generation sequencing for undiagnosed genetic disorders. Genet Med 2014;16(2):176–82.

21. Survey of the delay in diagnosis for 8 rare diseases in Europe ('Eurordiscare2'). 2007; Available at: http://www.eurordis.org/sites/default/files/publications/Fact_Sheet_Eurordiscare2.pdf. Accessed February 22, 2017.

22. Graungaard AH, Skov L. Why do we need a diagnosis? A qualitative study of parents' experiences, coping and needs, when the newborn child is severely disabled. Child Care Health Dev 2007;33(3):296–307.

23. Grimbly C, Caluseriu O, Metcalfe P, et al. 46,XY disorder of sex development due to 17-beta hydroxysteroid dehydrogenase type 3 deficiency: a plea for timely genetic testing. Int J Pediatr Endocrinol 2016;2016(1):1–5.

24. Perry RJ, Novikova E, Wallace AM, et al. Pitfalls in the diagnosis of 5α-Reductase Type 2 deficiency during early infancy. Horm Res Paediatr 2011;75(5):380–2.

25. Barseghyan H, Delot E, Vilain E. New genomic technologies: an aid for diagnosis of disorders of sex development. Horm Metab Res 2015;47(5):312–20.

26. Baxter RM, Vilain E. Translational genetics for diagnosis of human disorders of sex development. Annu Rev genomics Hum Genet 2013;14:371–92.

27. Jaillard S, Bashamboo A, Pasquier L, et al. Gene dosage effects in 46, XY DSD: usefulness of CGH technologies for diagnosis. J Assist Reprod Genet 2015; 32(2):287–91.

28. Ledig S, Hiort O, Scherer G, et al. Array-CGH analysis in patients with syndromic and non-syndromic XY gonadal dysgenesis: evaluation of array CGH as diagnostic tool and search for new candidate loci. Hum Reprod 2010;25(10):2637–46.

29. Tannour-Louet M, Han S, Corbett ST, et al. Identification of de novo copy number variants associated with human disorders of sexual development. PLoS One 2010;5(10):e15392.

30. White S, Ohnesorg T, Notini A, et al. Copy number variation in patients with disorders of sex development due to 46,XY gonadal dysgenesis. PLoS One 2011; 6(3):e17793.

31. Amarillo IE, Nievera I, Hagan A, et al. Integrated small copy number variations and epigenome maps of disorders of sex development. Hum Genome var 2016;3:16012.

32. Lee H, Deignan JL, Dorrani N, et al. Clinical exome sequencing for genetic identification of rare Mendelian disorders. JAMA 2014;312(18):1880–7.

33. Dong Y, Yi Y, Yao H, et al. Targeted next-generation sequencing identification of mutations in patients with disorders of sex development. BMC Med Genet 2016; 17(1):1–9.

34. Farwell KD, Shahmirzadi L, El-Khechen D, et al. Enhanced utility of family-centered diagnostic exome sequencing with inheritance model-based analysis: results from 500 unselected families with undiagnosed genetic conditions. Genet Med 2015;17(7):578–86.

35. Sawyer SL, Hartley T, Dyment DA, et al. Utility of whole-exome sequencing for those near the end of the diagnostic odyssey: time to address gaps in care. Clin Genet 2016;89(3):275–84.
36. Soden SE, Saunders CJ, Willig LK, et al. Effectiveness of exome and genome sequencing guided by acuity of illness for diagnosis of neurodevelopmental disorders. Sci Transl Med 2014;6(265):265ra168.
37. Yang Y, Muzny DM, Reid JG, et al. Clinical whole-exome sequencing for the diagnosis of mendelian disorders. N Engl J Med 2013;369(16):1502–11.
38. Yang Y, Muzny DM, Xia F, et al. Molecular findings among patients referred for clinical whole-exome sequencing. JAMA 2014;312(18):1870–9.
39. Biesecker LG, Green RC. Diagnostic clinical genome and exome sequencing. N Engl J Med 2014;370(25):2418–25.
40. Christensen DK, Dukhovny D, Siebert U, et al. Assessing the costs and cost-effectiveness of genomic sequencing. J Pers Med 2015;5(4):470–86.
41. Baxter RM, Arboleda VA, Lee H, et al. Exome sequencing for the diagnosis of 46,XY disorders of sex development. J Clin Endocrinol Metab 2015;100(2): E333–44.
42. Liehr T, Weise A. Frequency of small supernumerary marker chromosomes in prenatal, newborn, developmentally retarded and infertility diagnostics. Int J Mol Med 2007;19(5):719–31.
43. Hipp LE, Mohnach LH, Wei S, et al. Isodicentric Y mosaicism involving a 46, XX cell line: implications for management. Am J Med Genet A 2016;170(1):233–8.
44. Amaral RC, Inacio M, Brito VN, et al. Quality of life of patients with 46,XX and 46,XY disorders of sex development. Clin Endocrinol 2015;82(2):159–64.
45. McNamara ER, Swartz JM, Diamond DA. Initial management of disorders of sex development in newborns. Urology 2016. [Epub ahead of print].
46. Arboleda VA, Lee H, Sánchez FJ, et al. Targeted massively parallel sequencing provides comprehensive genetic diagnosis for patients with disorders of sex development. Clin Genet 2013;83(1):35–43.
47. Tobias ES, McElreavey K. Next generation sequencing for disorders of sex development. Endocr Dev 2014;27:53–62.
48. Wenger AM, Guturu H, Bernstein JA, et al. Systematic reanalysis of clinical exome data yields additional diagnoses: implications for providers. Genet Med 2017;19(2):209–14.
49. Williams E, Retterer K, Cho M, et al. Diagnostic yield from reanalysis of whole exome sequencing data. 2016; Available at: http://www.genedx.com/wp-content/uploads/2016/04/ACMG-2016-Reanalysis-of-WES-Data.pdf. Accessed February 22, 2017.
50. Cummings BB, Marshall JL, Tukiainen T, et al. Improving genetic diagnosis in Mendelian disease with transcriptome sequencing. bioRxiv 2016. Available at: http://biorxiv.org/content/early/2016/09/09/074153.
51. Parikshak NN, Gandal MJ, Geschwind DH. Systems biology and gene networks in neurodevelopmental and neurodegenerative disorders. Nat Rev Genet 2015; 16(8):441–58.
52. Berg JS. Genome-scale sequencing in clinical care: establishing molecular diagnoses and measuring value. JAMA 2014;312(18):1865–7.

Genetics of Lipodystrophy

Marissa Lightbourne, MD, MPH[a], Rebecca J. Brown, MD, MHSc[b],*

KEYWORDS

- Lipodystrophy • Leptin • Berardinelli-Seip syndrome • Dunnigan syndrome
- Kobberling syndrome

KEY POINTS

- Lipodystrophy syndromes are inherited or acquired disorders of missing body fat, with metabolic complications, including insulin resistance, diabetes, and dyslipidemia.
- There are many genetic causes of lipodystrophy. Most genes encode proteins involved in adipocyte differentiation/survival, or lipid droplet formation; however, there remain unknown genetic causes.
- Congenital generalized lipodystrophy is caused by recessive mutations in *AGPAT2*, *BSCL2*, *CAV1*, and *PTRF*.
- Most familial partial lipodystrophy is caused by autosomal dominant mutations in *LMNA*, *PPARγ*, *PLIN1*, and *AKT2*; recessive mutations can occur in *CIDEC* and *LIPE*.
- Acquired lipodystrophies are related to presumed autoimmune destruction of adipocytes; acquired partial lipodystrophy has been linked to mutations in *LMNB*.

BACKGROUND

The lipodystrophy syndromes are genetic or acquired disorders characterized by selective loss of adipose tissue that may involve the entire body (generalized) or only certain adipose depots (partial). More than 1000 cases have been reported, with prevalence less than 1:1,000,000, although underreporting is likely.[1] The characterization of the various phenotypes has been evolving and many molecular defects have been elucidated. The diagnosis is dependent on regional or generalized lack of adipose tissue on physical examination, potentially including body composition analysis, combined with supportive data from history, laboratory testing, imaging, and molecular genetic testing in some cases.

The major subtypes of lipodystrophy include congenital generalized lipodystrophy (CGL), familial partial lipodystrophy (FPLD), acquired generalized lipodystrophy

Disclosure Statement: The authors have nothing to disclose.
[a] Eunice Kennedy Shriver National Institute of Child Health and Human Development, National Institutes of Health, 10-CRC/1-3330, MSC 1103, 10 Center Drive, Bethesda, MD 20892, USA; [b] National Institute of Diabetes and Digestive and Kidney Diseases, National Institutes of Health, Building 10-CRC, Room 6-5942, 10 Center Drive, Bethesda, MD 20892, USA
* Corresponding author.
E-mail address: brownrebecca@mail.nih.gov

(AGL), and acquired partial lipodystrophy (APL) (**Fig. 1**). There also are other systemic disorders associated with lipodystrophy, such as the progeroid disorders (**Fig. 2**) and autoinflammatory disorders. Localized forms of lipodystrophy and lipodystrophy in patients infected with the human immunodeficiency virus are the more

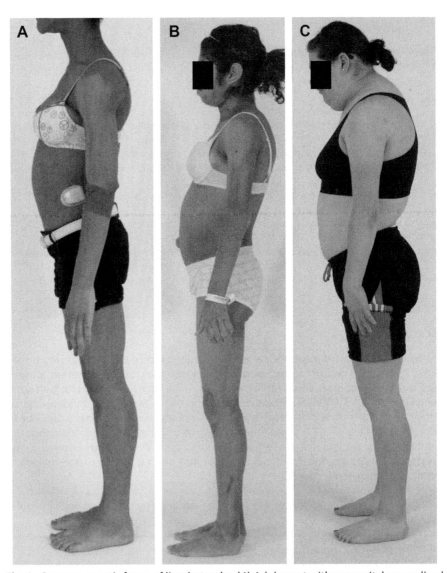

Fig. 1. Common genetic forms of lipodystrophy. (*A*) Adolescent with congenital generalized lipodystrophy due to recessive mutation in *AGPAT2*, demonstrating generalized lack of subcutaneous fat with prominent muscularity, acromegaloid hands and feet, and insulin pump use. (*B*) Adolescent with congenital generalized lipodystrophy due to recessive mutation in *BSCL2*, demonstrating generalized lack of fat, including the face, hands, and feet, prominent umbilicus, and severe acanthosis nigricans. (*C*) Adolescent with familial partial lipodystrophy due to *LMNA* mutation, demonstrating lack of fat in the buttocks and extremities, preserved truncal fat, and increased fat in the head, neck, and dorsocervical area.

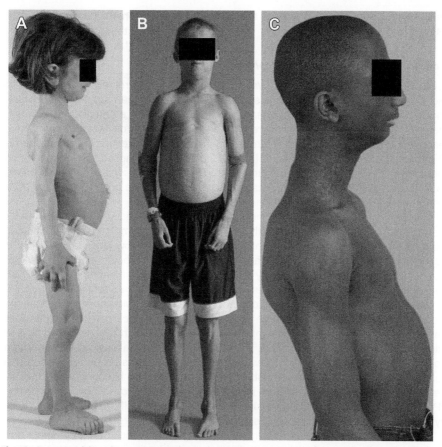

Fig. 2. Progeroid lipodystrophy syndromes. (*A*) Two-year-old child with atypical progeria due to de novo mutation in *LMNA*, demonstrating generalized lack of fat and mandibular hypoplasia. (*B*) Twelve-year-old boy with mandibulo-acral dysplasia type B due to recessive mutation in *ZMPSTE24*, demonstrating generalized lack of fat with prominent veins, mandibular hypoplasia, and joint contractures. Subcutaneous calcifications also were present. (*C*) Twelve-year-old boy with atypical progeria due to de novo mutation in LMNA, demonstrating generalized lack of fat, mandibular hypoplasia, and mottled skin pigmentation on the neck.

common acquired forms of lipodystrophy, but are beyond the scope of this discussion.

Metabolic complications of lipodystrophy are key factors in morbidity and mortality. The deficiency in adipose mass results in leptin deficiency, leading to hyperphagia and ectopic lipid storage, causing insulin resistance. Insulin resistance and associated complications include diabetes mellitus, hypertriglyceridemia, nonalcoholic fatty liver disease, polycystic ovaries, acanthosis nigricans, and premature atherosclerosis.[2]

Although genetic testing is not necessary for the diagnosis, it is very helpful for identifying subtypes of the familial lipodystrophies. Genetic testing can help identify at-risk family members, especially for lipodystrophy subtypes associated with subtle physical phenotypes or those with high risk of morbidity and mortality (eg, cardiomyopathy and arrhythmias found in the LMNA mutations). A negative genetic test does not rule out a genetic condition, as there are forms of lipodystrophy for which the genetic mutations are unknown.

Congenital Generalized Lipodystrophy

CGL (Berardinelli-Seip syndrome) was first reported by Berardinelli[3] from Brazil and Seip[4] from Scandinavia in the 1950s. Patients have since been reported worldwide, including patients of African, European, Middle Eastern, Native American, and Latino descent.[5] CGL is a rare autosomal recessive disorder, and 4 distinct mutations have been reported. CGL1, the most common variant, is due to mutations in 1-acylglycerol-3-phosphate O-acyltransferase 2 (AGPAT2),[6] CGL2 is caused by mutations in Berardinelli-Seip congenital lipodystrophy 2 (BSCL2),[7] CGL3 is caused by mutations in caveolin 1 (CAV1),[8] and CGL4 is caused by mutations in the polymerase I and transcript release factor (PTRF) gene.[9]

Although each mutation has distinct features, they share many similar characteristics that can be used to phenotypically identify CGL. These common features include a near-total lack of body fat, prominent muscularity, and very low leptin levels.[5] CGL is recognizable at birth or soon after based on the paucity of subcutaneous adipose tissue. In infancy, hepatosplenomegaly and umbilical prominence or hernia[5,10] often are present. During childhood, patients often have voracious appetites, accelerated growth, advanced bone age, and acanthosis nigricans.[5,11] Metabolic complications become more prevalent as children age, and by adolescence many have diabetes mellitus with severe hyperinsulinemia and dyslipidemia (high triglycerides and low high-density lipoprotein cholesterol).[5,6,12] Hypertriglyceridemia may be severe enough to cause acute pancreatitis.[5,11] Nonalcoholic fatty liver disease is common, and can lead to cirrhosis.[13] Female individuals with CGL may develop hirsutism, menstrual irregularity, polycystic ovaries, and infertility similar to polycystic ovary syndrome (PCOS), with occasional clitoromegaly.[1] Clinical features specific to each genetic subtype are discussed in the following sections.

Morbidity and mortality are usually associated with metabolic derangements and include complications of diabetes mellitus, hyperlipidemia (eg, acute pancreatitis), and cirrhosis. Depending on the mutation, patients may also have cardiomyopathy and rhythm disturbances.

Congenital generalized lipodystrophy type 1

Genetics CGL1 is caused by recessive mutations in 1-acylglycerol-3-phosphate O-acyltransferase 2 (AGPAT2) on chromosome 9q34.[6] It was identified via genome-wide linkage analysis with positional cloning.[6] Although equal sex distribution is expected based on the inheritance pattern, there is a female predominance of reported patients,[5] and it has been postulated that less severe fat loss in patients with AGPAT2 mutations can result in the diagnosis being missed in some male individuals. It has been described in many diverse pedigrees (with origins in Europe, Africa, Pakistan, Argentina, Germany, Mexico, and the United Arab Emirates). Most patients with CGL of African origin have CGL1.[5]

Phenotype Phenotypic characteristics that distinguish CGL1 from other forms of generalized lipodystrophy include absent bone marrow fat and preserved mechanical adipose tissue in the retro-orbital and periarticular regions, palms, and soles. Patients also can develop enlargement of the hands, feet, and mandible, resulting in an acromegaloid appearance[14] and hyperhidrosis.[5] The onset of diabetes is at a median age of 12.5 years.[5] Focal lytic lesions in the appendicular bones have been almost exclusively linked to the AGPAT2 mutation.[5,14]

Mechanism AGPATs are critical enzymes involved in the biosynthesis of triglycerides and phospholipids from glycerol-3-phosphate. There are 11 known AGPAT isoforms, each encoded by different genes, with distinct tissue expression and biochemical properties. AGPAT2 catalyzes the acylation of lysophosphatidic acid to phosphatidic acid.[15] There is high expression of AGPAT2 mRNA in adipose tissue and deficiency may cause lipodystrophy by limiting triglyceride biosynthesis and decreasing the bioavailability of phosphatidic acid and glycerophospholipids.

Congenital generalized lipodystrophy type 2

Genetics CGL2 is caused by recessive mutations in Berardinelli-Seip congenital lipodystrophy 2 (BSCL2) on chromosome 11q13.[7] It was identified via genome-wide linkage analysis with positional cloning. Patients have been identified with origins from Turkey, Brazil, India, Pakistan, China, Japan, Europe, North America (indigenous peoples), United Kingdom, Portugal, Norway, and Lebanon. Most patients of Lebanese and Norwegian origin have CGL2 due to founder mutations.[5]

Phenotype CGL2 is considered to be the most severe variety of CGL. Infants are born without any body fat. In addition to lack of metabolically active adipose tissue in the subcutaneous, intra-abdominal, and intrathoracic depots, patients lack mechanical adipose tissue and bone marrow fat. Consistent with the severe deficiency of body fat, patients with BSCL2 mutations have very low leptin levels.[5] Patients with CGL2 have earlier onset of lipoatrophic diabetes mellitus compared with those with CGL1, with median age of onset of 10 years (range 8–30 years).[5] Half of patients with CGL2 have mild mental retardation, which is not a feature of other lipodystrophy subtypes.[5,11,12] Cardiomyopathy is 3 times more frequent in patients with CGL2 compared with CGL1.[16,17]

Mechanism BSCL2 encodes the protein, seipin. The function of seipin is complex and incompletely understood, but it appears to be involved in lipid droplet assembly, particularly the fusion of nascent lipid droplets.[18] Seipin also may aid in trafficking of lipids or proteins between the lipid droplet and the endoplasmic reticulum, and also may play a role in phospholipid and triglyceride synthesis via interactions with AGPAT2.[19]

Congenital generalized lipodystrophy type 3

Genetics CGL3 has been reported only in a single patient, and is caused by autosomal recessive mutations in CAV1 on chromosome 7q31, which encodes the protein caveolin-1.[8] The gene was identified via a candidate gene approach and is a nonsense mutation in which a nucleotide change c.112G3T leads to substitution of the glutamic acid residue at position 38, resulting a stop codon (p.Glu38X). Heterozygous mutations in CAV1 have been linked to an atypical partial lipodystrophy[20] and neonatal progeroid syndrome.[21,22]

Phenotype Mechanical adipose tissue and bone marrow fat are preserved in CGL3. The patient had the typical metabolic complications of lipodystrophy (insulin resistance, hypertriglyceridemia, hyperandrogenism, and hepatic steatosis) in addition to some unique features, including short stature and presumed vitamin D resistance.[8]

Mechanism Caveolin-1 is a highly conserved 22-kDa protein and an integral component of plasma membrane invaginations known as caveolae. Caveolae are abundant on adipocyte membranes, and act to bind fatty acids and translocate them to lipid droplets.[20]

Congenital generalized lipodystrophy type 4

Genetics CGL4 is caused by autosomal recessive mutations in PTRF on chromosome 17q21.2, encoding the protein cavin-1.[9] It was identified via a candidate gene approach, and has been reported in approximately 30 patients.[19]

Phenotype Patients may have some body fat present at birth, but progress to generalized lipodystrophy during infancy, with preservation of mechanical and bone marrow fat.[19,23] In addition to metabolic complications of lipodystrophy, there can be associated cardiac, neuromuscular, gastrointestinal, and skeletal diseases. Clinical features unique to CGL4 include congenital myopathy with percussion-induced muscle mounding and elevated creatine kinase levels, pyloric stenosis, atlantoaxial instability, cardiac rhythm disturbances including prolonged QT interval and exercise-induced ventricular tachycardia, and sudden death.[11,23]

Mechanism PTRF is involved in biogenesis of caveolae and regulates expression of caveolins 1 and 3.[9] Also important for lipid traffic, it assists in the proper formation of membrane caveolae.

Familial Partial Lipodystrophy

Most cases of FPLD are autosomal dominant. Phenotypically, patients with FPLD lack extremity and gluteal subcutaneous fat. In most cases, body fat distribution is normal during infancy and early childhood, with onset of fat redistribution occurring around puberty. Adipose tissue in the face, neck, and intra-abdominal areas is preserved, and may be increased, leading to a Cushingoid appearance. Patients also may have acanthosis nigricans and muscular hypertrophy.[24] Diabetes and metabolic complications occur in adulthood. Men are less likely to be recognized phenotypically because the fat distribution of partial lipodystrophy overlaps with normal male habitus. Men are also less likely to be recognized because metabolic disease is less severe.[25] Women may have reduced fertility with irregular menses and hirsutism.[26] Metabolic complications are common and include coronary artery disease.[27,28]

Familial partial lipodystrophy type 1

Genetics Familial partial lipodystrophy type 1 (FPLD1),[29] otherwise known as the Kobberling type of familial partial lipodystrophy, is usually autosomal dominant but the genetic cause is unknown. It is possible that FPLD1 is actually a group of disorders with multiple genetic etiologies.

Phenotype Patients exhibit loss of fat to the extremities, including the buttocks; increased fat in the face, neck, and abdomen resulting in a Cushingoid appearance; and increased waist-to-hip ratio with high body mass index. The classic fat distribution typically develops during childhood, although there is a single report of fat redistribution occurring after menopause.[29] There is classically a prominent ledge of fat above the gluteal area, upper medial thigh, and upper arm over the deltoid and upper triceps. Extremities can be muscular with phlebomegaly or thin without phlebomegaly (supporting the concept that there are multiple genetic causes). Patients have typical metabolic complications of lipodystrophy, which may include severe hypertriglyceridemia and acute pancreatitis, and early coronary artery disease.[29] FPLD1 has been described only in female individuals to date, which may be due to mild or lethal forms in men.[30]

Familial partial lipodystrophy type 2

Genetics FPLD2, also known as the Dunnigan variety of FPLD, is caused by autosomal dominant mutations in the *LMNA* gene on chromosome 1q21 to 22.[31,32] *LMNA* encodes nuclear lamin A/C. The most common mutation is the R482Q mutation.

Phenotype Onset of fat loss typically occurs at puberty, with loss of fat in the buttocks and limbs, and gain of fat to the face, neck, abdominal viscera, and labia. Patients have acanthosis nigricans, muscle hypertrophy, phlebomegaly, eruptive xanthomata, lipomas, and hirsutism. Cardiovascular complications include coronary artery disease and hypertension, and metabolic complications include insulin resistance, diabetes mellitus, hypertriglyceridemia with resultant pancreatitis, and hepatic steatosis, which tend to increase with age.[33,34] Women also can have PCOS, breast hypoplasia, pre-eclampsia, and miscarriages. Men with FPLD2 have a less obvious physical phenotype and milder metabolic abnormalities.[25]

Mechanism The mechanism by which LMNA mutations result in partial lipodystrophy is discussed under Laminopathies, later in this article.

Familial partial lipodystrophy type 3
Genetics FPLD3 is caused by autosomal dominant mutations in the peroxisome proliferator-activated receptor gene (PPARγ) on chromosome 3p25.[35–38]

Phenotype The onset of fat loss is usually in the second decade, with loss of fat to the trunk, buttocks, and limbs. There is no increase in head and neck fat (in contrast to FPLD2). There may be gain of fat to the abdomen.[39] FPLD3 is associated with typical metabolic complications of lipodystrophy, and also may have an increased risk of hypertension.[38]

Mechanism PPARγ is highly expressed in adipocytes and is considered a master regulator of adipocyte differentiation.[40] It is not clear how germline mutations in PPARγ lead to region-specific loss of adipose tissue.

Familial partial lipodystrophy types 4, 5, and 6, and AKT2-linked lipodystrophy
Genetics and mechanism FPLD4 is caused by autosomal dominant mutations in PLIN1, encoding perilipin-1.[41] FPLD5 has been reported in only a single case, caused by an autosomal recessive mutation in CIDEC.[42] Perilipin-1 and CIDEC are involved in the structure and function of adipocyte lipid droplets. FPLD6 is caused by autosomal recessive mutations in LIPE, encoding hormone-sensitive lipase, which is involved in regulation of lipolysis.[43,44] Akt2-linked lipodystrophy was described in a single family, and is caused by autosomal dominant mutations in AKT2, which is a key mediator of insulin signaling downstream of the insulin receptor.[45]

Phenotype FPLD4, FPLD 5, FPLD 6, and Akt2-linked lipodystrophy share common phenotypes. The typical onset is at puberty with loss of fat to the buttocks and limbs and a gain of fat to the face, neck, and abdomen. Skin changes include acanthosis nigricans, phlebomegaly, eruptive xanthomata, and hirsutism. Patients also can have calf hypertrophy. Metabolic complications include insulin resistance, diabetes mellitus, and hypertriglyceridemia. Cardiovascular complications include hypertension and coronary artery disease.

ACQUIRED LIPODYSTROPHIES

Acquired lipodystrophies are only briefly discussed, as they are thought to be autoimmune in origin rather than genetic.

Patients with AGL, or Lawrence syndrome, are born with normal body fat, and experience a progressive loss of fat that eventually affects almost all fat depots, including mechanical fat.[46] In some cases, fat in the face, neck, and axillae may be preserved. Onset is most commonly in childhood, but can occur at any age. There is a 3-to-1 female-to-male ratio. Patients experience typical metabolic complications of lipodys-trophy, including insulin resistance, diabetes, hypertriglyceridemia, and nonalcoholic steatohepatitis. In addition, patients frequently have other associated autoimmune diseases (juvenile dermatomyositis, type 1 diabetes, autoimmune hepatitis, and others) and complement abnormalities.

APL, or Barraquer Simons syndrome, is a unique form of lipodystrophy in which loss of fat occurs in a cranio-caudal direction, beginning in the face, and variably progress-ing to include the neck, shoulders, arms, and trunk.[47] Excess fat accumulation may occur in the lower body, including the hips, buttocks, and legs. Onset of fat loss typi-cally occurs in childhood or adolescence, and there is a 4 to 1 female preponderance. APL is associated with other autoimmune conditions, including membranoproliferative glomerulonephritis in 20% of cases, low serum C3, and the presence of C3 nephritic factor.[47,48] Unlike other forms of lipodystrophy, metabolic complications are infre-quent, perhaps due to the preservation of fat in the lower body. A single study has linked APL to mutations in *LMNB* (see Laminopathies, later in this article).[49]

AUTOINFLAMMATORY DISORDERS

Three distinct but overlapping recessive autoinflammatory disorders associated with lipodystrophy are caused by mutations in the proteasome subunit beta type 8 (*PSMB8*) on chromosome 6. These syndromes include the joint contractures, muscle atrophy, microcytic anemia (JMP) panniculitis-induced lipodystrophy syndrome,[50] the Nakajo-Nishimura syndrome,[51] and chronic atypical neutrophilic dermatosis with lipodystrophy and elevated temperature (CANDLE) syndrome.[52] *PSMB8* encodes the immunoproteasome subunit β5i. Abnormal incorporation of β5i mutants into the immu-noproteasome results in decreased proteasome activity, leading to cellular accumula-tion of ubiquitinated and oxidized proteins and increased sensitivity to apoptosis. The mechanism by which dysfunction of the immunoproteasome leads to lipodystrophy and other features of the autoinflammatory syndromes remains to be elucidated; how-ever, the autoinflammatory response may result in infiltration of adipose tissue with lym-phocytes and other immune cells, leading to loss of nearby adipocytes.

JMP was initially described in 3 patients belonging to 2 pedigrees from Portugal and Mexico.[53] Features of the disease include lipodystrophy beginning in childhood, mus-cle atrophy, joint contractures, skin lesions, microcytic anemia, hepatosplenomegaly, and hypergammaglobulinemia. Nakajo-Nishimura syndrome has been reported in more than 20 Japanese patients, and presents in infancy with rash, periodic fevers, nodular erythematous skin eruptions, and myositis.[51] Atrophy of the subcutaneous fat and muscles is progressive, with joint contractures. Additional features include hepatosplenomegaly, hypergammaglobulinemia, and basal ganglia calcifications.

CANDLE syndrome typically presents in the first year of life, with recurrent fevers, annular violaceous plaques, arthralgias, anemia, lipodystrophy, and elevated acute phase reactants.[52] Lipodystrophy is variable, but usually begins in infancy with loss of subcutaneous fat from the face, with loss of fat from upper (and occasionally lower) limbs later in childhood.[52]

PROGEROID DISORDERS

Many progeroid disorders include lipodystrophy as a manifestation, and a detailed discussion of each of these is beyond the scope of this article. A list of progeroid dis-orders, including their causative gene and its function, inheritance, and lipodystrophic regions, is in **Table 1**. There is further discussion of progeroid disorders with lipodys-trophy related to genetic defects in nuclear lamins (Laminopathies) later in this article.

Table 1
Progeroid disorders

Disorder	Gene (Protein)	Gene Function	Inheritance	Lipodystrophic Areas	Reference
Hutchinson-Gilford progeria syndrome	*LMNA* (lamin A/C)	Structure and functions of nuclear lamina	De novo	Almost all fat lost (intra-abdominal fat spared)	Eriksson et al,[57] 2003; De Sandre-Giovannoli et al,[58] 2003
Mandibulo-acral dysplasia type A (with partial lipodystrophy)	*LMNA* (lamin A/C)	Structure and functions of nuclear lamina	AR	Upper and lower limbs	Novelli et al,[59] 2002
Mandibulo-acral dysplasia type B (with generalized lipodystrophy)	*ZMPSTE24* (zinc metalloproteinase)	Prelamin A processing	AR	Almost all fat lost	Agarwal et I,[60] 2003
Atypical progeria	*LMNA* (lamin A/C)	Structure and functions of nuclear lamina	AD, de novo	Partial or generalized fat loss Normal mechanical fat	Chen et al,[61] 2003
Néstor-Guillermo progeria syndrome	*BANF1* (Barrier to autointegration factor)	Assembly of emerin and A-type lamins at the reforming nuclear envelope	AR	Almost all fat lost	Cabanillas et al,[62] 2011

(continued on next page)

Table 1
(continued)

Disorder	Gene (Protein)	Gene Function	Inheritance	Lipodystrophic Areas	Reference
Werner syndrome	RECQL2 (WRN)	DNA helicase, DNA repair	AR	Limbs	Donadille et al,[63] 2013
Bloom syndrome	BLM	DNA repair	AR	Limbs	Ellis et al,[64] 1995
Mandibular hypoplasia, deafness and progeroid features (MDP) syndrome	POLD1 (subunit of DNA polymerase δ)	DNA polymerization and repair	De novo	Almost all fat lost	Weedon et al,[65] 2013
Neonatal Marfan progeroid syndrome	FBN1 (fibrillin 1)	Connective tissue	De novo	Almost all fat lost	Graul-Neumann et al,[66] 2010
Neonatal progeroid syndrome	CAV1 (Caveolin-1)	Caveolin-1, formation of membrane caveolae, lipid traffic	De novo	Face, distal extremities	Garg et al,[21] 2015
Keppen-Lubinsky syndrome (KCNJ6)	KCNJ6 (G protein-activated inward rectifier potassium channel 2)	Inwardly rectifying potassium channel	De novo	Almost all fat lost	Masotti et al,[67] 2015
Cockayne syndrome	ERCC6, ERCC8	DNA repair and transcription	AR	Almost all fat lost	Laugel et al,[68] 2010
Ruijs-Aalfs syndrome (SPRTN)	SPRTN (SprT-like N-terminal domain protein)	DNA repair	AR	Almost all fat lost	Lessel et al,[69] 2014

Abbreviation: AR, autosomal recessive.

OTHER SYNDROMES ASSOCIATED WITH LIPODYSTROPHY

Mutations in *PCYT1a*, which cause either generalized or partial lipodystrophy, and the short stature, hyperextensibility, hernia, ocular depression, Rieger anomaly, and teething delay (SHORT) syndrome, caused by mutations in *PIK3R1*, are briefly discussed in **Table 2**.

LAMINOPATHIES

Several lipodystrophy syndromes fall in the class of disorders known as "laminopathies." The laminopathies are heterogeneous disorders caused by mutations in genes encoding nuclear lamina proteins (*LMNA*, *LMNB1*, *LMNB2*), posttranslational processing of these proteins (*ZMPSTE24*), or that interact with lamins (eg, *EMD*, encoding the protein emerin).[54] There are 4 categories of diseases associated with lamin dysfunction, including lipodystrophies, progeroid disorders (many of which are associated with lipodystrophy), muscle diseases, and neuropathies. The Dunnigan variety of familial partial lipodystrophy, described previously, is caused by mutations in *LMNA*. APL (Barraquer Simons syndrome) has been linked to *LMNB* mutations in a single study, but it is not inherited as a Mendelian trait, and expression is likely linked to other genes and/or environmental factors.[49] Progeroid laminopathies include Hutchinson-Gilford progeria syndrome, atypical Werner syndrome, restrictive dermopathy, mandibulo-acral dysplasia type A, and atypical progeroid syndrome. The most common laminopathies are muscle-related diseases, including Emery-Dreifuss muscular dystrophy (autosomal dominant, autosomal recessive, and X-linked), limb-girdle muscular dystrophy type 1B, dilated cardiomyopathy 1A with conduction defect, and heart-hand syndrome (Slovenian type).[54] Neuropathies include Charcot-Marie-Tooth disease type 2B1, and adult-onset autosomal dominant leukodystrophy.[54]

The laminopathies are of particular interest from a genetic perspective due to both the diversity of phenotypes, and the relatively poor genotype-phenotype correlation. Most laminopathy syndromes can be caused by multiple mutations, and the same mutation can result in different clinical syndromes, possibly due to other genetic variants. Even different missense mutations of the same amino acid residue can cause different syndromes (eg, *LMNA* mutations R527H and R527C cause mandibulo-acral dysplasia [a progeroid lipodystrophy], but R527P causes Emery-Dreifuss muscular dystrophy). Moreover, overlap syndromes exist, such as Dunnigan familial partial lipodystrophy combined with muscular dystrophy and/or cardiomyopathy or cardiac conduction defects.[55]

SUMMARY

There continues to be progress to uncover the genetic causes of lipodystrophy syndromes, but more genetic mutations remain to be discovered. For example, FPLD1 is usually autosomal dominant with no known genetic cause, and the phenotypic heterogeneity suggests that there may be multiple genetic etiologies. Although APL has been linked to mutations in *LMNB*, the acquired lipodystrophies are not inherited in a Mendelian manner, and are presumed to be caused by autoimmune destruction of adipocytes.

Progress in the field of the genetics of lipodystrophy also has led to increased understanding of the physiology of these disorders, and has the potential to lead to advancements in treatment. Leptin replacement has become a critical factor resulting in decreased morbidity.[56] Early identification of the genetic cause of lipodystrophy may

Table 2
Other lipodystrophic disorders

Disorder	Gene (Protein)	Gene Function	Inheritance	Lipodystrophic Areas	Reference
PCYT1-linked lipodystrophy	PCYT1A (phosphate cytidylyltransferase 1 alpha)	Synthesis of phosphatidylcholine	AR	Either generalized or partial loss of fat	Payne et al,[70] 2014
Short stature, hyperextensibility, ocular depression, Rieger anomaly, and teething delay (SHORT) syndrome	PIK3R1 (regulatory subunits of the phosphatidyl inositol-3 kinase)	Insulin signaling	AD, de novo	Almost all fat lost (most cases)	Thauvin-Robinet et al,[71] 2013

Abbreviations: AD, autosomal dominant; AR, autosomal recessive.

lead to early treatment and better outcomes; for example, in patients identified to have the *BSCL2* mutation who may develop cirrhosis in the first decade of life, early diagnosis and treatment may halt or delay the advancement of liver disease.[13] Genetic screening and counseling also may allow patients to make informed decisions regarding family planning and early management of disease in their children.

REFERENCES

1. Garg A. Acquired and inherited lipodystrophies. N Engl J Med 2004;350(12): 1220–34.

2. Brown RJ, Gorden P. Leptin therapy in patients with lipodystrophy and syndromic insulin resistance. In: Dagogo-Jack S, editor. Leptin: regulation and clinical applications. Switzerland: Springer International Publishing; 2015. p. 225–36.

3. Berardinelli W. An undiagnosed endocrinometabolic syndrome—report of 2 cases. J Clin Endocrinol Metab 1954;14(2):193–204.

4. Seip M. Lipodystrophy and gigantism with associated endocrine manifestations. A new diencephalic syndrome? Acta Paediatr 1959;48:555–74.

5. Agarwal AK, Simha V, Oral EA, et al. Phenotypic and genetic heterogeneity in congenital generalized lipodystrophy. J Clin Endocrinol Metab 2003;88(10): 4840–7.

6. Agarwal AK, Arioglu E, De Almeida S, et al. AGPAT2 is mutated in congenital generalized lipodystrophy linked to chromosome 9q34. Nat Genet 2002;31(1): 21–3.

7. Magre J, Delépine M, Khallouf E, et al. Identification of the gene altered in Berardinelli-Seip congenital lipodystrophy on chromosome 11q13. Nat Genet 2001;28(4):365–70.

8. Kim CA, Delépine M, Boutet E, et al. Association of a homozygous nonsense caveolin-1 mutation with Berardinelli-Seip congenital lipodystrophy. J Clin Endocrinol Metab 2008;93(4):1129–34.

9. Hayashi YK, Matsuda C, Ogawa M, et al. Human PTRF mutations cause secondary deficiency of caveolins resulting in muscular dystrophy with generalized lipodystrophy. J Clin Invest 2009;119(9):2623–33.

10. Garg A. Clinical review: Lipodystrophies: genetic and acquired body fat disorders. J Clin Endocrinol Metab 2011;96(11):3313–25.

11. Akinci B, Onay H, Demir T, et al. Natural history of congenital generalized lipodystrophy: a nationwide study from Turkey. J Clin Endocrinol Metab 2016;101(7): 2759–67.

12. Van Maldergem L, Magré J, Khallouf TE, et al. Genotype-phenotype relationships in Berardinelli-Seip congenital lipodystrophy. J Med Genet 2002;39(10):722–33.

13. Safar Zadeh E, Lungu AO, Cochran EK, et al. The liver diseases of lipodystrophy: the long-term effect of leptin treatment. J Hepatol 2013;59(1):131–7.

14. Fleckenstein JL, Garg A, Bonte FJ, et al. The skeleton in congenital, generalized lipodystrophy: evaluation using whole-body radiographic surveys, magnetic resonance imaging and technetium-99m bone scintigraphy. Skeletal Radiol 1992;21(6):381–6.

15. Leung DW. The structure and functions of human lysophosphatidic acid acyltransferases. Front Biosci 2001;6:D944–53.

16. Bhayana S, Siu VM, Joubert GI, et al. Cardiomyopathy in congenital complete lipodystrophy. Clin Genet 2002;61(4):283–7.

17. Bjornstad PG, Semb BK, Trygstad O, et al. Echocardiographic assessment of cardiac function and morphology in patients with generalised lipodystrophy. Eur J Pediatr 1985;144(4):355–9.

18. Szymanski KM, Binns D, Bartz R, et al. The lipodystrophy protein seipin is found at endoplasmic reticulum lipid droplet junctions and is important for droplet morphology. Proc Natl Acad Sci U S A 2007;104(52):20890–5.

19. Patni N, Garg A. Congenital generalized lipodystrophies–new insights into metabolic dysfunction. Nat Rev Endocrinol 2015;11(9):522–34.

20. Cao H, Alston L, Ruschman J, et al. Heterozygous CAV1 frameshift mutations (MIM 601047) in patients with atypical partial lipodystrophy and hypertriglyceridemia. Lipids Health Dis 2008;7:3.

21. Garg A, Kircher M, Del Campo M, et al. Whole exome sequencing identifies de novo heterozygous CAV1 mutations associated with a novel neonatal onset lipodystrophy syndrome. Am J Med Genet A 2015;167A(8):1796–806.

22. Schrauwen I, Szelinger S, Siniard AL, et al. A frame-shift mutation in CAV1 is associated with a severe neonatal progeroid and lipodystrophy syndrome. PLoS One 2015;10(7):e0131797.

23. Rajab A, Straub V, McCann LJ, et al. Fatal cardiac arrhythmia and long-QT syndrome in a new form of congenital generalized lipodystrophy with muscle rippling (CGL4) due to PTRF-CAVIN mutations. PLoS Genet 2010;6(3):e1000874.

24. Ji H, Weatherall P, Adams-Huet B, et al. Increased skeletal muscle volume in women with familial partial lipodystrophy, Dunnigan variety. J Clin Endocrinol Metab 2013;98(8):E1410–3.

25. Jackson SN, Howlett TA, McNally PG, et al. Dunnigan-Kobberling syndrome: an autosomal dominant form of partial lipodystrophy. QJM 1997;90(1):27–36.

26. Vantyghem MC, Vincent-Desplanques D, Defrance-Faivre F, et al. Fertility and obstetrical complications in women with LMNA-related familial partial lipodystrophy. J Clin Endocrinol Metab 2008;93(6):2223–9.

27. Hegele RA. Premature atherosclerosis associated with monogenic insulin resistance. Circulation 2001;103(18):2225–9.

28. Bidault G, Garcia M, Vantyghem MC, et al. Lipodystrophy-linked LMNA p.R482W mutation induces clinical early atherosclerosis and in vitro endothelial dysfunction. Arterioscler Thromb Vasc Biol 2013;33(9):2162–71.

29. Herbst KL, Tannock LR, Deeb SS, et al. Kobberling type of familial partial lipodystrophy: an underrecognized syndrome. Diabetes Care 2003;26(6):1819–24.

30. Kobberling J, Dunnigan MG. Familial partial lipodystrophy: two types of an X linked dominant syndrome, lethal in the hemizygous state. J Med Genet 1986;23(2):120–7.

31. Shackleton S, Lloyd DJ, Jackson SN, et al. LMNA, encoding lamin A/C, is mutated in partial lipodystrophy. Nat Genet 2000;24(2):153–6.

32. Cao H, Hegele RA. Nuclear lamin A/C R482Q mutation in Canadian kindreds with Dunnigan-type familial partial lipodystrophy. Hum Mol Genet 2000;9(1):109–12.

33. Schmidt HH, Genschel J, Baier P, et al. Dyslipemia in familial partial lipodystrophy caused by an R482W mutation in the LMNA gene. J Clin Endocrinol Metab 2001;86(5):2289–95.

34. Speckman RA, Garg A, Du F, et al. Mutational and haplotype analyses of families with familial partial lipodystrophy (Dunnigan variety) reveal recurrent missense mutations in the globular C-terminal domain of lamin A/C. Am J Hum Genet 2000;66(4):1192–8.

35. Agarwal AK, Garg A. A novel heterozygous mutation in peroxisome proliferator-activated receptor-gamma gene in a patient with familial partial lipodystrophy. J Clin Endocrinol Metab 2002;87(1):408–11.
36. Hegele RA, Cao H, Frankowski C, et al. PPARG F388L, a transactivation-deficient mutant, in familial partial lipodystrophy. Diabetes 2002;51(12):3586–90.
37. Savage DB, Tan GD, Acerini CL, et al. Human metabolic syndrome resulting from dominant-negative mutations in the nuclear receptor peroxisome proliferator-activated receptor-gamma. Diabetes 2003;52(4):910–7.
38. Barroso I, Gurnell M, Crowley VE, et al. Dominant negative mutations in human PPARgamma associated with severe insulin resistance, diabetes mellitus and hypertension. Nature 1999;402(6764):880–3.
39. Hegele RA. Lessons from human mutations in PPAR[gamma]. Int J Obes Relat Metab Disord 2005;29(S1):S31–5.
40. Rosen ED, Sarraf P, Troy AE, et al. PPAR gamma is required for the differentiation of adipose tissue in vivo and in vitro. Mol Cell 1999;4(4):611–7.
41. Gandotra S, Le Dour C, Bottomley W, et al. Perilipin deficiency and autosomal dominant partial lipodystrophy. N Engl J Med 2011;364(8):740–8.
42. Rubio-Cabezas O, Puri V, Murano I, et al. Partial lipodystrophy and insulin resistant diabetes in a patient with a homozygous nonsense mutation in CIDEC. EMBO Mol Med 2009;1(5):280–7.
43. Albert JS, Yerges-Armstrong LM, Horenstein RB, et al. Null mutation in hormone-sensitive lipase gene and risk of type 2 diabetes. N Engl J Med 2014;370(24):2307–15.
44. Farhan SM, Robinson JF, McIntyre AD, et al. A novel LIPE nonsense mutation found using exome sequencing in siblings with late-onset familial partial lipodystrophy. Can J Cardiol 2014;30(12):1649–54.
45. George S, Rochford JJ, Wolfrum C, et al. A family with severe insulin resistance and diabetes due to a mutation in AKT2. Science 2004;304(5675):1325–8.
46. Misra A, Garg A. Clinical features and metabolic derangements in acquired generalized lipodystrophy: case reports and review of the literature. Medicine (Baltimore) 2003;82(2):129–46.
47. Misra A, Peethambaram A, Garg A. Clinical features and metabolic and autoimmune derangements in acquired partial lipodystrophy: report of 35 cases and review of the literature. Medicine (Baltimore) 2004;83(1):18–34.
48. Savage DB, Semple RK, Clatworthy MR, et al. Complement abnormalities in acquired lipodystrophy revisited. J Clin Endocrinol Metab 2009;94(1):10–6.
49. Hegele RA, Cao H, Liu DM, et al. Sequencing of the reannotated LMNB2 gene reveals novel mutations in patients with acquired partial lipodystrophy. Am J Hum Genet 2006;79(2):383–9.
50. Agarwal AK, Xing C, DeMartino GN, et al. PSMB8 encoding the beta5i proteasome subunit is mutated in joint contractures, muscle atrophy, microcytic anemia, and panniculitis-induced lipodystrophy syndrome. Am J Hum Genet 2010;87(6):866–72.
51. Arima K, Kinoshita A, Mishima H, et al. Proteasome assembly defect due to a proteasome subunit beta type 8 (PSMB8) mutation causes the autoinflammatory disorder, Nakajo-Nishimura syndrome. Proc Natl Acad Sci U S A 2011;108(36):14914–9.
52. Liu Y, Ramot Y, Torrelo A, et al. Mutations in proteasome subunit beta type 8 cause chronic atypical neutrophilic dermatosis with lipodystrophy and elevated temperature with evidence of genetic and phenotypic heterogeneity. Arthritis Rheum 2012;64(3):895–907.

53. Garg A, Hernandez MD, Sousa AB, et al. An autosomal recessive syndrome of joint contractures, muscular atrophy, microcytic anemia, and panniculitis-associated lipodystrophy. J Clin Endocrinol Metab 2010;95(9):E58–63.
54. Zaremba-Czogalla M, Dubinska-Magiera M, Rzepecki R. Laminopathies: the molecular background of the disease and the prospects for its treatment. Cell Mol Biol Lett 2011;16(1):114–48.
55. Vantyghem MC, Pigny P, Maurage CA, et al. Patients with familial partial lipodystrophy of the Dunnigan type due to a LMNA R482W mutation show muscular and cardiac abnormalities. J Clin Endocrinol Metab 2004;89(11):5337–46.
56. Diker-Cohen T, Cochran E, Gorden P, et al. Partial and generalized lipodystrophy: comparison of baseline characteristics and response to metreleptin. J Clin Endocrinol Metab 2015;100(5):1802–10.
57. Eriksson M, Brown WT, Gordon LB, et al. Recurrent de novo point mutations in lamin A cause Hutchinson-Gilford progeria syndrome. Nature 2003;423(6937):293–8.
58. De Sandre-Giovannoli A, Bernard R, Cau P, et al. Lamin a truncation in Hutchinson-Gilford progeria. Science 2003;300(5628):2055.
59. Novelli G, Muchir A, Sangiuolo F, et al. Mandibuloacral dysplasia is caused by a mutation in LMNA-encoding lamin A/C. Am J Hum Genet 2002;71(2):426–31.
60. Agarwal AK, Fryns JP, Auchus RJ, et al. Zinc metalloproteinase, ZMPSTE24, is mutated in mandibuloacral dysplasia. Hum Mol Genet 2003;12(16):1995–2001.
61. Chen L, Lee L, Kudlow BA, et al. LMNA mutations in atypical Werner's syndrome. Lancet 2003;362(9382):440–5.
62. Cabanillas R, Cadiñanos J, Villameytide JA, et al. Nestor-Guillermo progeria syndrome: a novel premature aging condition with early onset and chronic development caused by BANF1 mutations. Am J Med Genet A 2011;155A(11):2617–25.
63. Donadille B, D'Anella P, Auclair M, et al. Partial lipodystrophy with severe insulin resistance and adult progeria Werner syndrome. Orphanet J Rare Dis 2013;8:106.
64. Ellis NA, Groden J, Ye TZ, et al. The Bloom's syndrome gene product is homologous to RecQ helicases. Cell 1995;83(4):655–66.
65. Weedon MN, Ellard S, Prindle MJ, et al. An in-frame deletion at the polymerase active site of POLD1 causes a multisystem disorder with lipodystrophy. Nat Genet 2013;45(8):947–50.
66. Graul-Neumann LM, Kienitz T, Robinson PN, et al. Marfan syndrome with neonatal progeroid syndrome-like lipodystrophy associated with a novel frameshift mutation at the 3' terminus of the FBN1-gene. Am J Med Genet A 2010;152A(11):2749–55.
67. Masotti A, Uva P, Davis-Keppen L, et al. Keppen-Lubinsky syndrome is caused by mutations in the inwardly rectifying K+ channel encoded by KCNJ6. Am J Hum Genet 2015;96(2):295–300.
68. Laugel V, Dalloz C, Durand M, et al. Mutation update for the CSB/ERCC6 and CSA/ERCC8 genes involved in Cockayne syndrome. Hum Mutat 2010;31(2):113–26.
69. Lessel D, Vaz B, Halder S, et al. Mutations in SPRTN cause early onset hepatocellular carcinoma, genomic instability and progeroid features. Nat Genet 2014;46(11):1239–44.
70. Payne F, Lim K, Girousse A, et al. Mutations disrupting the Kennedy phosphatidylcholine pathway in humans with congenital lipodystrophy and fatty liver disease. Proc Natl Acad Sci U S A 2014;111(24):8901–6.
71. Thauvin-Robinet C, Auclair M, Duplomb L, et al. PIK3R1 mutations cause syndromic insulin resistance with lipoatrophy. Am J Hum Genet 2013;93(1):141–9.

Index

Note: Page numbers of article titles are in **boldface** type.

Endocrinol Metab Clin N Am 46 (2017) 555–592
http://dx.doi.org/10.1016/S0889-8529(17)30027-0
0889-8529/17

endo.theclinics.com

Moving?

Make sure your subscription moves with you!

To notify us of your new address, find your **Clinics Account Number** (located on your mailing label above your name), and contact customer service at:

Email: journalscustomerservice-usa@elsevier.com

800-654-2452 (subscribers in the U.S. & Canada)
314-447-8871 (subscribers outside of the U.S. & Canada)

Fax number: 314-447-8029

Elsevier Health Sciences Division
Subscription Customer Service
3251 Riverport Lane
Maryland Heights, MO 63043

ELSEVIER

Printed and bound by CPI Group (UK) Ltd, Croydon, CR0 4YY

08/05/2025

01864699-0006